AF848844

NEW DEVELOPMENTS IN MEDICAL RESEARCH

CUTANEOUS SCARS

BIOLOGY, CLINICS AND MANAGEMENT

New Developments in Medical Research

Additional books and e-books in this series can be found
on Nova's website under the Series tab.

NEW DEVELOPMENTS IN MEDICAL RESEARCH

CUTANEOUS SCARS

BIOLOGY, CLINICS AND MANAGEMENT

BERNA AKSOY
HASAN METE AKSOY
ASLI TATLIPARMAK
AND
EROL KOÇ
EDITORS

nova
Medicine & Health
New York

Copyright © 2019 by Nova Science Publishers, Inc.

All rights reserved. No part of this book may be reproduced, stored in a retrieval system or transmitted in any form or by any means: electronic, electrostatic, magnetic, tape, mechanical photocopying, recording or otherwise without the written permission of the Publisher.

We have partnered with Copyright Clearance Center to make it easy for you to obtain permissions to reuse content from this publication. Simply navigate to this publication's page on Nova's website and locate the "Get Permission" button below the title description. This button is linked directly to the title's permission page on copyright.com. Alternatively, you can visit copyright.com and search by title, ISBN, or ISSN.

For further questions about using the service on copyright.com, please contact:
Copyright Clearance Center
Phone: +1-(978) 750-8400 Fax: +1-(978) 750-4470 E-mail: info@copyright.com.

NOTICE TO THE READER

The Publisher has taken reasonable care in the preparation of this book, but makes no expressed or implied warranty of any kind and assumes no responsibility for any errors or omissions. No liability is assumed for incidental or consequential damages in connection with or arising out of information contained in this book. The Publisher shall not be liable for any special, consequential, or exemplary damages resulting, in whole or in part, from the readers' use of, or reliance upon, this material. Any parts of this book based on government reports are so indicated and copyright is claimed for those parts to the extent applicable to compilations of such works.

Independent verification should be sought for any data, advice or recommendations contained in this book. In addition, no responsibility is assumed by the Publisher for any injury and/or damage to persons or property arising from any methods, products, instructions, ideas or otherwise contained in this publication.

This publication is designed to provide accurate and authoritative information with regard to the subject matter covered herein. It is sold with the clear understanding that the Publisher is not engaged in rendering legal or any other professional services. If legal or any other expert assistance is required, the services of a competent person should be sought. FROM A DECLARATION OF PARTICIPANTS JOINTLY ADOPTED BY A COMMITTEE OF THE AMERICAN BAR ASSOCIATION AND A COMMITTEE OF PUBLISHERS.

Additional color graphics may be available in the e-book version of this book.

Library of Congress Cataloging-in-Publication Data

ISBN: 978-1-53615-657-7

Published by Nova Science Publishers, Inc. † New York

This book is dedicated to our precious princess Elifsu Aksoy and her loving grandmother Muazzez Aksoy…

Berna & H. Mete Aksoy

CONTENTS

PREFACE

When a skin injury occurs, the wound heals via a dynamic series of physiological wound healing events, including hemostasis, proliferation and remodeling. The final remodeling stage can take many months, yet the newly formed scar never achieves the flexibility and resistance of the original skin. When the wound healing process is regulated correctly, the resultant physiological scar is thin and hardly visible. In certain circumstances the wound healing proceeds improperly and the resultant scar is far beyond what we expected. This time the result is a pathological scar; atrophic, hypertrophic or a keloidal scar.

The question "will there be a scar?" is one of the most common questions that physicians come across in everyday practice. Many patients having scars are affected both physically and psychologically due to cosmetic and/or functional problems, sometimes with subjective symptoms. Patients having especially extensive scars or scars located in visible areas report a severe adverse effect on quality of life.

So related to these concerns our book aims to review biology, clinical aspects and management of cutaneous scar formation.

Berna Aksoy, MD

In: Cutaneous Scars: Biology, Clinics and Management ISBN: 978-1-53615-657-7
Editors: Berna Aksoy, Hasan Mete Aksoy et al. © 2019 Nova Science Publishers, Inc.

Chapter 1

INTRODUCTION AND HISTORICAL PERSPECTIVES

F. Elif Yildirim*
Department of Dermatology,
Faculty of Medicine, SANKO University, Gaziantep, Turkey

ABSTRACT

This chapter is an introductory section of this updated cutaneous scars book, and includes a short journey of the history of medical literature on scars.

Keywords: cutaneous scar, history of scars, scar formation, cutaneous wound, wound healing

1. INTRODUCTION

Healing of injured tissue does not always proceed perfectly in human beings. It is often associated with scar formation, as opposed to other species such as lower vertebrates, salamanders, and invertebrates that possess the ability to regenerate injured or missing tissue. Mammalian fetuses prior to midgestation are also capable of rapid wound repair in the absence of scar formation. For cutaneous wounds which evolve beyond the second trimester of fetal development, only the epidermis is able to regenerate; any injury that extends into the dermis after this stage, always heal with the formation of a scar.

*Corresponding Author's Email: elifalper27@gmail.com.

When an injury occurs, the cutaneous wound heals via a dynamic series of physiological events, including coagulation, granulation tissue formation, re-epithelialization, and extracellular matrix (ECM) remodeling. The final stage can take many months, during which the new ECM forms a scar that never achieves the flexibility and resistance of the original tissue. When the wound healing process is precisely regulated, the resultant scar is thin and hardly visible. In some instances, the wound healing is improper, and the original tissue then fails to achieve normal flexibility or strength. Thus, it is replaced by a pathological tissue in the form of atrophic, hypertrophic or a keloid scar [1].

Cutaneous scar formation is often one of the major challenges of patient-related concerns, and the question they commonly asked during physician consultation is, "will there be a scar?" Most dermatologists, plastic surgeons or doctors performing invasive surgical procedures are confronted with this enigma in their everyday practice. This is because patients' living with scars are affected both physically and psychologically due to cosmetic worries, disfiguring of body parts, and functional problems, including contractures, and subjective symptoms, such as pruritus, pain, anxiety or depression. These predicaments result in severe negative impacts on the quality of life of such individuals [1, 2].

2. Historical Perspectives

The history and medical literature on cutaneous scar formation go as far back as 2500-3000 BC in the era of Smith papyrus [3]. Among the events documented in the Smith Papyrus case number 45, is the description of the existence of swellings on his breast; large, spreading, hard, and touching them felt like touching a ball of wrappings, which might have been the description of excessive wound healing [3].

Literature from the Yoruba tribe in Nigeria, around the tenth century and beyond, indicates that the Yorubas not only knew about keloids but understood some of the specifics of their characteristics and presentation [4].

The first full medical description of scar tissue, however, was probably the account made by Retz (1790) in his book "Treatise on Skin Diseases and Things of the Mind", where he reported the case of a woman with hypertrophic scars and a thick contracture band on her left arm. Retz described the lesion as "dartre de graisse" meaning fatty hernia in his book, which was probably a misnomer since the clinical description was suggestive of a keloid [5].

Nonetheless, it was Alibert (1806, 1816 and 1817) who coined the name, cancroid or cheloide or keloide, derived from the Greek chele or crab's claw, to describe the lateral growth of tissue which arises from an unaffected skin and then differentiates into lesions of malignant neoplasms. Also, Alibert introduced the differences between keloids arising spontaneously (true keloids) and those arising after trauma (false keloids) [6]. Many years later Mancini (1962) and Peacock (1970) classified excessive scarring into hypertrophic and keloid scar formation. According to their definition, although both scar types rise above skin level, hypertrophic scars do not extend beyond the initial site of injury, while keloids typically project beyond the original wound margins [7, 8]. This distinction led to the controversy of keloids and hypertrophic scars that has been ongoing. Today, keloids and hypertrophic scars are defined as uncontrolled proliferation of fibrous tissue after injury or trauma to the skin [9].

Conclusion

Cutaneous scars develop as a response to cutaneous injury and affect patients' psychological and physical well-being. History of medical literature on abnormal scarring extends as far back as 3000 BC. However, the controversy on the nomenclature of proliferative scars continues, and there are still no effective, proven methods of prevention and treatment of abnormal cutaneous scar formation. This book aimed to give current knowledge of biology, clinical, and treatment methods of cutaneous scars.

References

[1] Bayat, A. and D. A. McGrouther, M. W. J. Ferguson. 2003. "Skin scarring". *British Medical Journal,* 326:88 - 92.

[2] Bock, Oliver and Gerhard Schmid-Ott, Peter Malewski, Ulrich Mrowietz. 2006. "Quality of life of patients with keloid and hypertrophic scarring". *Archives of Dermatological Research,* 297:433 - 8.

[3] Breasted, J. H. 1930. "Bulging tumors on the breast". In: *The Edwin Smith surgical papyrus, Volume 1: Hieroglyphic text translation and commentary*, 403 - 406. Chicago: University of Chicago Press.

[4] Omo-Dare, P. 1973. "Yoruban contributions to the literature on keloids". *Journal of the National Medical Association,* 65:367 - 72.

[5] Child, F. J. and L. C. Fuller, E. M. Higgins, D. U. Vivier. 1999. "A study of the spectrum of skin disease occurring in a black population in South-East London". *British Journal of Dermatology,* 141:512 - 7.

[6] Alibert, J. L. 1817. "Quelques recherches sur la cheloide". *Mem. Soc. Med. d'Emul.,* 8:744 - 52.

[7] Peacock, Jr, E. E. and J. W. Madden, W. C. Trier. 1970. “Biologic basis for the treatment of keloids and hypertrophic scars”. *Southern Medical Journal,* 63: 755 - 60.

[8] Mancini, R. E. and J. V. Quaife. 1962. “Histogenesis of experimentally produced keloids”. *Journal of Investigative Dermatology,* 38:143 - 81.

[9] From, L. and D. Assaad. 1993. “Neoplasms, pseudoneoplasms, and hyperplasia of supporting tissue origin”. In: *Dermatology in General Medicine,* edited by Fitzpatrick, T. B. and A. Z. Eisen AZ, K. Wolff, I. M. Freedberg, K. F. Austen, 1196 - 209, New York: McGraw-Hill.

In: Cutaneous Scars: Biology, Clinics and Management ISBN: 978-1-53615-657-7
Editors: Berna Aksoy, Hasan Mete Aksoy et al. © 2019 Nova Science Publishers, Inc.

Chapter 2

THE SIGNIFICANCE OF SCARS: PATIENT AND CLINICIAN PERSPECTIVES

***Emin Ozlu*[1] *and Ayse S. Karadag*[2,*]**
[1]Department of Dermatology, Faculty of Medicine,
Duzce University, Duzce, Turkey
[2]Department of Dermatology, Faculty of Medicine,
Istanbul Medeniyet University, Istanbul, Turkey

ABSTRACT

The formation of a scar represents the extension of regenerative wound repair mechanisms. On the one hand, scar tissue helps in wound closure by supporting wound contracture and reepithelization. There is no doubt that the scar formation developed in response to an injury facilitates the organism's survival process directly and effectively. On the other hand, the effect of the pathologically developed scarring on the global disease burden has still not been accurately defined. There are three basic subtypes of scars, namely simple, atrophic, and hypertrophic/pathological (hypertrophic scars and keloids), and they have different histopathological features, development, dispersion patterns, and remission phases. There are important consequences when scars' global and individual effects are considered. Patients with scars face long-term functional and psychological problems. In interpreting scars for both individuals and society, individual, cultural, psychological, and social effects and prejudices play a crucial role. Both the psychosocial and financial aspects of the scars, as well as the effects on the patient and society, should be considered.

Keywords: global burden, psychosocial effect

[*]Corresponding Author's Email: karadagaserap@gmail.com.

1. Introduction

A scar is a finding that occurs during the wound healing process after an injury or surgical intervention; it is characterized by the displacement of normal functional skin with a scar tissue, and it is a normal and inevitable result of the tissue repair. Scars on the skin have a wide spectrum, ranging from a normal thin line to atrophic or abnormally enlarged hypertrophic/keloidal lesions, and even contractures. Scar development is not expected when the skin damage is limited to the epidermis. However, if the dermis and lower layers of the skin are damaged, structural and functional scar development is seen. The developing scar tissue lacks elasticity and tensile strength of normal skin. For this reason, the questions that patients ask most frequently when undergoing surgical procedures are; "Will this cause a scar?" and "What kind of a scar will it cause?" However, scar development differs from person to person, and the outcome of this process is difficult to anticipate [1].

The process of normal wound healing consists of three consecutive and intertwined steps, as follows: hemostasis/inflammation, proliferation, and remodeling. To achieve hemostasis after trauma, the coagulation cascade is rapidly activated and then inflammation is triggered. Granulation tissue starts to form during the proliferation phase, 2–3 days after trauma. In the remodeling phase, the extracellular matrix is reorganized as the immature collagen is replaced by organized and mature collagen [2].

Although various factors affecting scar formation are currently known, the cause is still unclear. Genetic predisposition, wound-related regional features, and environmental factors play an important role in the development of hypertrophic scars. Features like the patient's age, skin type, genetic and hormonal factors, anatomical characteristics, type of surgical operation, presence of inflammation and infection, wound tension and depth all affect wound healing [3].

Typically, the scars that develop after burns or surgery introduce a *global burden* to both the individuals and societies. Children are frequently affected by scars, and this can lead to long-term physical dysfunction and *psychosocial effects.* In the United States, approximately 500,000 patients receive burn injury treatment annually, and most of these injuries leave painful contractures and scarring that require major surgery. Approximately $7.5 billion is spent every year on treatment, and the clear majority of this money is spent on scar and contracture treatment [4].

Excessive scars can have unpleasant physical, aesthetic, psychological, and social consequences. Physical symptoms, such as pruritus, stiffness, contractures, pain, and tenderness may be present in scarred patients, as well as psychological problems like decreased self-esteem, social stigma, deterioration of daily activities, anxiety, and depression [5]. This chapter focuses on the epidemiology, risk factors, *global burden,* and *psychosocial effects* of scars in the context of the current literature.

2. Classification of Scars

Cutaneous scars have a wide spectrum, ranging from mature linear scars to atrophic or proliferative hypertrophic scars (HTSs) and major keloids. HTSs do not extend beyond the borders of the primary lesion and tend to spontaneously regress over time. These scars can be divided into two subgroups, namely linear and widespread HTSs. Linear HTSs often develop after surgery or trauma, whereas widespread HTSs frequently arise after burn injury, extensive soft tissue trauma, and/or infection. Keloids are lesions that extend beyond the limits of the primary injury, do not tend to spontaneously regress, and can recur. Histologically, HTSs contain well-organized type 3 collagen bundles, while keloids contain disorganized type 1 and type 3 collagen bundles [5].

3. Risk Factors for Scarring

The underlying mechanism for HTS development is still not fully understood. There are also limited studies to date on the risk factors that may be associated with HTS emergence. In their review, Butzelaar et al. [2] claimed that a genetic predisposition, young age, presence of allergies, bacterial colonization on the wound, and tension on the skin facilitate HTS development; whereas chemotherapy, cigarette use, and local administration of statins protect against HTSs. In addition, Stella et al. [6] suggested that female sex, young age, neck and upper extremity burns, >1 surgical operation, meshed grafts, burn severity, and longer duration of healing are risk factors for HTS development. In a study conducted on 703 burn patients, 44% of the patients had HTS, 28% had scarring with contracture and 5% had scarring without developing contracture [7]. In addition to these factors, it has been suggested that dark-skinned individuals may develop HTSs more easily than light-skinned individuals do; however, the extent of supporting evidence for this claim is weak [2].

Due to their nature, HTSs are dynamic. It is thought that HTSs go through three phases, as follows: the initial phase, characterized by active growth; intermediate phase, characterized by contractures; and finally, the regressive phase. Several factors, such as age, gender, etiology, and retention area play a role in the progression of these phases. Although pathologic scars are thought to occur with the same incidence in both genders, women are somewhat more prone to HTS development. Burn injuries are one of the most important factors contributing to pathological scar development. However, genetics, familial predisposition, and race have long been accepted as risk factors for pathological scar development [8].

Like that of HTSs, the process of keloid development is not well understood, but it is known to be induced by skin damage in susceptible individuals. There are many theories concerning the keloid etiology, but most of them are related to fibroblast dysfunction. The fibroblasts present in the keloids synthesize more collagen, fibronectin, elastin, and proteoglycans. In addition, the rate of apoptosis is lower in the keloid cells. Many factors play an important role in the development of keloids. Perhaps the most important of these is a genetic predisposition. Autosomal recessive, autosomal dominant with incomplete penetrance and variable expression are among the proposed inheritance patterns. Several genes are considered responsible for the development of keloids, but until now, no single gene mutation has been identified. It has also been suggested that those with blood type A are more likely to develop keloids than individuals with other blood types do [9].

Melanin is the pigment that plays the most important role in determining skin color in different races around the world. Predisposition to keloid development is known to be associated with skin color. It has been suggested that black patients are twice as likely to develop keloids compared with Hispanic and Asian people [10]. Spontaneous keloids are extremely rare; keloids may develop after any type of skin damage, but it has been reported that the most common cause is burns. The anatomical site plays an extremely important role in keloid development. The anterior chest, shoulders, earlobes, upper arms, and cheeks are the most vulnerable areas for keloid development. It is accepted that the incidence of keloids is often the same in both men and women, but it is higher in women in some anatomical sites due to factors like ear piercing. Age is an important factor in the development of keloids. While they are rare in the first decade of life, their incidence reaches its highest level during the second and third decades and then decreases in older ages. Delayed wound healing and increased wound tension are other modifying factors associated with keloid development [9].

4. The Global Burden of Cutaneous Scarring

The total *global burden* of pathologically developed scars is not well defined. Discussions related to the *global burden* often include patients in scarring subgroups, such as scars that occur after burns, trauma, or elective surgical procedures. In addition, most studies on this topic are limited to a small number of institutions and geopolitically similar socioeconomic regions. The most relevant data on trauma-related scars concerns burns. While the data on the incidence of burns is increasing due to the databases established in developed countries, unfortunately, epidemiological data are extremely limited in developing and underdeveloped countries. While patients in countries with a high socioeconomic status can rapidly and easily access burn wound care treatment, patients in countries with a low socioeconomic status face challenges regarding wound care. Patients may experience delays in terms of their ability to reach wound care treatment, and such delays may prolong the wound-healing process or cause patients who can benefit from surgery to lose this opportunity. Injuries that are poorly treated in the inflammatory phase contribute to the development of pathological scars. Scarring is a chronic, long-term problem for each affected patient [8].

Determining scarring prevalence is a more accurate approach for assessing *global burden* than evaluating incidence of cases of scarring. Most of the data on burn scarring relates to countries with a high socioeconomic level. It is estimated that approximately 100 million people develop scarring due to surgical procedures, burns, and trauma in developed countries [11]. Cutaneous scarring develops in approximately 11 million patients after elective surgery and in approximately 25 million patients after trauma. Moreover, it has been found that approximately 91% of postoperative patients desire an improvement in wound healing, while 15% are dissatisfied with excessive or non-aesthetic scarring. Scars lead to a heterogeneous group of problems that affect many organ systems. In this respect, although the most distinct one is cutaneous scars, scar-related internal problems constitute an important part of scar-related pathological processes [12].

In their review, Mirastschijski et al. [13] evaluated the acute phase, early rehabilitation period and reconstructive care costs of burn victims. They found that reconstructive and rehabilitation care costs were 4.4 times greater than the acute phase costs. According to 2006 data, this cost was calculated to be 245 billion Euros worldwide. This cost included psychiatric care, workforce loss, and other social costs. The real *global burden* of burn injuries has not yet been determined. In 2004, 11 million burn cases needed medical care, 300,000 cases lost their lives, and 90% of these cases were in low socioeconomic countries where it was difficult to access medical and surgical care [8]. The application of conservative approaches in cases with prolonged inflammation and deep partial or full-thickness burns often results in pathological scarring [8].

5. Epidemiology for Cutaneous Scarring

The most relevant data on epidemiology of pathological scarring is related to burn injuries. The risk of developing pathological scarring after burns is higher than it is for other types of trauma or surgical injuries. The incidence of HTS after burn injuries ranges from 32 to 94%, and it is estimated that the cost of treatment of these scars in the United States exceeds $4 billion [8]. In a retrospective cohort study performed by Hop et al. [14], it was reported that 13% of 1,768 patients in three Dutch burn centers were treated with reconstructive surgery within 10 years; the average number of reconstructive procedures applied per patient was 3.6, and the most commonly reconstructed regions were the hand and head–neck region. They also found that the most common indication was scar contracture and that the average medical cost per patient was 8,342 Euros for a period of 10 years.

In developing countries, approximately 52% of burn injuries are seen in children under the age of 5. Here, the etiology is comparable to that in developed countries, and the most common reason is unintentional scalding. Children aged 1–4 years are more likely to suffer from burns than older children and adults are. Intentional burn injuries account for about 5% of all burn injuries in the United States [8]. In their study conducted with more than 700 children under 15 years of age, Dedovic et al. [15] found that the prevalence of pathological scarring after burn injury was 32%.

Worldwide, more than 200 million incisions are made every year in the context of surgery that result in scarring, while only 170,000 scar revisions were made in the United States in 2011 [16]. The prevalence of HTS has been reported to be between 15% and 63% in the Caucasian population. It has been reported that approximately 350,000 scarring-related surgical procedures are performed every year in Hong Kong. Li-Tsang et al. [17] conducted a study on 154 patients who underwent surgical operations in the Department of Orthopedics and Traumatology and found that 74.67% of the patients had HTS symptoms.

Contractures are a pathological consequence of excessive scar development and a well-known complication that develop after burns. Scar contractures restrict joint movements and limit daily activities. Oosterwijk et al. [18] reported that the prevalence of post-burn scar contracture varied in the range of 38–54% at discharge, but this was lower in the long term after burns. They also suggested that contractures were more likely in severe burns and flame burns, in children and women, and in cervical spine and upper extremity burns. The type of surgical operation performed may also play an important role in the development of contracture. Although the studies in this regard are limited, it has been suggested that full-thickness skin grafts result in fewer contractures than partial-thickness skin grafts or spontaneously healing scars do [7].

The data from countries with low socioeconomic status on burn sequalae reveals the actual situation. In a cross-sectional study on 1,400 households in Ethiopia, it was reported that burns were observed in 1.2% of the population annually. Eighty percent of these burns take place at home; 90% of patients recover without complications, while 1% loses their lives [19]. In Bangladesh, the permanent sequela development due to childhood burns has been reported to be 5.7/100,000 with a mortality rate of 0.6/100,000 [20].

A recent study found that only 4.3% of cases treated in emergency care units were directed to burn centers when the ratio of patients hospitalized among all burn cases were examined [21]. The frequency of admittance rate for burns was reported to be 20.6/100,000 per year on average. For children, it was estimated that the incidence of hospitalization for burn treatment was 8/100,000 in the community [22].

A decline has been observed in mortality rates due to burns. From 1982 to 2002, it was found that burn-related mortality decreased from 1.5/100,000 to 0.7/100,000 in Australia and from 1.1/100,000 to 0.5/100,000 in Brazil. However, the decline in the incidence of mortality due to burn injuries in the last three decades has not been observed in all countries. Individual factors, such as alcohol consumption and changes in social, political, and environmental factors can play an important role in national variations in burn-related mortality rates. Most burn-related mortalities worldwide are seen in countries with low-to-moderate or low socioeconomic status. Childhood burn injury mortality is 11 times higher in countries with a low socioeconomic level than those with a high socioeconomic level [22].

6. Psychosocial Effects of Cutaneous Scarring

Patients complaining of scarring, especially those who have history of facial trauma, suffer from severe negative functional and social effects [8]. A study reported that a significant decrease in life expectancy and significant increases in the incidence of negative body image, post-traumatic stress disorder (PTSD), alcoholism, and depression were observed in patients aged 8–45 years with a laceration of 3 cm or longer or a facial bone fracture requiring surgery. Furthermore, it was shown that the incidence of unemployment, marital problems, imprisonment, and reduction in attractiveness scores were higher in this group of patients [23]. It has been suggested that routine psychiatric screening tests should be performed to detect patients at risk of *psychosocial effects* and arrange psychiatric treatment, especially among patients with facial trauma [8].

Burn injury is a devastating event that often has long-lasting physical and *psychosocial effects*. Burn scars that develop after deep dermal injuries force the individual to cope with changes in body appearance. Furthermore, the traumatic nature of burn injuries and painful treatment processes can trigger psychopathological effects. The most frequently researched psychopathologies in burn patients are depression and PTSD, and their prevalence rates are 13–23% and 13–45%, respectively. Risk factors for PTSD include pre-burn depression, severity of symptoms, pain-related anxiety, and the appearance of lesions. In these patients, difficulties can also be seen in sexual life and social relations. The quality of life is lower in these patients compared with the normal population [24].

Psychological and social factors in children with scarring and the scar's effect on quality of life are often ignored. In these patients, the clinician's scar severity scoring may not correlate with the patient's psychosocial distress. Sometimes, other people's reaction to scarring can play an important role in development of stigmatization and discrimination in the individual. Such behaviors can lead to major problems, such as a sense of rejection, loneliness, isolation, and "social death" [25]. It has been shown that burn traumas, followed by troublesome treatment processes and resulting in subsequent malformations and dysfunction, lead to depression, anxiety disorder, and PTSD in children. Therefore, a multidisciplinary team effort in the treatment of children with disfiguring and debilitating scars will be more beneficial [26].

The number of randomized studies on the treatment of *psychosocial effects* of scarring is limited. Blakeney et al. [27] investigated the effect of an intensive, short-term social skills training program on improving patients' psychosocial adjustment in adolescent patients with burn injuries. It was determined that there was significantly higher improvement in the group that received 1 year of training compared with the group that did not receive any training. In another study, sexuality, body image, affect, and relationships were evaluated in burn patients over time following injury. It was found that there was no significant improvement in these patients with time in terms of any of these four factors, regardless of good physical and functional recovery [28]. Similarly, Berg et al. [29] conducted a study on burn patients and divided them into four groups according to the time period passed since the burn. Quality of life, anxiety, depression, PTSD, stigmatization, and social support were evaluated. There were no significant differences between the groups with regard to the factors evaluated in this study, and it was suggested that the psychosocial burden in burn patients persisted without any decrease in time.

Conclusion

In conclusion, scar development is an undesired condition after trauma. There are many risk factors associated with the development of cutaneous scarring; knowing these risk factors may contribute to the development of scar-preventive approaches. In addition, cutaneous scars are an important cause of morbidity and place a tremendous burden on the healthcare system. The overall dimensions of the global burden caused by cutaneous scarring are still not fully known, and the most relevant data in this respect comes from burn scars. Cutaneous scarring can cause serious physical problems in patients; however, psychosocial problems that may occur in these patients should not be ignored.

References

[1] Ferahbas, Ayten. 2005. "Skar oluşumunu etkileyen faktörler." *Turkiye Klinikleri Journal of Internal Medical Sciences* 1: 127-31.

[2] Butzelaar, L., M. M. W. Ulrich, A. B Mink van der Molen, F. B. Niessen, R. H. J. Beelen. 2016. "Currently known risk factors for hypertrophic skin scarring: A

review." *Journal of Plastic, Reconstructive & Aesthetic Surgery* 69:163-9. doi: 10.1016/j.bjps.2015.11.015.

[3] Kelekci, Kıymet H. 2015. "Risk factors for scar formation after surgical incision." *Turkderm* 49: 213-7.

[4] Marshall, Clement D., and Michael S. Hu, Tripp Leavitt, Leandra A. Barnes, H. Peter Lorenz, Michael T. Longaker. 2018. "Cutaneous Scarring: Basic Science, Current Treatments, and Future Directions." *Advances in Wound Care* (New Rochelle) 7:29-45. doi: 10.1089/wound.2016.0696.

[5] Monstrey, S., and E. Middelkoop, J. J. Vranckx, F. Bassetto, U. E. Ziegler, S. Meaume, L. Téot. 2014. "Updated scar management practical guidelines: non-invasive and invasive measures." *Journal of Plastic, Reconstructive & Aesthetic Surgery* 67:1017-25. doi: 10.1016/j.bjps.2014.04.011.

[6] Stella, Maurizio, and Carlotta Castagnoli, Ezio N. Gangemi. 2008. "Postburn scars: an update." *International Journal of Lower Extremity Wounds* 7:176-81. doi: 10.1177/1534734608323057.

[7] Gangemi, Ezio N., and Dario Gregori, Paola Berchialla, Enrico Zingarelli, Monica Cairo, Daniele Bollero, Jamal Ganem, Roberto Capocelli, Franca Cuccuru, Pompeo Cassano, Daniela Risso, Maurizio Stella. 2008. "Epidemiology and risk factors for pathologic scarring after burn wounds." *Archives of Facial Plastic Surgery* 10:93-102. doi: 10.1001/archfaci.10.2.93.

[8] Tenenhaus, Mayer, and Hans-Oliver Rennenkhampff, Bruce M. Potenza. 2017. "The Global Impact of Scars." In: *The Scar Book: Formation, Mitigation, Rehabilitation, and Prevention,* edited by Krakowski, Andrew C., and Peter R. Shumaker, 61-75. Philadelphia: Wolters Kluwer.

[9] Shaheen, Abeer A. 2017. "Risk Factors of Keloids: A Mini Review." *Austin Journal of Dermatology* 4: 1074.

[10] Desmoulière, Alexis, and Christine Chaponnier, Giulio Gabbiani. 2005. "Tissue repair, contraction, and the myofibroblast." *Wound Repair and Regeneration* 13:7-12.

[11] Walmsley, Graham G., and Zeshaan N. Maan, Victor W. Wong, Dominik Duscher, Michael S. Hu, Elizabeth R. Zielins, Taylor Wearda, Ethan Muhonen, Adrian McArdle, Ruth Tevlin, David A. Atashroo, Kshemendra Senarath-Yapa, H. Peter Lorenz, Geoffrey C. Gurtner, Michael T. Longaker. 2015. "Scarless wound healing: chasing the holy grail." *Plastic and Reconstructive Surgery* 135:907-17. doi: 10.1097/PRS.0000000000000972.

[12] Young, V. Leroy, and John Hutchison. 2009. "Insights into patient and clinician concerns about scar appearance: semiquantitative structured surveys." *Plastic and Reconstructive Surgery* 124:256-65. doi: 10.1097/PRS.0b013e3181a80747.

[13] Mirastschijski, Ursula, and Jan-Thorben Sander, Birgit Weyand, Hans-Oliver Rennekampff. 2013. "Rehabilitation of burn patients: an underestimated socio-economic burden." *Burns* 39:262-8. doi: 10.1016/j.burns.2012.06.009.

[14] Hop, M. J., and L. C. Langenberg, J. Hiddingh, C. M. Stekelenburg, M. B. van der Wal, C. J. Hoogewerf, M. L. J. van Koppen, S. Polinder, P. P. van Zuijlen, M. E. van Baar, E. Middelkoop. 2014. "Reconstructive surgery after burns: a 10-year follow-up study." *Burns* 40:1544-51. doi: 10.1016/j.burns.2014.04.014.

[15] Dedovic, Z., and I. Koupilová, P. Brychta. 1999. "Time trends in incidence of hypertrophic scarring in children treated for burns." *Acta Chirurgica Plasticae* 41:87-90.

[16] Lim, Angeline F., and Jennifer Weintraub, Ernest N. Kaplan, Michael Januszyk, Christy Cowley, Peggy McLaughlin, Bill Beasley, Geoffrey C. Gurtner, Michael T. Longaker. 2014. "The embrace device significantly decreases scarring following scar revision surgery in a randomized controlled trial." *Plastic and Reconstructive Surgery* 133:398-405. doi: 10.1097/01.prs.0000436526.64046.d0.

[17] Li-Tsang, Cecilia W. P., and Joy C. M. Lau, Chetwyn C. H. Chan. 2005. "Prevalence of hypertrophic scar formation and its characteristics among the Chinese population." *Burns* 31:610-6.

[18] Oosterwijk, Anouk M., and Leonora J. Mouton, Hennie Schouten, Laurien M. Disseldorp, Cees P. van der Schans, Marianne K. Nieuwenhuis. 2017. "Prevalence of scar contractures after burn: A systematic review." *Burns* 43:41-49. doi: 10.1016/j.burns.2016.08.002.

[19] Nega, Kidanu E., and Bernt Lindtjjorn. 2002. "Epidemiology of burn injuries in Mekele Town, Northern Ethiopia: a community based study." *Ethiopian Journal of Health Development* 16:1-7.

[20] Mashreky, S. R., and A. Rahman, S. M. Chowdhury, S. Giashuddin, L. SvanstrOm, M. Linnan, S. Shafinaz, I. J. Uhaa, F. Rahman. 2008. "Epidemiology of childhood burn: yield of largest community based injury survey in Bangladesh." *Burns* 34:856-62. doi: 10.1016/j.burns.2007.09.009.

[21] DeKoning, Elisha P., and Anne Hakenewerth, Timothy F. Platts-Mills, Judith E. Tintinalli. 2009. "Epidemiology of burn injuries presenting to North Carolina emergency departments in 2006-2007." *Burns* 35:776-82. doi: 10.1016/j.burns.2008.09.012.

[22] Peck, Michael D. 2011. "Epidemiology of burns throughout the world. Part I: Distribution and risk factors." *Burns* 37:1087-100. doi: 10.1016/j.burns.2011.06.005.

[23] Levine, Elie, and Linda Degutis, Thomas Pruzinsky, Joseph Shin, John A. Persing. 2005. "Quality of life and facial trauma: psychological and body image effects." *Annals of Plastic* Surg*ery* 54:502-10.

[24] Van Loey, N. E., and M. J. Van Son. 2003. "Psychopathology and psychological problems in patients with burn scars: epidemiology and management." American *Journal of Clinical Dermatology* 4:245-72.

[25] Krakowski, Andrew C., and Christine R. Totri, Matthias B. Donelan, Peter R. Shumaker. 2016. "Scar Management in the Pediatric and Adolescent Populations." *Pediatrics* 137:e20142065. doi: 10.1542/peds.2014-2065.

[26] Langeland, Willie, and Miranda Olff. 2008. "Psychobiology of posttraumatic stress disorder in pediatric injury patients: a review of the literature." *Neuroscience & Biobehavioral Reviews* 32:161-74.

[27] Blakeney, Patricia, and Christopher Thomas, Charles Holzer, Mary Rose, Frances Berniger, Walter J. Meyer. 2005. "Efficacy of a short-term, intensive social skills training program for burned adolescents." *Journal of Burn Care & Rehabilitation* 26:546-55.

[28] Connell, K. M., and M. Phillips, R. Coates, M. Doherty-Poirier, F. M. Wood. 2014. "Sexuality, body image and relationships following burns: analysis of BSHS-B outcome measures." *Burns* 40:1329-37. doi: 10.1016/j.burns.2014.01.006.

[29] Berg, Lea, and Stefanie Meyer, Ramin Ipaktchi, Peter M. Vogt, Astrid Müller, Martina de Zwaan. 2017. "Psychosocial Distress at Different Time Intervals after Burn Injury." *Psychotherapie, Psychosomatik, Medizinische Psychologie* 67:231-239. doi: 10.1055/s-0042-111006.

In: Cutaneous Scars: Biology, Clinics and Management ISBN: 978-1-53615-657-7
Editors: Berna Aksoy, Hasan Mete Aksoy et al. © 2019 Nova Science Publishers, Inc.

Chapter 3

BIOLOGY OF WOUND HEALING AND SCAR FORMATION

Timuçin Avsar[1,2,*], Alihan Sursal[2], Berfu Nur Yigit[2] and Deniz Altunsu[2]
[1]Department of Medical Biology, Bahcesehir University, School of Medicine, Istanbul, Turkey
[2]Neuroscience Program, Bahcesehir University, Health Sciences Institute, Istanbul, Turkey

ABSTRACT

Wound healing is a complex physiologic process in which tissue repairs itself upon an injury. This physiological phenomenon includes successive and sequential biological processes like hemostasis, inflammatory response, proliferation of involved cells, and remodeling of the tissue. In this chapter molecules and cell types taking part in these processes are summarized.

Keywords: angiogenesis, apoptosis, contraction, fibrin clot, granulation tissue, hemostasis, inflammation, maturation, MMPs, PDGF, proliferation, re-epithelization, remodeling, TGF, wound healing

1. Introduction

Skin is the largest and partially regenerative multifunctional organ of the body. Skin acts as a physical barrier and an immune protective layer. It maintains homeostasis in terms of body temperature, preserves water inside the body and produces vitamin D [1].

Cutaneous *wound healing* can be defined as a complex physiological process starting after skin injury. Management of wound healing is becoming less problematic as a resort of an increasing number of studies focused on new therapeutic approaches and the development of new technologies for both acute and chronic wound treatment. Cutaneous *wound healing* mechanism is regulated via complex molecular signaling pathways which result in recruitment of a number of different cells. A variety of proteins, proteases, growth factors, and extracellular matrix components are involved in wound healing process.

Cellular and biochemical events in *wound healing* can be divided into four different stages: Maintaining the *hemostasis*, initiating the inflammatory reaction, *proliferation* of required cells with synthesis of extracellular matrix elements, and the final *remodeling* phase.

2. Maintaining Hemostasis

In case of a skin injury, the first phase of *wound healing* includes prevention of blood outflow and fluid loss as a result of vascular injury. The *hemostasis* phase begins at the onset of wound formation and lasts till the end of blood clot formation. Sequential events of platelet aggregation, clotting and complement cascade activation prevent further blood, fluid and electrolyte loss from the wound within seconds after injury. The components of hemostasis phase are cross linked fibrin along with fibronectin, vitronectin and thrombospondin and they create a blood clot [2]. Blood clot acts as a temporary protective shield for the injury site and attracts the inflammatory cells, endothelial cells, keratinocytes and fibroblasts to the injury area [3]. Fibrin clot can also provide a niche for the cells and harbor a variety of growth factors that contribute to the formation of new blood vessels and extracellular matrix [4]. One exception to the formation of fibrin clot is the case with burn injury which causes coagulation necrosis of blood vessels.

2.1. Vasoconstriction of Blood Vessels

The first reaction to the wounding trauma including dermal blood vessel injury is the secretion of vasoactive amines from the exposed dermal cells of the skin. Nervous system releases epinephrine into the blood circulation and additionally peripheral sympathetic nervous system releases norepinephrine into wound site and these also contribute to vasoconstriction of blood vessels. Finally, local cells secrete prostaglandins for additional contribution to the response to blood vessel injury [5].

2.2. Platelet Aggregation

Injured cells at the wound site secrete tissue factors to stimulate platelet aggregation. Aggregated platelets have two major functions in hemostasis stage. First, they secrete one of the serine protease enzymes called as thrombin [6]. Conversion of soluble plasma fibrinogen into an insoluble *fibrin clot* is catalyzed by thrombin enzyme and this conversion is the key factor for clotting.

The second role of platelets takes place when they are trapped in the fibrin net. These trapped cells release their granules which are reservoirs for biologically active proteins like, RANTES, CCL5, transforming growth factor (*TGF*)-Beta, hepatocyte growth factor (HGF), insulin like growth factor (IGF), platelet derived growth factor (*PDGF*) and vascular endothelial growth factor (VEGF) [7]. In addition to the growth factors which are necessary for proliferation of cells to repair the gap formed as a result of injury, chemoattractant molecules are also released from platelets and they attract the inflammatory cells into the wound site [8]. CCL5 is one of the major attractant molecules for monocytes and MCP-1 (CCL2), MIP-1 alpha (CCL3), *TGF* alpha, fibronectin, C5a and C3a are the other important molecules to induce native inflammatory response.

PDGF released from granules not only induces differentiation of cells and attracts immune cells, but also enhances *proliferation* of fibroblasts and increases the healing capacity [4]. However, increased release of *PDGF* from the platelets can cause formation of hypertrophic scars [9].

2.3. Coagulation Cascade Formation

There are two independent pathways responsible for coagulation cascade formation; *contact activated* (intrinsic) and *tissue factor* (extrinsic) pathways. For the initiation of healing process, extrinsic pathway always needs to be activated, but there is no obligation for activation of intrinsic one [10].

When the blood vessel is injured, surrounding fibroblasts and leukocytes release Factor VII or Factor VIIa to activate extrinsic pathway [5]. On the other hand, intrinsic pathway is triggered when the blood is exposed to the external surfaces, which causes secretion of Faxtor XII (Hageman factor). Both pathways work together for the production of thrombin that converts fibrinogen to fibrin. Fibrin is crucial for increasing permeability of blood vessels and supports the migration of inflammatory cells to the wound site [11]. But, fibrin needs to be stabilized in wound area to provide a meshwork network system of platelet plug. Fibrin molecule is then coated with a serum derived protein called vitronectin. This action results in attraction of fibronectin produced by epithelial cells and fibroblasts and of thrombospondin coming from granules of platelets [12]. Together, they form *fibrin clot* which acts as a scaffold and supports growth factors and cytokines needed for the wound healing. Following wound closure, fibronectin expression decreases within a few days, but in some scars its expression continues at a high level for months and hence this results in higher fibroblast density seen in hypertrophic scars [12].

After *fibrin clot* is formed and blood flow is regulated, endothelial cells start to degrade the clot by releasing plasminogen activator (tPA), the major fibrinolytic protease [13]. Degraded fibrin molecules also act as chemotactic signals for neutrophils and monocytes. As a result, various cells and proteins in hemostasis stage are part of both the clotting and inflammatory response and regulate cell adhesion.

3. Inflammation in Wound Healing

Inflammation can be defined as a complex response of body to the damaged cells or other immunological abnormality. Increased permeabilization in venules and migration of leukocytes to extravascular space result in inflammatory response in wounding injuries. The main function of *inflammation* is to provide nonspecific and then specific defense against pathogens, as well as to clean-up various cell debris by releasing lysozomal enzymes and reactive oxygen species, so that the repair process can proceed [14, 15].

In the first 24 hours after injury, inflammatory response mediated by cells is established. This initiation time of inflammation may be delayed up to two days in some cases. In the wound site, neutrophils are the first to appear as inflammatory cells, subsequently macrophages are seen within 48-72 hours and afterward fibroblasts become dominant cell types at the wound site [16]. This quick activation of immune system at the location of injury can proceed by the help of mastocytes, Langerhans cells and gamma-delta T cells that secrete cytokines and chemokines.

3.1. Neutrophils

Neutrophils are the first immune cells travelling to the site of wound within hours after injury. The stimulation of neutrophil migration into the area is triggered by collagen, bacterial products, complement factors, immunomodulatory factors like TNF-a, PAF, *TGF*-β, platelet factor IV [5]. The main purpose of these cells is to clean up foreign substances, necrotic tissue and bacteria through secretion of pro-inflammatory cytokines and antimicrobial substances such as cationic peptides, proteases and reactive oxygen species (ROS). After completion of their function, remaining neutrophils become senescent and undergo *apoptosis* or phagocytozed by macrophages [17].

3.2. Monocytes-Macrophages

Monocytes start to migrate from neighboring blood vessels in response to chemotactic stimuli and accumulate within avascular hypoxic area of wound site 48 hours after injury. They are capable of binding to certain proteins like cell adhesion molecules (CAMs) present in the extracellular matrix [18]. In the extracellular matrix, monocytes are exposed to many cytokines like IFN-γ, IL-4, IL-10, IL-13 and bacterial products and differentiate into macrophages. This differentiation reaches a peak nearly 2 to 3 days after wounding [19]. In this differentiation, macrophages undergo many changes resulting in alterations in their gene expression. According to this activation system, they can be classified into two types; alternatively activated (pro-angiogenic and anti-inflammatory, M2, promoting wound healing) and classically activated (pro-inflammatory, M1, promoting chronic inflammation) macrophages [20]. This activation is crucial for the adaptation of macrophages to be fully functional at wound site.

The macrophages are multipurpose cells involved in many aspects of immunological functions like phagocytosis, antigen presentation, and wound healing responses by releasing numerous growth factors and they are also involved in regulation of healing processes like collagen deposition. First role of macrophages is to recognize, bind and engulf foreign substances, senescent cells and necrotic debris within the wound. The α-domain of β2 integrin CR3 (CD11b-CD18) and cluster of differentiation 14 (CD14), Toll-like receptors, Fc receptors and complement receptors are binding receptors that provide recognition of pathogen-associated *molecular* patterns like lipoteichoic acid [21]. The digestion of these unwanted molecules is achieved by hydrolytic enzymes and oxygen radicals following the engulfment process. Macrophages that are involved in cleaning necrotic tissues drag into apoptosis. Remaining macrophages contribute to regulation of collagen production by releasing matrix metalloproteinases (MMPs). In this way, these cells not only contribute to elimination of unwanted molecules but also support and control transition from inflammatory stage to proliferation stage in the wound site [22].

Other important feature of macrophages is continued synthesis and secretion of growth factors and cytokines into the wound environment. There are many growth factors that regulate cellular proliferation and support synthesis of ECM by participating cells of wound healing, and these are basic fibroblast growth factor (bFGF), vascular endothelial growth factor (VEGF), platelet-derived growth factor (PDGF), TGF-α, and TGF-β (Table 1) [23].

Macrophages can remain in the wound site up till the 7th day and then they diminish in number if there is no inflammatory stimuli [23].

Table 1. Growth factors involved in wound healing (Table is adapted from [25])

Growth Factor	Effect	Released From
Epidermal growth factor (EGF)	Stimulation of epidermal and dermal regeneration [26]	Platelets
Fibroblast growth factor (FGF)	Promotion of fibroblast proliferation and neovascularization [27]	Endothelial cells, Macrophages
Transforming growth factor-alpha (TGF-α)	Enhances cell proliferation and cell migration [28]	Macrophages, Keratinocytes
Transforming growth factor- beta 1 and 2 (TGF-β)	Induces secretion of protease inhibitors and promotes chemotaxis of fibroblasts and macrophages	Macrophages, Plateles
Vascular endothelial growth factor (VEGF)	Increases vascular permeability and stimulates vasodilation [29]	Macrophages, Keratinocytes
Keratinocyte growth Factor (KGF)	Regulates migration and differentiation of epithelial cells [30]	Fibroblasts
Hepatocyte growth factor (HGF)	Induces angiogenesis [31]	Platelets
Insulin-like growth factor (IGF)	Enhances proliferation of fibroblasts and endothelial cells	Platelets and plasma
Platelet derived growth factors (AA, AB, BB) (PDGFs)	Induces chemotaxis of fibroblasts and macrophages and enhances fibroblast proliferation	Platelets, Macrophages Keratinocytes
Tumor necrosis factor-alpha (*TNF-α)*	Activates growth factor expression in keratinocytes, fibroblasts and macrophages	Neutrophils
Interleukin-1alpha and beta (*IL*-1 family)	Activates growth factor expression in keratinocytes, fibroblasts and macrophages	Neutrophils

3.3. T Lymphocytes

Although T cells are present at the wound site 5 to 7 days after injury, their crucial role has a place in wound healing process rather than inflammatory response, because local infection problem has already been overcome by neutrophils and macrophages. T cells especially CD4+ ones over CD8+ cells are important sources of cytokines; fibroblast activating factor, EGF, *TGF*-β, TNF-α, IL-1 and IL-2 [24]. By releasing cytokines, they regulate and control microenvironment at the wound site. Inflammatory responses of T lymphocytes can be seen in the case of presence of virus infected cells at the wound site.

4. Proliferation Phase

The proliferative stage follows the initial inflammatory response upon injury and provides the formation of scar structure necessary for the subsequent production of a new functional skin barrier. Important events during this phase are the creation of a permeability barrier i.e., re-epithelialization process, establishment of blood supply i.e., angiogenesis, and fortification of the injured dermal tissue i.e., fibroplasia.

The cutaneous wound healing in proliferative phase can also be referred to as granulation phase. It includes the angiogenic sprouting (angiogenesis), fibroplasia (fibroblast proliferation & migration, and collagen & extracellular matrix synthesis), regeneration of epidermis (re-epithelization), and wound contraction [32].

4.1. Angiogenesis in Wound Healing

Angiogenesis is generally brought about by the process of endothelial cell *proliferation*, rearrangement of the basal membrane and cell migration [32]. Angiogenesis is a significant process for optimal *wound healing* considering nutritional requirement of cells to migrate and proliferate. There is a huge controversy in the scientific literature about the level and status of angiogenic molecules during wound healing. Here, the recent information on angiogenic factors having role in *wound healing* will be summarized:

There are several angiogenic growth factors in *wound healing*, each has different roles. Fibroblast growth factor-2 (FGF-2) is synthesized by macrophages and damaged endothelial cells while vascular endothelial growth factor (VEGF) production is induced in wound-edge keratinocytes and macrophages [25]. If FGF-2 is depleted, the process of *angiogenesis* in the wound will be blocked. Similar to fibroblasts and keratinocytes, the endothelial cells additionally need to upregulate specific integrins ($\alpha v\beta 3$) on their surface to keep themselves respondant to angiogenic signals. All these signals induce *proliferation*, migration and phenotypic expression in endothelial cells but these issues have not been completely understood yet. It is evident that angiogenesis is a complex process and depends on the availability of extracellular matrix in the wound [25].

4.2. Extra-Cellular Matrix Synthesis

Extracellular matrix (ECM) is a complex structure formed by various protein subunits such as collagen, proteoglycans, glycosaminoglycans and specific glycoproteins. Not only does ECM support the cell network but also it maintains other cellular activities such as induction of proliferation of fibroblasts, chemotaxis and apoptosis of unnecessary cells alongside with controlled degradation of ECM proteins [33]. ECM proteins are mainly synthesized by fibroblasts and can be stimulated by mechanical tension which may emerge during an acute injury [34]. Apoptosis and controlled degradation of ECM proteins are crucial to improve the scar tissue during wound remodeling phase [35]. ECM also participates in various signalling cascades, an example is that completion of the ECM production allows fibroblasts to differentiate into myofibroblasts, enabling the progress of the wound healing process to its final phase [36]. Moreover, ECM also indirectly regulates synthesis of proteolytic enzymes and cytokines [37].

4.3. Fibroblast Migration and Proliferation

After an acute injury, fibroblast excitation is stimulated by cytokine signalling, mostly by *TGF*-β and *PDGF*, produced by the *fibrin clot* structure formed in *hemostasis* phase. Hemostatic clot is the result of thrombin directed fibrinogen cleavage which renders the fibrinogen proteins suitable to form a polymer structure, the fibrin plug [38]. Fibroblast excitation stimulates their *proliferation* around the wound space. Increased fibroblast *proliferation* results in enhanced production of ECM proteins such as proteoglycans, fibronectins, vitronectins, collagens and hyaluronans.

The enhanced angiogenesis along with fibroblast proliferation brings about the formation of *granulation tissue*. *Granulation tissue* is mostly composed of type III collagen. Fibroblast to myofibroblast differentiation occurs following ECM production. Myofibroblasts will play a major role during wound contraction by producing cytoplasm-filled projections targeting fibronectins and collagens and afterwards they contract the newly formed tissue. Wound contraction helps to achieve the required tensile strength [36].

4.4. Collagen Deposition

Collagen is the primary protein of ECM and plays major roles in every step of *wound healing*. Collagen can form strong structures with high tensile strength. In addition to its supportive properties, collagen is a strong chemotactic agent that maintains the motility during cellular migration of fibroblasts and keratinocytes [39]. Fibroblasts also synthesize collagen proteins to advance fortification. There is a systematic degradation and synthesis of collagen molecules during *wound healing*. The synthesis of collagen molecules is mainly executed by fibroblasts. The degradation of collagen molecules is catalyzed by proteolytic enzymes such as matrix metalloproteinases (*MMPs*), plasminogens (PAs) and collagenase [40]. PAs are the precursors of plasmin enzyme that also degrades blood proteins including fibrin clot [41]. MMPs on the other hand are specific for degradation of ECM proteins [35].

Deposition of collagen proteins reaches the peak level around 3 weeks. Degradation of the collagenous structure is crucial for preventing excessive deposition as seen in hypertrophic scarring. Opposite to hypertrophic scar formation, chronic wound is the result of abnormally high levels of proteolytic enzymes which consistently degrade required ECM structures, so wound healing enters a lag phase [42].

4.5. Re-Epithelization

Re-epithelization is one of the earliest events after wound formation since the epithelial cell proliferation and migration starts directly after acute injury [5]. *Re-epithelization* occurs from the wound edges and remaining lower parts of skin appendages. *Re-epithelization* occurs at a slower rate in the case of total tissue disruption. In the absence of the basal dermal layers, the starting point of *re-epithelization* process remains at the edges of the injury and this limits the proliferation rate and cell migration. *Re-epithelization* is very important as the outermost layer of the skin, epidermis, acts as a protective layer against infection during incoming phases of the wound healing process. Moreover this layer acts like a sheath.

During *re-epithelization*, cell migration and ECM degradation play crucial roles together with cell proliferation and differentiation. Both mechanisms require proper environmental signalling in order to achieve proper re-epithelization. Like other biological mechanisms, *re-epithelization* has specific signalling cascades that are not completely known [43]. Via these signalling cascades, epidermal cells localized at the edge of the wounded area start to proliferate, remove their adhesions to facilitate migration and migrate in the direction of more central sites of the injury [43, 44]. Numerous cytokines play diverse roles during the *re-epithelization* process such as *PDGF*, KGF, EGF, *TGF*-α, *TGF*-β and IL-1 [9, 44]. Moreover, epidermal cell migration is mainly controlled via transmembranous participation of different integrin receptor proteins, vitronectins and fibronectins. Mainly, αvβ6 and α5β1 fibronectin receptors in cooperation with αvβ5 vitronectin receptor play major roles during epithelial migration [5, 43]. Besides the sole epithelial cell translocation, emerging mechanisms promoting the epithelial migration also force the *granulation tissue* to move away from the fibrinogen polymer (*fibrin clot*) [45]. Keratinocytes offer a proper environment by synthesizing various cytokines such as interleukins and growth factors for *wound healing* and they also release proteolytic enzymes for separation of the *granulation tissue* [46]. The capacity of epithelial migration depends on the controlled disruption of the links between the fibrin plug and the granulation tissue and this separation is the result of MMP and PA synthesis. As the regulation of the cell migration process is controlled by enzymatic and signalling processes, it is inhibited by physical contact of the migrating cells to each other. At the contact area, cell proliferation followed by cell differentiation forms the new epidermis [5, 44].

5. Wound Remodeling

Remodeling is the final phase of the *wound healing* process and takes longer time to be completed in comparison with previous stages. It generally continues for months or even years contrary to the median three weeks time duration required by previous phases [47]. The *remodeling* process is more complicated when the damage involves the deeper layers of the skin and scar tissue is more noticeable when the new collagen molecules laid down for rebinding the damaged skin forming wound edges. Scar formation continues to ameliorate over two years as collagenous tissue and blood vessel remodeling progress further [48]. There is a clinical association between the depth of cutaneous injury and the cutaneous scarring since the critical depth for fibrous scar formation has been quantified as 33.1% of the thickness of the skin [49].

Three sub-events occur during *remodeling* phase and can be described as degradation and re-synthesis of the ECM proteins, particularly collagen, and apoptosis of unnecessary cells like fibroblasts. Collagen proteins are remodeled into wider and more durable form while cell proliferation slows down. Due to reduced proliferation, diminished nutritional requirement allows the blood capillaries to shrink. Thus, the redness of the scar tissue fades over time [50]. In normal conditions, during *remodeling* phase, scar tissue is shielded against external environment. Therefore, there is no need for immune cells such as macrophages, so hence they undergo apoptosis or rejected from the wounded area via emigration process [50]. As the *remodeling* of the scar continues, the highly cellular and vascular granulation tissue diminishes, leaving its place to less cellularized and vascularized scar tissue with enhanced collagenous structure.

5.1. Collagen Remodeling and Proteoglycans

Collagen is main protein of the connective tissue and it is the principal element of the *granulation tissue* and mature scar tissue as well as the normal skin [5]. Additionally, collagen synthesis and organization is the principal event involved in fibrillogenesis. Collagen protein synthesis continues during all 3 stages of *wound healing* process. Destruction of the collagen protein is executed at the same velocity with its synthesis during the remodeling phase. Synthesis of procollagen, which is the precursor form of collagen, depends on oxygen, L-ascorbic acid, 2-oxoglutaric acid and hydroxylase enzymes. Hydroxylases maintain the proline and lysine hydroxylation that contributes to covalent bond formation during fibrillogenesis. Insufficient lysine and proline hydroxylation prevents the collagen to form stable and thick fibrils [5]. The increased strength and diameter of the collagen fibrils allows the scar tissue to gain more tensile strength during the remodeling phase [51].

Hyaluronic acid and fibronectin diminish during the maturation of the scar tissue. Hyaluronic acid is a glycosaminoglycan and acts on cell proliferation and migration during early phases of the *wound healing* process. Reduced need for cell proliferation allows hyaluronic acid destruction during *maturation* by the help of metalloproteinase enzymes and particular cells. Hyaluronic acid induces lymphocyte activation via its primary receptor, CD44.

So this enhances cytokine signaling and localization [52]. In addition, remaining hyaluronic acid plays an inhibitory role on ECM degradation by catalyzing protease-inhibitor relationships to help prevention of over-degradation. Decreased hyaluronic acid concentration in the later phases is replaced by sulfated glycosaminoglycans in the order of versican, decorin and biglycan. Sulfated properties of these proteoglycans enhance the ECM protein relations. Thus, they increase elasticity and tensile strength [52, 53]. Vitronectin is another proteoglycan that acts on collagen proteins during scar contraction and aids ECM organization in order to increase the tensile strength of contracted area [51]. Besides the increased activity during hemostasis, the relationship between vitronectin and its receptor from integrin family promotes cellular binding to ECM, and induces cell adhesion.

Collagen type I is the most abundant form of collagen protein during *maturation* stage of the *wound healing* process [5]. Despite the fact that collagen type III is more abundant during initial phases of the wound healing process, destruction rate of type III collagen is higher than that of collagen type I during the *maturation* phase. Collagen synthesis is affected by physical stress and cytokines, particularly *TGF*-β and FGF, which are strong activators of collagen synthesis via gene transcription activation and inhibition of protease activity [42]. In addition to the generalized increase in collagen synthesis, different scar types have different collagen molecule synthesis not only during *maturation* phase but also in the first stages of *wound healing* process. Besides the morphological appearance of the scar tissue, collagen fiber orientation of the *granulation tissue* may give prognostic hints whether hypertrophic scar will develop or not [54].

5.2. Scar Contraction

In addition to the cytokines, the decreased number of unnecessary cells via emigration and apoptosis allows the scar tissue to recover to its normal shape over time. The remaining fibroblasts in the *granulation tissue* undergo specific differentiation in order to express actin protein by the help of positive regulatory signaling cascade. The actin expressing fibroblasts are called myofibroblasts and have a smooth muscle cell-like phenotype that aids the scar contraction process [55]. The scar *contraction* starts from the outer side of the scar by the help of actin and other ECM proteins like collagen, fibrin, fibronectin, glycoprotein and vitronectin [55]. Although cytokine activation is much lower compared to the inflammation phase of the *wound healing* process, scar *contraction* is stimulated via cytokines such as *PDGF*, *TGF*-β1 and *TGF*-β2. In addition to cytokine signaling, eukaryotic initiation factor 6 (EIF6), which is an upstream modulator of *TGF*-β response, have a role of fine tuning of myofibroblast differentiation. These growth factors additionally induce remaining fibroblasts and differentiated myofibroblasts to bind the collagenous matrix in order to create a cross-linked network. This network allows the boundaries of the scar contracted via increased tension and make the scar tissue more durable against tension. In addition, myofibroblasts have increased collagen type III synthesis and aid in the ECM organization [16]. Myofibroblast differentiation also originates from epidermal stem cells via transdifferentiation. Upregulation of *TGF*-β signaling have an important role during this transdifferentiation process [56].

5.3. Matrix Metalloproteinases (MMPs) and ECM Remodeling

ECM *remodeling* involves systematic degradation of collagen fibrils. As a result, thickness, texture and color of the scar tissue ameliorate. Controlled degradation process indirectly involves IFN-γ and TNF-α signaling which repress collagen synthesis. IFN-γ induces macrophage activation resulting in TNF-α production which is mainly produced by macrophages [5, 57]. This direct degradation process is steered mainly by *MMPs*. MMPs, matrixins, are calcium dependent zinc containing endopeptidases and have a strong proteolytic activity. MMPs are mainly synthesized by fibroblasts, endothelial cells, macrophages and epidermal cells. Some important *MMPs* are hyaluronidase that maintains hyaluronic acid degradation and urokinase, which is the activator of serine protease enzymes such as collagenase and elastase. These enzymes play important roles in collagen and elastin degradation respectively. Gelatinase A, gelatinase B and MMP-3 mainly promote degradation of collagens type I, II, III, X, XIII and IV, V, XI respectively. Moreover, plasmin is another MMP, which mainly promotes the degradation of fibrin clots formed by blood plasma proteins and activates collagenase.

MMP-13 and MMP-14 also prevent excess collagen formation in the scar tissue [58-60]. These enzymes are major modulators of degradation of ECM proteins during *remodeling* of the scar tissue [61]. The activities of *MMPs* are inhibited by tissue inhibitor of metalloproteinases (TIMPs). All together, these enzymes maintain controlled degradation of the ECM proteins and specific membrane macromolecules to smaller molecules in order to reorganize the scar tissue. MMPs have controlling effects on capillary regression in addition to ECM *remodeling* [35]. Macrophages are the major source of *MMPs* and serine proteases. During wound *remodeling*, macrophages express MMP-2 and MMP-9 which are also named as gelatinase A and B respectively [58]. MMP-12, also known as macrophage-specific metalloelastase, is also expressed by macrophages and mostly maintains capillary regression [62]. Since the wound *remodeling* requires both controlled degradation and synthesis of ECM proteins, collagen synthesis occurs at the same rate with the rate of degradation. Besides the degradation mechanism, collagen type VIII production is one of the re-synthesis mechanisms of macrophages contributing to ECM integrity together with fibroblasts [62].

5.4. Apoptosis

The decreased number of macrophages during *maturation* phase via *apoptosis* and emigration allows the scar tissue to decrease in size and prevents abnormal scarring. Endothelial cells are the first to undergo *apoptosis* during wound *remodeling* phase followed by fibroblasts as the proper scar *contraction* process needs actin containing myofibroblasts. Approximately 3 weeks after proper scar *contraction*, myofibroblasts are eradicated completely by *apoptosis* from the scar tissue [5]. *Apoptosis* allows terminal differentiation of newly formed scar tissue and derogates the cellularity of the *granulation tissue* as the *remodeling* phase continues. Proteins such as c-myc, DAD-1, TRADD and p53 are apoptotic signal proteins and have a modulatory role in apoptotic cascade. According to a study, *apoptosis* also occurs during the first stages of *wound healing* process in order to eliminate stressed cells from the wound area [63].

Wound healing process depends on the factors which are intrinsically and extrinsically modulated by scar environment. Additionally, exogenous as well as endogenous elements have regulatory roles on scar environment. Thus, smoking, nutrition or corticosteroid therapy may disrupt the *remodeling* phase. They may also disrupt *inflammation* step, *angiogenesis* and causing insufficient immunologic activity, increased risk of infection, slower *proliferation* due to reduced nutrient flow and prolonged time for completion of the *wound healing* process. Systemic diseases such as venous stasis, immunosuppression and diabetes are endogenous factors causing aberrant *wound healing* process [64].

5.5. Fetal Wound Healing

Fetal tissue can heal completely upon injury without any remaining scar owing to its strong regeneration capacity. The complete mechanism of how fetuses can heal by eliminating scar formation during the beginning of the gestation is unknown [48]. Scarring process in adult tissues involves disturbances of the ECM and excessive connective tissue formation resulting in distorted surface texture of the skin. However, fetal scarring process regenerates the natural ECM network and maintains the original elasticity of the skin. As a result, skin texture remains intact after *wound healing* process. Despite the lowered concentration of collagen type I in the fetal skin, hyaluronic acid and collagen type III are more abundant compared to adult skin. Moreover, MMP-1 and MMP-9 upregulation emerges much faster during fetal wound *remodeling* process. These slightly different environments are associated with tremendous effects on scarless healing of fetal tissues [65].

5.6. Epithelial-Mesenchymal Transdifferentiation

Epithelial-mesenchymal transition is a transdifferentiation process. It causes the epithelial cell to lose its properties and gain mesenchymal characteristics. There are 3 types of transition between epithelial and mesenchymal cells. Type I occurs in the embryogenesis and the type III occurs during the acquisition of motility by a cancer cell prior to metastasis [3]. Type II plays a role during *wound healing* process and it promotes fibrosis. Myofibroblast transdifferentiation from epithelial cells is an example of type II transition [66]. Type II transition requires morphogenic factors and factors that maintain terminal differentiation and resulting from particular signaling pathways such as Wnt, Notch, Bmp and Hedgehog during *wound healing* [66].

5.7. Hedgehog Signaling Pathway

Hedgehog signaling pathway regulates many biological processes such as development, differentiation, homeostasis, and *wound healing* [32]. It was first discovered by using the saturation mutagenesis technique applied on Drosophila, as it was found that specific genes were activated during the progression of body segmentation. There are 3 homologous hedgehog genes discovered in vertebrates named as Sonic hedgehog, Indian hedgehog and Desert hedgehog [67]. Sonic-hedgehog signaling cascade is required for proper *wound healing* process and it enhances the *wound healing* process via increased nitrous oxide function in the skin. *Wound healing* processes have similarities with the developmental stage because the need for differentiation and *proliferation* increases during *wound healing* [68].

6. Abnormal Scarring and Repigmentation

Normal scarring process involves numerous productive and destructive processes regulated by scar tissue environment. Four overlapping phases have both similar and distinctive signaling patterns which not only contribute to proper synthesis of necessary proteins but also to their degradation during wound *remodeling* phase [48]. Final texture or color of the scar can be a sign of how accurate the scarring process has happened. Unproper *remodeling* or unsuccessful repigmentation causes abnormal scar texture. Proper repigmentation is based on melanocyte migration targeting the scar tissue. The migrated melanocytes induce melanin synthesis, which is also named as melanogenesis, and this is followed by melanin transportation targeting keratinocytes [69]. In addition to the melanocyte precursor and stem cells, pilosebaceous units localized in the wound bed contribute to melanocyte repopulation of the target scar area [70]. Anti-scarring agents can be used as preventive or therapeutic measures in order to eliminate abnormal scar formation. Activated protein C (APC) treatment during myocardial healing shows its preventive effect on extreme scarring as well as expediting the healing process, since prolongation of the scarring process may cause abnormal scarring [65]. APC is an anticoagulant which is present naturally during *wound healing* [71]. Another study mentions that APC contributes to keratinocyte *proliferation* in culture conditions via mitogen activated protein kinase (MAPK) activity. In addition to its keratinocyte *proliferation* enhancement property, it decreases the rate of keratinocyte *apoptosis* and enhances the ability of migration of keratinocytes [72].

Conclusion

Inflammatory cells, endothelial cells, keratinocytes and fibroblasts responding to a complex cascade of signals with a coordinated effort enable proper wound healing process to occur. Many of these events are initiated and terminated by the controlled expression of molecules in response to wounding. There are start and stop signals. Further developments in understanding the biology of wound healing will enable us to prevent and treat the unhealed wounds more effectively.

References

[1] Proksch, E., and J. M. Brandner, J. M. Jensen. 2008. "The skin: an indispensable barrier." *Experimental Dermatology* 17:1063-72.

[2] Midwood, Kim S., and Leyla V. Williams, Jean E. Schwarzbauer. 2004. "Tissue repair and the dynamics of the extracellular matrix." *International Journal of Biochemistry & Cell Biology* 36:1031-7. Doi: 10.1016/j.biocel.2003.12.003.

[3] Martin, P. 1997. "Wound healing--aiming for perfect skin regeneration." *Science* 276 (5309): 75-81.

[4] Werner, Sabine, and Richard Grose. 2003. "Regulation of wound healing by growth factors and cytokines." *Physiological Reviews* 83:835-70. Doi: 10.1152/physrev.2003.83.3.835.

[5] Monaco, J. L., and W. T. Lawrence. 2003. "Acute wound healing an overview." *Clinics in Plastic Surgery* 30 (1): 1-12.

[6] He, Shu, and Margareta Blombäck, Niklas Bark, Hans Johnsson, N. Hakan Wallen. 2010. "The direct thrombin inhibitors (argatroban, bivalirudin and lepirudin) and the indirect Xa-inhibitor (danaparoid) increase fibrin network porosity and thus facilitate fibrinolysis." *Thrombosis and Haemostasis* 104:1076-84.

[7] Frank, Stefan, and Heiko Kämpfer, Christian Wetzler, Birgit Stallmeyer, Josef Pfeilschifter. 2000. "Large induction of the chemotactic cytokine RANTES during cutaneous wound repair: a regulatory role for nitric oxide in keratinocyte-derived RANTES expression." *Biochemical Journal* 347:265-73.

[8] Maraganore, J. M. 1993. "Thrombin, thrombin inhibitors, and the arterial thrombotic process." *Thrombosis and Haemostasis* 70:208-11.

[9] Niessen, F. B., and P. H. Spauwen, J. Schalkwijk, M. Kon. 1999. "On the nature of hypertrophic scars and keloids: a review." *Plastic and Reconstructive Surgery* 104:1435-58.

[10] Carter, SB. 1970. "Cell movement and cell spreading: A passive or an active process?" *Nature* 225(5235):858.

[11] Stiernberg, J., and W. R. Redin, W. S. Warner, D. H. Carney. 1993. "The role of thrombin and thrombin receptor activating peptide (TRAP-508) in initiation of tissue repair." *Thrombosis and Haemostasis* 70:158-62.

[12] Tamkun, John W., and Douglas W. DeSimone, Deborah Fonda, Ramila S. Patel, Clayton Buck, Alan F. Horwitz, Richard O. Hynes. 1986. "Structure of integrin, a glycoprotein involved in the transmembrane linkage between fibronectin and actin." *Cell* 46:271-82.

[13] Cesarman-Maus, Gabriela, and Katherine A. Hajjar. 2005. "Molecular mechanisms of fibrinolysis." *British Journal of Haematology* 129:307-21.

[14] Medrado, Alena R. A. P., and Lívia S. Pugliese, Sílvia Regina A. Reis, Zilton A. Andrade. 2003. "Influence of low level laser therapy on wound healing and its

biological action upon myofibroblasts." *Lasers in Surgery and Medicine* 32:239-44.

[15] Majno, Guido, and Stephen M. Shea, Monika Leventhal. 1969. "Endothelial contraction induced by histamine-type mediators: an electron microscopic study." *The Journal of Cell Biology* 42:647-72.

[16] Peled, Ziv M., and Gyu S. Chin, W. Liu, Robert Galliano, Michael T. Longaker. 2000. "Response to tissue injury." *Clinics in Plastic Surgery* 27:489-500.

[17] Clarke, R. A. 1988. "Overview and general considerations of wound repair." *The Molecular and Cellular Biology of Wound Repair* 18-22.

[18] Brown, Eric J. 1995. "Phagocytosis." *Bioessays* 17:109-17.

[19] Eming, Sabine A., and Thomas Krieg, Jeffrey M. Davidson. 2007. "Inflammation in wound repair: molecular and cellular mechanisms." *Journal of Investigative Dermatology* 127:514-25.

[20] Rodero, Mathieu P., and Kiarash Khosrotehrani. 2010. "Skin wound healing modulation by macrophages." *International Journal of Clinical and Experimental Pathology* 3:643.

[21] Karin, Michael, and Toby Lawrence, Victor Nizet. 2006. "Innate immunity gone awry: linking microbial infections to chronic inflammation and cancer." *Cell* 124:823-835.

[22] Baum, Christian L., and Christopher J. Arpey. 2005. "Normal cutaneous wound healing: clinical correlation with cellular and molecular events." *Dermatologic Surgery* 31:674-86.

[23] DiPietro, L.A., and P.J. Polverini. 1993. "Role of the macrophage in the positive and negative regulation of wound neovascularization." *Behring Institute Mitteilungen* 92:238-47.

[24] Minchenko, A., and S. Salceda, T. Bauer, J. Caro. 1994. "Hypoxia regulatory elements of the human vascular endothelial growth factor gene." *Cellular & Molecular Biology Research* 40:35-9.

[25] Aukhil, Ikramuddin. 2000. "Biology of wound healing." *Periodontology* 22:44-50.

[26] Bodnar, Richard J. 2013. "Epidermal growth factor and epidermal growth factor receptor: the yin and yang in the treatment of cutaneous wounds and cancer." *Advances in Wound Care* 2:24-9. Doi: 10.1089/wound.2011.0326.

[27] Matsumoto, Shigeru, and Rica Tanaka, Kayoko Okada, Kayo Arita, Hiko Hyakusoku, Masaaki Miyamoto, Yasuhiko Tabata, Hiroshi Mizuno. 2013. "The effect of control-released basic fibroblast growth factor in wound healing: histological analyses and clinical application." *Plastic and Reconstructive Surgery Global Open* 1:e44. doi: 10.1097/GOX.0b013e3182a88787.

[28] Cheng, Chieh-Fang, and Jianhua Fan, Mark Fedesco, Shengxi Guan, Yong Li, Balaji Bandyopadhyay, Alexandra M Bright, Dalia Yerushalmi, Mengmeng Liang, Mei Chen. 2008. "Transforming growth factor α (TGFα)-stimulated secretion of

HSP90α: using the receptor LRP-1/CD91 to promote human skin cell migration against a TGFβ-rich environment during wound healing." *Molecular and Cellular Biology* 28:3344-58. doi: 10.1128/MCB.01287-07.

[29] Ku, David D., and Joanne K. Zaleski, Siyu Liu, Tommy A. Brock. 1993. "Vascular endothelial growth factor induces EDRF-dependent relaxation in coronary arteries." *American Journal of Physiology-Heart and Circulatory Physiology* 265:H586-H592.

[30] Yen, T. T., and D. T. Thao, T. L. Thuoc. 2014. "An overview on keratinocyte growth factor: from the molecular properties to clinical applications." *Protein and Peptide Letters* 21:306-17.

[31] Fan, Tai-Ping, and Richard Warn, Ermanno Gherardi. 1998. "Hepatocyte growth factor (HGF) and wound healing." *Pathophysiology* 1001:169.

[32] Gonzalez, A. C. O. 2016. "*Wound healing - A literature review.*" 91: 614-20. Doi: 10.1590/abd1806-4841.20164741.

[33] Maquart, F. X., and J. C. Monboisse. 2014. "Extracellular matrix and wound healing." *Pathologie Biologie* 62:91-5. Doi: 10.1016/j.patbio.2014.02.007.

[34] Chiquet, M., and M. Matthisson, M. Koch, M. Tannheimer, R. Chiquet-Ehrismann. 1996. "Regulation of extracellular matrix synthesis by mechanical stress." *Biochemistry and Cell Biology* 74:737-44.

[35] Madlener, M., and W. C. Parks, S. Werner. 1998. "Matrix metalloproteinases (MMPs) and their physiological inhibitors (TIMPs) are differentially expressed during excisional skin wound repair." *Experimental Cell Research* 242:201-10. Doi: 10.1006/excr.1998.4049.

[36] Young, Alistair, and Clare-Ellen McNaught. 2011. "The physiology of wound healing." *Surgery (Oxford)* 29:475-9. Doi: 10.1016/j.mpsur.2011.06.011.

[37] Maquart, F. X., and J. C. Monboisse. 2014. "Extracellular matrix and wound healing." *Pathologie Biologie* 62:91-5.

[38] Wolberg, A. S., and R. A. Campbell. 2008. "Thrombin generation, fibrin clot formation and hemostasis." *Transfusion and Apheresis Science* 38:15-23. Doi: 10.1016/j.transci.2007.12.005.

[39] Bosanquet, D. C., and A. Rangaraj, A. J. Richards, A. Riddell, V. M. Saravolac, K. G. Harding. 2013. "Topical steroids for chronic wounds displaying abnormal inflammation." *The Annals of The Royal College of Surgeons of England* 95:291-6.

[40] Swirski, Filip K., and Matthias Nahrendorf, Martin Etzrodt, Moritz Wildgruber, Virna Cortez-Retamozo, Peter Panizzi, Jose-Luiz Figueiredo, Rainer H. Kohler, Aleksey Chudnovskiy, Peter Waterman, Elena Aikawa, Thorsten R. Mempel, Peter Libby, Ralph Weissleder, Mikael J. Pittet. 2009. "Identification of Splenic Reservoir Monocytes and Their Deployment to Inflammatory Sites." *Science (New York, N.Y.)* 325(5940):612-6. Doi: 10.1126/science.1175202.

[41] Law, R. H., and T. Caradoc-Davies, N. Cowieson, A. J. Horvath, A. J. Quek, J. A. Encarnacao, D. Steer, A. Cowan, Q. Zhang, B. G. Lu, R. N. Pike, A. I. Smith, P. B. Coughlin, J. C. Whisstock. 2012. "The X-ray crystal structure of full-length human plasminogen." *Cell Reports* 1:185-90. Doi: 10.1016/j.celrep.2012.02.012.

[42] Burns, J. L., and J. S. Mancoll, L. G. Phillips. 2003. "Impairments to wound healing." *Clinics in Plastic Surgery* 30:47-56.

[43] Singer, A. J., and R. A. Clark. 1999. "Cutaneous wound healing." *New England Journal of Medicine* 341:738-46. Doi: 10.1056/NEJM199909023411006.

[44] Lawrence, W. T. 1998. "Physiology of the acute wound." *Clinics in Plastic Surgery* 25:321-40.

[45] Bailey, K., and F. R. Bettelheim, L. Lorand, W. R. Middlebrook. 1951. "Action of Thrombin in the Clotting of Fibrinogen." *Nature* 167:233. Doi: 10.1038/167233a0.

[46] Mustoe, T. A., and G. F. Pierce, C. Morishima, T. F. Deuel. 1991. "Growth factor-induced acceleration of tissue repair through direct and inductive activities in a rabbit dermal ulcer model." The *Journal of Clinical Investigation* 87:694-703. Doi: 10.1172/jci115048.

[47] Mahdavian Delavary, B., and W. M. van der Veer, M. van Egmond, F. B. Niessen, R. H. Beelen. 2011. "Macrophages in skin injury and repair." *Immunobiology* 216:753-62. Doi: 10.1016/j.imbio.2011.01.001.

[48] Baker, R., and F. Urso-Baiarda, C. Linge, A. Grobbelaar. 2009. "Cutaneous scarring: a clinical review." *Dermatology Research and Practice* 2009:625376. Doi: 10.1155/2009/625376.

[49] Dunkin, C. S., and J. M. Pleat, P. H. Gillespie, M. P. Tyler, A. H. Roberts, D. A. McGrouther. 2007. "Scarring occurs at a critical depth of skin injury: precise measurement in a graduated dermal scratch in human volunteers." *Plastic and Reconstructive Surgery* 119:1722-32. Doi: 10.1097/01.prs.0000258829.07399.f0.

[50] Gurtner, G. C., and S. Werner, Y. Barrandon, M. T. Longaker. 2008. "Wound repair and regeneration." *Nature* 453(7193):314-21. Doi: 10.1038/nature07039.

[51] Goncalves, R. V., and J. M. Mezencio, G. P. Benevides, S. L. Matta, C. A. Neves, M. M. Sarandy, E. F. Vilela. 2010. "Effect of gallium-arsenide laser, gallium-aluminum-arsenide laser and healing ointment on cutaneous wound healing in Wistar rats." *Brazilian Journal of Medical and Biological Research* 43:350-5. Doi: 10.1590/s0100-879x2010007500022.

[52] Shaffer, J. J., and S. C. Taylor, F. Cook-Bolden. 2002. "Keloidal scars: a review with a critical look at therapeutic options." *Journal of the American Academy of Dermatology* 46:S63-S97.

[53] McCarty, S. M., and S. L. Percival. 2013. "Proteases and Delayed Wound Healing." *Advances in Wound Care (New Rochelle)* 2:438-47. Doi: 10.1089/wound.2012.0370.

[54] Linares, Hugo A., and Duane L. Larson. 1974. "Early Differential Diagnosis Between Hypertrophic and Nonhypertrophic Healing." *Journal of Investigative Dermatology* 62:514-6. Doi: 10.1111/1523-1747.ep12681048.

[55] Herascu, N., and B. Velciu, M. Calin, D. Savastru, and C. Talianu. 2005. "Low-level laser therapy (LLLT) efficacy in post-operative wounds." *Photomedicine and Laser Surgery* 23:70-3. Doi: 10.1089/pho.2005.23.70.

[56] McGonigle, S., and M. J. Beall, E. J. Pearce. 2002. "Eukaryotic initiation factor 2 alpha subunit associates with TGF beta receptors and 14-3-3 epsilon and acts as a modulator of the TGF beta response." *Biochemistry* 41:579-87.

[57] Gahring, L. C., and N. G. Carlson, R. A. Kulmar, S. W. Rogers. 1996. "Neuronal expression of tumor necrosis factor alpha in the murine brain." *Neuroimmunomodulation* 3:289-303. Doi: 10.1159/000097283.

[58] Rohani, M. G., and W. C. Parks. 2015. "Matrix remodeling by MMPs during wound repair." *Matrix Biology* 44-46:113-21. Doi: 10.1016/j.matbio.2015.03.002.

[59] Bieth, J. G. 2001. "The elastases." *Journal de la Societe de Biologie* 195:173-9.

[60] Parsons, S. L., and S. A. Watson, P. D. Brown, H. M. Collins, R. J. Steele. 1997. "Matrix metalloproteinases." *British Journal of Surgery* 84:160-6.

[61] Verma, R. P., and C. Hansch. 2007. "Matrix metalloproteinases (MMPs): chemical-biological functions and (Q)SARs." *Bioorganic & Medicinal Chemistry* 15:2223-68. Doi: 10.1016/j.bmc.2007.01.011.

[62] Shapiro, S. D., and D. K. Kobayashi, T. J. Ley. 1993. "Cloning and characterization of a unique elastolytic metalloproteinase produced by human alveolar macrophages." The *Journal of Biological Chemistry* 268: 23824-9.

[63] Nagata, M., and H. Takenaka, R. Shibagaki, S. Kishimoto. 1999. "Apoptosis and p53 protein expression increase in the process of burn wound healing in guinea-pig skin." *The British Journal of Dermatology* 140:829-38.

[64] Kumar, Vinay, and Abul K. Abbas, Nelson Fausto, Jon C. Aster. 2014. *Robbins and Cotran pathologic basis of disease, professional edition e-book*. USA: Elsevier health sciences.

[65] Xue, M., and C. J. Jackson. 2015. "Extracellular Matrix Reorganization During Wound Healing and Its Impact on Abnormal Scarring." *Advances in Wound Care (New Rochelle)* 4:119-136. Doi: 10.1089/wound.2013.0485.

[66] Kalluri, R., and R. A. Weinberg. 2009. "The basics of epithelial-mesenchymal transition." The *Journal of Clinical Investigation* 119:1420-8. Doi: 10.1172/jci39104.

[67] Arthur, Wallace. 2002. "The emerging conceptual framework of evolutionary developmental biology." *Nature* 415: 757. Doi: 10.1038/415757a.

[68] Luo, J. D., and T. P. Hu, L. Wang, M. S. Chen, S. M. Liu, A. F. Chen. 2009. "Sonic hedgehog improves delayed wound healing via enhancing cutaneous nitric

oxide function in diabetes." *American Journal of Physiology, Endocrinology and Metabolism* 297:E525-31. Doi: 10.1152/ajpendo.00308.2009.

[69] Chadwick, S. L., and C. Yip, M. W. J. Ferguson, M. Shah. 2013. "Repigmentation of cutaneous scars depends on original wound type." *Journal of Anatomy* 223:74-82. Doi: 10.1111/joa.12052.

[70] Staricco, R. J., and H. Pinkus. 1957. "Quantitative and qualitative data on the pigment cells of adult human epidermis." The *Journal of Investigative Dermatology* 28:33-45.

[71] Jackson, C. J., and M. Xue, P. Thompson, R. A. Davey, K. Whitmont, S. Smith, N. Buisson-Legendre, T. Sztynda, L. J. Furphy, A. Cooper, P. Sambrook, L. March. 2005. "Activated protein C prevents inflammation yet stimulates angiogenesis to promote cutaneous wound healing." *Wound Repair and Regeneration* 13:284-94. Doi: 10.1111/j.1067-1927.2005.00130311.x.

[72] McKelvey, K., and C. J. Jackson, M. Xue. 2014. "Activated protein C: A regulator of human skin epidermal keratinocyte function." *World Journal of Biological Chemistry* 5:169-79. Doi: 10.4331/wjbc.v5.i2.169.

In: Cutaneous Scars: Biology, Clinics and Management ISBN: 978-1-53615-657-7
Editors: Berna Aksoy, Hasan Mete Aksoy et al. © 2019 Nova Science Publishers, Inc.

Chapter 4

THE BIOLOGY OF PROLIFERATIVE SCARS: HYPERTROPHIC SCAR AND KELOIDS

Ezgi Ozkur*
Department of Dermatology, Health Science University,
Şişli Etfal Training and Research Hospital, Istanbul, Turkey

ABSTRACT

Hypertrophic scars and keloids are conditions with excessive fibrosis caused by injury to the skin. Our understanding of this process has increased significantly, but their pathogenesis has not yet been well established and treatment strategies are not always satisfactory.

Keywords: decorin, fibroblasts, genetic predisposition, hypertrophic scar, hypoxia inducible factors, keloid, matrix metalloproteinases (MMPs), MicroRNAs, periostin, myofibroblasts, PDGF, SMADs, TGF-β, thymic stromal lymphopoietin, tissue inhibitors of metalloproteinases (TIMPs), TNF–α; VEGF

1. INTRODUCTION

Hypertrophic scars and *keloids* are excessive scar tissue caused by injury to the skin [1]. They may lead to cosmetic disfigurement or functional loss and also may become

*Corresponding Author's Email: ezgierdal@hotmail.com.

symptomatic with the occurrence of pruritus and pain. Disfigurement and contractures affect patients' quality of life and physchological status [2]. Keloids most commonly occur on the head, neck (especially on ears), upper chest, shoulder, and upper back. The prevalence and incidence of keloids and hypertrophic scars are not known precisely. The annual incidence of 15 per 10,000 has been reported in the Taiwanese population [3]. The biology of these conditions has a complex process, especially at the molecular level, and remains incompletely understood.

2. Hypertrophic Scar Versus Keloid

The term *'keloid'* comes from a Greek word meaning "crab's claw" and tends to extend beyond the original area of injury. *Hypertrophic scars* do not extend beyond the boundaries of the original wound. Moreover, hypertrophic scars can resolve spontaneously over time and occur earlier after injury (generally within 4 weeks), whereas keloids rarely regress or may enlarge progressively over time and may occur later, even years after injury [4]. Both show excessive collagen formation in histopathologic examination. In *hypertrophic scars,* collagen fibers are arranged in a wavy pattern, form nodules, and mostly run parallel to the surface. In contrast, in *keloids,* collagen bundles show a thickened, eosinophilic pattern, and are randomly oriented to the surface [4].

3. The Classic Pathways of Wound Healing

The classic wound healing model is described in three phases: the inflammatory phase, proliferative phase, and remodeling phase. The inflammatory phase starts at the time of injury. Cytokines are released as a result of the coagulation cascade and stimulate immune cell migration to the wound area.

After 2-3 days, the proliferative phase starts and *fibroblasts* and endothelial cells migrate to the wound site to form granulation tissue, which lasts 3 to 6 weeks. In the late proliferative phase, fibroblasts differentiate into *myofibroblasts,* synthesize collagen, and form most of the eventual scar. After the wound is closed, the remodeling phase starts, which may last several months, even a year or more. Excessive extracellular matrix (ECM) is subject to remodeling in this phase [5].

4. The Biology of Hypertrophic Scars and Keloids

4.1. Role of Fibroblasts

In *keloids,* it has been shown that collagen synthesis is 20 times greater than that of normal skin and 3 times greater than that of *hypertrophic scars* [6]. Dermal *fibroblasts* play a major role in collagen synthesis and scar formation. In vitro studies showed that *keloid fibroblasts* continued to produce high levels of collagen, fibronectin, elastin, and proteoglycan in response to metabolic modulators such as glucocorticoids, hydrocortisone, growth factors, and phorbol esters in comparison with normal *fibroblasts* [7]. It has been suggested that these keloidal *fibroblasts* show increased receptors to growth factors such as transforming growth factor *(TGF)-β* and platelet-derived growth factor (PDGF) [8]. *Fibroblasts* from *hypertrophic scars* also display a slight elevation in collagen production in vitro; however, their response to these metabolic modulators is similar to *fibroblasts* in normal skin [9]. It also was found that fibronectin synthesis was four times higher in *keloid fibroblasts* [10]. Fibrin degradation occurs through plasmin-mediated fibrinolysis, which is started by fibroblast-secreted urokinase plasminogen activator (uPA). Normal *fibroblasts* exhibit high uPA, but low plasminogen activator inhibitor-1 (PAI-1) activities to control the equilibrium between matrix synthesis and fibrin degradation. TGF- β1 prevents fibrinolysis by normal *fibroblasts* via upregulating PAI-1 while downregulating uPA activities. In contrast, *keloid fibroblasts* produce high levels of PAI-1 and a low level of uPA. This change in the ratio of activator and inhibitor activities results in a decreased capacity for fibrinolysis and, therefore, decreased fibrin degradation [11]. Also, increased PAI-1 activity results in a reduction of plasmin generation, which may subsequently result in a reduction in plasmin-mediated collagenase activation and collagen degradation by collagenases [12]. In other words, *keloids* might result from a reduction in collagen degradation and removal during scar remodeling and not solely from increased collagen production by *fibroblasts*. Moreover, it has been shown that normal skin *fibroblasts* have higher rates of apoptosis than keloidal *fibroblasts* [13]. Increased numbers of mast cells have been reported during scar formation. Mast cells have been shown to promote *fibroblast* proliferation by the release of histamine, heparin, and cytokines [14].

Overproduction of extracellular matrix (ECM) by *fibroblasts* in the wound and persistence of *myofibroblasts* causes scar contractures. This can lead to joint contracture, loss of range-of-motion or body disfigurement. Scar contracture is mostly seen in *hypertrophic scars*, not in *keloids.* This may be the result of hypertrophic scar *fibroblasts* showing a consistently higher basal level of fibrin matrix gel (FMG) contraction than other *fibroblasts* [15]. Moreover, *hypertrophic scars* contain *myofibroblasts* with alpha-smooth muscle actin (α-SMA). In vitro studies showed that TGF-*β*1 induced α-SMA expression by *fibroblasts* [16]. In turn, tension may subsequently develop in the matrix through stimulation by the over-abundant growth factors. Contrarily, *fibroblasts* in *keloids* represent a unique phenotype that is genetically predisposed to changes in ECM production.

4.2. Proteins and Cytokines in Hypertrophic Scars and Keloids

Recent studies found various growth factors contributing to *hypertrophic scar* and *keloid* formation. *TGF-β* and *PDGF* seem to play the most important roles. *TGF-β* induces chemotaxis of fibroblasts to the wound area. In healthy skin, *TGF-β* is normally turned off after healing is completed, but in *keloids, TGF-β* is overexpressed and the autocrine signaling mechanism is not regulated. Overexpression of *TGF-β1* and *-β2* has been found in keloid and keloid-derived fibroblasts, with significantly lower TGF-β3 mRNA expression [17]. Another hypothesis is over expression of *TGF-β* and *PDGF* receptors on fibroblasts in *keloids* [18, 19]. Also, overexpression of vascular endothelial growth factor (*VEGF*) is related to increased capillary formation, which may additionally cause an increase in scar volume [20].

The matrix metalloproteinases (MMPs) family has a major role in ECM degradation and remodeling. MMP-2 and MMP-9 are active during remodeling; MMP-9 is active in the degradation of type IV and V collagens, fibronectin and elastin, and MMP-2 is responsible for the degradation of denatured collagen. *Tissue inhibitors of metalloproteinases (TIMPs)* are inhibitors of *MMPs*. Increased levels of *TIMPs* have been detected in *hypertrophic scars* [20]. There is another hypothesis that tumor necrosis factor *(TNF)-α* increases the *MMP/TIMP* ratio [21] and accelerates wound healing.

Another protein that has been blamed for the pathogenesis of *hypertrophic scar* and *keloids* is *Decorin. Decorin* is part of the proteoglycan component of dermal ECM tissue and has been shown to be decreased in *keloids and hypertrophic scars* [22]. *Decorin* decreases the stimulatory effects of *TGF-β* on collagen. *Decorin* also inhibits proangiogenic activity of *VEGF* by interacting with *VEGF* receptors [23].

T cells and interleukins (IL) also have a role in wound healing. CD4 T cells express Th1 and Th2 responses [24]. Th1 responses induce interferon-γ and IL-12 and they are thought to be antifibrotic. Th2 responses of CD4 cells and production of IL-4, IL-5, IL-6, and IL-13 are thought to be related to pro-fibrosis. On the other hand, IL-10 is thought to inhibit fibrosis. Also, endothelial cytokines including IL-8, insulin-like growth factor-1 (IGF-1), fibroblast growth factor (FGF)-β, and heparin promote angiogenesis and decrease fibroblast apoptosis [25].

4.3. Genetics

It has been reported that *keloids* mostly occur in Black, Hispanic, and Oriental skin types, and this observation suggests a *genetic predisposition* to keloid formation. Multiple genes were suggested to be involved in keloid pathogenesis and recently loci on chromosomes 1q41, 3q22.3-23, and 15q21.3 were described in the Japanese population [26]. Also genetic syndromes such as Rubinstein-Taybi syndrome and Goeminne syndrome were shown to be associated with *keloid* formation. In family studies, an autosomal dominant inheritance was suggested [27]. On the contrary, *hypertrophic scars* have no genetic association and such a link has not yet been described.

5. What's New in Scar Biology

5.1. SMADs Signaling Pathway

Hypoxia-inducible factors (HIFs) are a group of transcription factors that are rapidly activated in hypoxic cells [28]. It is already known that hypoxia plays a crucial role in *keloid* pathogenesis by increasing the expression of *VEGF* from keloidal fibroblasts. *SMADs* are a family of intracellular regulatory proteins that play a role in the cell's response to *TGF-β*. Once these *SMADs* are phosphorylated, they form a complex with the common mediator Co-SMAD4.

This SMAD complex translocates to the nucleus. SMAD intracellular signaling proteins can be categorized into receptor-regulated *SMADs* (R-SMADs), common-mediator Co-SMADs, and inhibitory *SMADs*. R-SMADs 3 and 4 have been identified as the predominant mediators of autocrine stimulation of *TGF-β* in *hypertrophic scar* fibroblasts [29]. In recent years, it has been postulated that hypoxia is able to drive the transition of human dermal fibroblasts into myofibroblasts by regulating the TGF-β1/SMAD3 pathway through HIFs [30].

5.2. Periostin

Periostin is a matrix protein that is abnormally found in fibrotic tissue. Recently, it has been reported that *periostin* promotes the persistence of myofibroblasts in *hypertrophic scars* and thus this finding makes *periostin* a potential therapeutic target for the reduction of scarring [31].

5.3. MicroRNAs

MicroRNAs (miRNAs) are a novel group of small non-coding RNAs that negatively regulate the expression of their target genes by complementary pairing with target genes and post-transcriptionally silencing the genes. The current literature shows that miRNAs might be responsible for many inflammatory and malignant skin diseases, including *keloids.* Investigators found that some of these miRNAs were upregulated and some were downregulated in *keloids* compared with normal skin. MiRNA-199a-5p [32], miRNA-21 [33,34], miRNA-146a [35], miRNA-1224-5p [36], and miRNA-31 [37] were investigated and thought to be involved in the occurrence and growth of *keloids;* accordingly, they have evolved as promising targets for treatment.

5.4. Thymic Stromal Lymphopoietin (TSLP)

Thymic stromal lymphopoietin (TSLP) was found to be increased in keloidal tissue compared with normal tissue, and it has been suggested that TSLP is a potent inducer of collagen and *TGF-β* production in *keloid* fibroblasts. In addition, it may activate the CXCR4/stromal cell-derived factor-1 axis to increase fibrocyte infiltration into keloidal tissue [38].

CONCLUSION

Hypertrophic scars and keloids are excessive scar tissue depositions caused by derangements of normal wound healing processes involving fibroblasts, extracellular matrix, cytokines, growth factors, intracellular signaling pathways, and miRNAs. Further developments in understanding the biology of proliferative scars will enable us to prevent and treat hypertrophic scars and keloids more effectively.

REFERENCES

[1] Nemeth, A. J. 1993. "Keloids and hypertrophic scars." *The Journal of Dermatologic Surgery and Oncology* 19:738-46.

[2] Chiang, Ryan S., and Anna A. Borovikova, Kassandra King, Derek A. Banyard, Shadi Lalezari, Jason D. Toranto, Keyianoosh Z. Paydar, Garrett A. Wirth, Gregory R. D. Evans, Alan D. Widgerow. 2016. "Current concepts related to hypertrophic

scarring in burn injuries." *Wound Repair and Regeneration* 24:466-77. doi: 10.1111/wrr.12432.

[3] Sun, L. M., and K. H. Wang, Y. C. Lee. 2014. "Keloid incidence in Asian people and its comorbidity with other fibrosis-related diseases: a nationwide population-based study." *Archieves of Dermatological Research* 306 (9):803-8. doi: 10.1007/s00403-014-1491-5.

[4] Mahdavian Delavary, B., and W. M. van der Veer, J. A. Ferreira, F. B. Niessen. 2012. "Formation of hypertrophic scars: evolution and susceptibility." *Journal of Plastic Surgery and Hand Surgery* 46:95-101. doi: 10.3109/2000656X.2012.669184.

[5] Wolfram, Dolores, and Alexandar Tzankov, Petra Pülzl, Hildegunde Piza-Katzer. 2009. "Hypertrophic scars and keloids—a review of their pathophysiology, risk factors, and therapeutic management." *Dermatologic Surgery* 35:171-81.

[6] Rockwell, W. Bradford, and I. Kelman Cohen, H. Paul Ehrlich. 1989. "Keloids and hypertrophic scars: a comprehensive review." *Plastic and Reconstructive Surgery* 84:827-37.

[7] Longaker, Michael T., and George K. Gittes, Howard Levinson, William J. H. Kim. 2016. "Molecular Mechanisms in Keloid Biology." In *Scarless Wound Healing* edited by, Garg, Hary G., and Michael T. Longaker. USA: CRC Press.

[8] Russell, Shirley B., and Joel S. Trupin, Rita Z. Kennedy, James D. Russell, Jeffrey M. Davidson. 1995. "Glucocorticoid regulation of elastin synthesis in human fibroblasts: down-regulation in fibroblasts from normal dermis but not from keloids." *Journal of Investigative Dermatology* 104:241-5.

[9] Younai, Soheil, and Larry S. Nichter, Tadeusz Wellisz, John Reinisch, Marcel E. Nimni, Tai-Lan Tuan. 1994. "Modulation of collagen synthesis by transforming growth factor-beta in keloid and hypertrophic scar fibroblasts." *Annals of Plastic Surgery* 33:148-51.

[10] Babu, M., and R. Diegelmann, N. Oliver. 1989. "Fibronectin is overproduced by keloid fibroblasts during abnormal wound healing." *Molecular and Cellular Biology* 9:1642-50.

[11] Tuan, Tai-Lan, and Judy Y. Zhu, Bo Sun, Larry S. Nichter, Marcel E. Nimni, Walter E. Laug. 1996. "Elevated levels of plasminogen activator inhibitor-1 may account for the altered fibrinolysis by keloid fibroblasts." *Journal of Investigative Dermatology* 106:1007-11.

[12] Montgomery, Anthony M. P., and Yves A. De Clerck, Keith E. Langley, Ralph A. Reisfeld, Barbara M. Mueller. 1993. "Melanoma-mediated dissolution of extracellular matrix: contribution of urokinase-dependent and metalloproteinase-dependent proteolytic pathways." *Cancer Research* 53:693-700.

[13] Messadi, Diana V., and Anh Le, Steve Berg, Anahid Jewett, Zhuang Wen, Paul Kelly, Charles N. Bertolami. 1999. "Expression of apoptosis-associated genes by human dermal scar fibroblasts." *Wound Repair and Regeneration* 7:511-7.

[14] Moyer, Kurtis E., and Gregory C. Saggers, H. Paul Ehrlich. 2004. "Mast cells promote fibroblast populated collagen lattice contraction through gap junction intercellular communication." *Wound Repair and Regeneration* 12:269-75.

[15] Younai, Soheil, and Gregory Venters, Steve Vu, Larry Nichter, Marcel E. Nimni, Tai-Lan Tuan. 1996. "Role of growth factors in scar contraction: an in vitro analysis." *Annals of Plastic Surgery* 36:495-501.

[16] Desmoulière, Alexis, and Antoine Geinoz, Franfoise Gabbiani, and Giulio Gabbiani. 1993. "Transforming growth factor-beta 1 induces alpha-smooth muscle actin expression in granulation tissue myofibroblasts and in quiescent and growing cultured fibroblasts." The *Journal of Cell Biology* 122:103-11.

[17] Xia, Wei, and Toan-Thang Phan, Ivor J. Lim, Michael T. Longaker, George P. Yang. 2004. "Complex epithelial–mesenchymal interactions modulate transforming growth factor-β expression in keloid-derived cells." *Wound Repair and Regeneration* 12:546-56.

[18] Haisa, Minoru, and Hitoshi Okochi, Gary R. Grotendorst. 1994. "Elevated levels of PDGF α receptors in keloid fibroblasts contribute to an enhanced response to PDGF." *Journal of Investigative Dermatology* 103:560-3.

[19] Yu, Haiyan, and Swantje Zitron, Ardeshir Bayat, Mark W. J. Ferguson, Ulrich Mrowietz. 2005. "Studies of transforming growth factors beta 1–3 and their receptors I and II in fibroblast of keloids and hypertrophic scars." *Acta Dermato-Venereologica* 85:216-20.

[20] Wang, Peng, and Li-Zhu Jiang, Bin Xue. 2016. "Recombinant human endostatin reduces hypertrophic scar formation in rabbit ear model through down-regulation of VEGF and TIMP-1." *African Health Sciences* 16:542-53. doi: 10.4314/ahs.v16i2.23.

[21] Chen, Xia, and Susan L. Thibeault. 2010. "Role of tumor necrosis factor–α in wound repair in human vocal fold fibroblasts." *The Laryngoscope* 120:1819-25.

[22] Järveläinen, Hannu, and Pauli Puolakkainen, Sari Pakkanen, Eric L. Brown, Magnus Höök, Renato V. Iozzo, E. Helene Sage, Thomas N. Wight. 2006. "A role for decorin in cutaneous wound healing and angiogenesis." *Wound Repair and Regeneration* 14:443-52.

[23] Sini, Patrizia, and Antonella Denti, M. Enrica Tira, Cesare Balduini. 1997. "Role of decorin on in vitro fibrillogenesis of type I collagen." *Glycoconjugate Journal* 14:871-4.

[24] Lee, Ho J., and Yong J. Jang. 2018. "Recent Understandings of Biology, Prophylaxis and Treatment Strategies for Hypertrophic Scars and Keloids." *International Journal of Molecular Sciences* 19:E711. doi: 10.3390/ijms19030711.

[25] Wick, Georg, and Cecilia Grundtman, Christina Mayerl, Thomas-Florian Wimpissinger, Johann Feichtinger, Bettina Zelger, Roswitha Sgonc, Dolores Wolfram. 2013. "The immunology of fibrosis." *Annual Review of Immunology* 31:107-35. doi: 10.1146/annurev-immunol-032712-095937.

[26] Nakashima, M., and S. Chung, A. Takahashi, N. Kamatani, T. Kawaguchi, T. Tsunoda, N. Hosono, M. Kubo, Y. Nakamura, and H. Zembutsu. 2010. "A genome-wide association study identifies four susceptibility loci for keloid in the Japanese population." *Nature Genetics* 42:768-71. doi: 10.1038/ng.645.

[27] Brown, J. J., and A. Bayat. 2009. "Genetic susceptibility to raised dermal scarring." *British Journal of Dermatology* 161:8-18.

[28] Zhang, Zhe, and Fangfei Nie, Chunfu Kang, Bin Chen, Zelian Qin, Jianxun Ma, Yongguang Ma, Xia Zhao. 2014. "Increased periostin expression affects the proliferation, collagen synthesis, migration and invasion of keloid fibroblasts under hypoxic conditions." *International Journal of Molecular Medicine* 34:253-61. doi: 10.3892/ijmm.2014.1760.

[29] Gauglitz, Gerd G., and Hans C. Korting, Tatiana Pavicic, Thomas Ruzicka, Marc G. Jeschke. 2011. "Hypertrophic scarring and keloids: pathomechanisms and current and emerging treatment strategies." *Molecular Medicine* 17:113-25. doi: 10.2119/molmed.2009.00153.

[30] Zhao, Bin, and Hao Guan, Jia-Qi Liu, Zhao Zheng, Qin Zhou, Jian Zhang, Lin-Lin Su, and Da-Hai Hu. 2017. "Hypoxia drives the transition of human dermal fibroblasts to a myofibroblast-like phenotype via the TGF-β1/Smad3 pathway." *International Journal of Molecular Medicine* 39:153-159. doi: 10.3892/ijmm.2016.2816.

[31] Crawford, Justin, and Karen Nygard, Bing S. Gan, David B. O'gorman. 2015. "Periostin induces fibroblast proliferation and myofibroblast persistence in hypertrophic scarring." *Experimental Dermatology* 24:120-6. doi: 10.1111/exd.12601

[32] Wu, Z. Y., and L. Lu, J. Liang, X. R. Guo, P. H. Zhang, S. J. Luo. 2014. "Keloid microRNA expression analysis and the influence of miR-199a-5p on the proliferation of keloid fibroblasts." *Genetics and Molecular Research* 13:2727-38. doi: 10.4238/2014.April.14.2.

[33] Li, Yan, and Juan Zhang, Yuying Lei, Lechun Lyu, Ruiling Zuo, Ting Chen. 2017. "MicroRNA-21 in Skin Fibrosis: Potential for Diagnosis and Treatment." *Molecular Diagnosis & Therapy* 21:633-42. doi: 10.1007/s40291-017-0294-8.

[34] Liu, Ying, and Yue Li, Ning Li, Wen Teng, Min Wang, Yingbo Zhang, Zhibo Xiao. 2016. "TGF-β1 promotes scar fibroblasts proliferation and transdifferentiation via up-regulating MicroRNA-21." *Scientific Reports* 6:32231. doi: 10.1038/srep32231.

[35] Liu, Zhen, and Cui-Ling Lu, Li-Ping Cui, Yong-Liang Hu, Qi Yu, Ying Jiang, Tian Ma, Da-Kai Jiao, Di Wang, Chi-Yu Jia. 2012. "MicroRNA-146a modulates TGF-

β1-induced phenotypic differentiation in human dermal fibroblasts by targeting SMAD4." *Archives of Dermatological Research* 304:195-202. doi: 10.1007/s00403-011-1178-0.

[36] Yao, Xiaodong, and Xiaomei Cui, Xiaoyan Wu, Pan Xu, Wenyan Zhu, Xiaodong Chen, Tianlan Zhao. 2018. "Tumor suppressive role of miR-1224-5p in keloid proliferation, apoptosis and invasion via the TGF-β1/Smad3 signaling pathway." *Biochemical and Biophysical Research Communications* 495:713-20. doi: 10.1016/j.bbrc.2017.10.070.

[37] Zhang, Juan, and Dan Xu, Na Li, Yan Li, Yongjing He, Xingbo Hu, Lechun Lyu, Li He. 2017. "Downregulation of microRNA-31 inhibits proliferation and induces apoptosis by targeting HIF1AN in human keloid." *Oncotarget* 8:74623-34. doi: 10.18632/oncotarget.20284.

[38] Shin, Jung U., and Seo H. Kim, Hyeran Kim, Ji Y. Noh, Shan Jin, Chang O. Park, Won J. Lee, Dong W. Lee, Ju H. Lee, Kwang H. Lee. 2016. "TSLP is a potential initiator of collagen synthesis and an activator of CXCR4/SDF-1 axis in keloid pathogenesis." *Journal of Investigative Dermatology* 136:507-15. doi: 10.1016/j.jid.2015.11.008.

In: Cutaneous Scars: Biology, Clinics and Management ISBN: 978-1-53615-657-7
Editors: Berna Aksoy, Hasan Mete Aksoy et al. © 2019 Nova Science Publishers, Inc.

Chapter 5

BIOLOGY OF SCAR COMPLICATIONS: UNSTABLE SCARS, CONTRACTURES AND SCAR MALIGNANCIES

Zehra Asiran Serdar [*] ***and Ezgi Aktas Karabay***
Department of Dermatology,
Faculty of Medicine, Bahcesehir University, Istanbul, Turkey

ABSTRACT

Abnormal wound healing is likely to induce pathologic scar formation, resulting in dysfunction, deformity, and psychological trauma in patients. Although important advances in understanding the processes of wound healing and scarring have been made, data on the pathophysiology of scar complications are still limited, and unfortunately, satisfactory treatment options have not yet been revealed. Despite advances in medical care and treatment, scar complications remain a challenge. The more we understand the pathogenesis of scar complications, the more the treatment options will improve.

In this chapter, we briefly describe the current pathophysiology of unstable scars, scar contracture, and scar malignancies and summarize the molecular events involved.

Keywords: contracture, hypoxia inducible factor, integrin, Marjolin's ulcers, MicroRNAs, myofibroblasts, PDGF, periostin, scar malignancy, TGF-β, unstable scar, wound healing

[*] Corresponding Author's Email: dr@drzehraserdar.com.

1. Introduction

Wound healing complications are considered as a pathologic wound healing response to injuries or surgeries. Hypertrophic scars and keloids that present with exuberant scar formation [1] do not pose a health risk. However, complications with the scar tissue, such as scar *contracture*, *unstable scar* and *scar malignancies*, may result in dysfunction and deformity and present an important health issue. Thus they still pose a challenge for treating physicians in clinical practice [2, 3].

Superficial partial thickness burns and wounds rarely lead to scarring with resultant complications. Wounds involving the destruction of epidermal appendages and extending deep into the dermis are more likely to lead to delayed healing and complicated scarring. Infection, smoking, suppressed immune system, age, poor circulation, and nutrition are well-known factors that cause delayed wound healing [4].

Scars may be immature/mature, atrophic/hypertrophic/keloid, stable/unstable, or depigmented (vitiligo)/hyperpigmented. The scars may also become malignant [5]. In this chapter, we discuss *unstable scars*, scar *contracture*s and *scar malignancies*.

2. Biology of Scar Complications

2.1. Unstable Scars

In cases where appropriate wound treatment is not recieved, healing may last for a prolonged period. New scar tissue is defined as an *unstable scar*. *Unstable scars* are usually single-cell layered and highly fragile. *Unstable scars*, particularly those on the extremities and near other areas of stress, are more likely to be damaged by minor traumas. They also show a tendency for repeated breakdowns. *Unstable scars* may heal initially but can be easily re-injured following minimal trauma. This cycle can go on for years and may ultimately result in the development of an aggressive skin cancer [6].

Unstable scars may occur due to involvement of deeper tissues (that were affected in the initial injury). They may also occur secondary to skin contracture present over a prolonged period of time, which may lead to shortening of musculotendinous units and neurovascular structures. The joints may be subluxated or dislocated, with joint capsules and ligaments becoming tight in the direction of the *contracture*. Furthermore, any unstable area in post-burn scars may also be associated with a Marjolin's ulcer [7].

Deformity of the bones may develop especially in growing children. In an *unstable scar*, the presence of *contracture* or a chronic non-healing ulcer is important and must be treated without delay. When dealing with an unstable scar, the surgical release of any accompanying *contracture* or the excision of the non-healing wound is mandatory.

Simply targeting the unstable scar will not be effective. The correct treatment will provide both functionally and aesthetically satisfactory outcomes. *Unstable scars* should be removed by excision/dermabrasion and should be covered with intermediate thickness split-skin grafts. Any associated contracting musculotendinous element should also be released along with the scar tissue [5].

2.2. Contractures

Scar *contracture* is a form of abnormal *wound healing*. Scars that cross joint creases are likely to develop shortening of the scar or *contracture* [8]. A scar *contracture* is the result of a contractile wound-healing process occurring in a scar that has already been reepithelialized and adequately healed [9]. Wound contraction must be distinguished from *contracture*.

Contracture is defined as tissue shortening or distortion resulting in decreased joint mobility and function. Scar *contracture* commonly refers to decreased function in the area, while scar contraction refers to shortening of the scar length (compared with the original wound) as a part of normal wound healing. Scar *contracture*s usually present as fixed, rigid scars that lead both to cosmetic and functional problems [10]. Scar *contracture*s are often hypertrophic and are typically disabling and dysfunctional [8]. The main reason for the functional morbidity of major hypertrophic scars, particularly of burn scars, is the *contracture* of the scar across joints [11, 12].

Wound contraction is an important part of healing. In normal scars, *myofibroblasts* undergo apoptosis after epithelialization is complete, and so contraction does not continue [13]. In hypertrophic scars, *myofibroblasts* still persist in the wound after re-epithelization is complete. Therefore wound contraction continues, leading to painful and functionally-limiting scar *contracture*s [14]. *Myofibroblasts* start to proliferate at the wound site, causing the edges of the wound to move towards each other. Unsutured wound edges in humans move toward each other at a rate of up to 0.75 mm per day due to the contractile force exerted by *myofibroblasts* [15, 16]. Delayed healing and scar formation lead to an over-proliferation of *myofibroblasts*, resulting in pathological *contracture*s [17].

The exact mechanism of the continuing contraction in hypertrophic scars has not been clarified, but the evidence suggests that continuous tension across a wound promotes continued production and activity of *myofibroblasts* [18]. This is consistent with the observation that scar *contracture*s are most common over the joints and mobile skin [19] and may be related to the finding that mechanical stress downregulates proapoptotic genes in fibroblasts [20].

The molecular basis/pathogenesis of scar *contracture*s is complicated and includes both cellular factors and environmental contributions. Normal wound healing proceeds through three overlapping stages. Once the injury occurs, the inflammatory stage begins, during which platelets, neutrophils, and macrophages release inflammatory mediators and cytokines which participate in the recruitment of inflammatory cells, fibroblasts, endothelial cells, and epithelial cells. The proliferative stage involves fibroblast activation, *myofibroblast* differentiation, and extracellular matrix (ECM) deposition. In this phase, the *myofibroblasts* present contractile properties that can contract the wound and promote re-epithelization. The third healing stage is remodeling, which includes scar tissue remodeling. During this stage, the persistent activation of *myofibroblasts*, imbalance of deposition and degradation of ECM, and poor arrangement of newly formed fibers, can lead to pathologic scar formation. *Myofibroblasts* are the principle cells in the formation of scar contraction [21, 22]. They differ from fibroblasts, and have been demonstrated to play a key role in the induction and maintenance of scar *contracture*s. Myofibroblasts are differentiated from fibroblasts at around one to two weeks after injury and express α-smooth muscle actin [23, 24]. Platelet-derived growth factor (*PDGF*) and transforming growth factor beta (*TGF-β*) are the cytokines promoting this transformation [22, 25, 26]. In the later stages of wound healing, *myofibroblast* activity leads a contractile response. Through their multiple collagen attachment points, these actin-rich cells contract and reduce the surface area of the scar [27]. In normal acute wound healing, the *myofibroblasts* are temporarily limited and cleared by apoptosis in the third healing phase when the tissue healing is complete. However, in hypertrophic scars and keloids, these *myofibroblasts* persist in high numbers for long periods and promote the synthesis of α-smooth muscle actin (α-SMA), transforming growth factor-β1 (*TGF-β*1), and other growth factors. Additionally, they have sustained contractile ability via the *TGF-β*1 positive loop [28, 29]. After fibrocytes and fibroblasts are activated in response to inflammatory factors, they migrate to the site of injury, based on the chemoattractant gradient, and differentiate into *myofibroblasts*. Most of the *myofibroblasts* are derived from fibroblast differentiation around the injury site [30], while some of them may originate from pericytes [31], smooth muscle cells from the vasculature [32], bone marrow-derived fibrocytes from peripheral blood [33], epithelial cells through the epithelial-mesenchymal transition (EMT) [34], epidermal stem cells [35, 36], local mesenchymal stem cells, and bone marrow-derived mesenchymal stem cells [37]. The *myofibroblasts* exhibit the characteristics of both fibroblasts and smooth muscle cells, containing high-contractile stress fibers. The α-SMA protein found in stress fibers can be used to differentiate between *myofibroblasts* and fibroblasts in tissues [29].

Several cytokines and mechanical microenvironment factors have been identified as contributing to scar *contracture*s [29]. *TGF-β*1 has been shown to be one of the most important factors in *myofibroblast* differentiation and function. *TGF-β* is found in all tissues and consists of three isoforms: β1, β2, and β3. The activation and recruitment of *TGF-β* receptor type I occurs when active *TGF-β*1 binds to *TGF-β* receptor type II. The active *TGF-β* receptor type I induces the phosphorylation of Smad2/3, followed by an association with Smad4. Then, the Smad complex translocates into the nucleus to enhance gene transcription of profibrotic molecules through binding with DNA gene promoters. In addition, the overproduction of α-SMA, collagen I, collagen III, fibronectin (FN), and profibrotic miRNA is induced [38]. As proteases (such as tissue inhibitor of metalloproteinases (TIMPs) I and II decrease, *TGF-β*1 reduces the activity of matrix metalloproteinases (MMPs) [39]. The *TGF-β*/Smads signaling pathway causes an increase in stress fiber stabilization and the stiffness of the microenvironment. This is a positive autocrine loop in both hypertrophic scars and keloid formation. It should be noted that TGF-β1 is an important inducer of *myofibroblast* differentiation. Additionally, TGF-β1 may also induce *myofibroblast* differentiation through other pathways, including the wnt, p38, and PI3K/PKA2 signaling pathways [40]. P311, which has been found to be involved in smooth muscle (SM) myogenesis, has been shown to be elevated in hypertrophic scars, and may induce a TGF-β1-independent, nonfibrogenic *myofibroblast* phenotype [23, 41]. Eukaryotic initiation factor 6 (eIF6), acting as a key binding protein of P311 [42], has also been demonstrated as a novel upstream regulator of the inhibition of *myofibroblast* differentiation. Its effects on downregulation of α-SMA and collagen I expression have also been demonstrated [43].

Several other growth factors have been shown to have positive roles in *myofibroblast* differentiation, such as connective tissue growth factor (CTGF), platelet-derived growth factor (*PDGF*), insulin growth factor (IGF), and vascular endothelial growth factor (VEGF) [44, 45]. CTGF may augment the activity of *TGF-β*, promoting ECM production and scar *contracture*s. Similarly, *PDGF* induces *myofibroblast* activation directly by itself or in synergy with TGF-β1. *PDGF* stimulates fibroblast proliferation and regulates collagen synthesis via extracellular signaling-regulated kinase (ERK) and the PI3K/JNK signaling pathway. The inhibition of *PDGF* receptors α and β have been shown to inhibit *myofibroblast* formation. IGF reduces the release of collagenase and also stimulates the expression of collagens I and III. VEGF can induce the expression of collagen I and promote scar formation [44]. Moreover, interleukin-6 (IL-6), interleukin-8 (IL-8), and nerve growth factor have also been shown to increase α-SMA transcription in fibroblasts [46-48].

Agonists of *myofibroblast* contraction, such as angiotensin-II, endothelin-1, and thrombin, can upregulate the expression of α-SMA [49].

In contrast to the above-mentioned cytokines, basic fibroblast growth factor (bFGF, FGF2), epidermal growth factor (EGF), interferon-γ (IFN-γ), interleukin-10 (IL-10), prostaglandin E2 (PGE2), eukaryotic translation initiation factor 6 (eIF6), and TGF-β3, have all been shown to suppress the expression of α-SMA and ECM synthesis [44, 50, 51].

The mechanical microenvironment also affects the activity of *myofibroblasts*. Stress fibers, fibronectin, and smooth muscle actin appear earlier in the inflammatory stage, which can increase mechanical tension by association with ECM. The α-SMA acts as a mechano-sensitive protein, which induces a rapid mechanism that controls the *myofibroblast* contractile function. A positive relationship exists between stress and α-SMA expression level. The exogenous mechanical force activates the Rho or mitogen-activated protein kinase (MAPK)/p38 signaling pathway, which induces the activation of serum response factor (SRF) and increases α-SMA transcription and incorporation into actin filaments. The continuous upregulation of α-SMA increases the intracellular tension, and the revealed force stimulates ECM contraction [51]. A decrease in the intracellular stress makes the *myofibroblasts* insensitive to external mechanical factors by interfering with α-SMA, inhibiting the Rho/Rho-associated kinase pathway's effect on myosin activity, interfering with megakaryoblastic leukemia factor 1 (MKL1) (which is linked with mechanical stress), and interfering with YAP/TAZ transcription factors that mediate mechano-responses [52-56].

Integrin, a mechano-transducer, is connected with stress fibers in cells and the ECM surrounding the cells [57]. These signal mediators are located on the cell surface and consist of two isoforms: α and β subunits. Integrin plays a role in the activation of latent *TGF-β*1 and the production of collagen, α-SMA and connective tissue growth factor (CTGF) via reactive FAK, RAC, NADPH oxidase and an oxygen species (ROS)-dependent mechanism [58]. *Integrin*s α1β1, α2β1, α3β1, αvβ5, α5β1, αvβ3, αvβ6, αvβ8, and α11β1 were demonstrated to participate in fibroblast proliferation, collagen contraction, and *myofibroblast* differentiation [59].

Some factors have been identified that maintain a profibrotic or fibrotic state in *wound healing*, which may result in *contracture*s. Zhao et. al [60] evaluated the level of *hypoxia inducible factor* (HIF)-1α in keloid and normal tissues and demonstrated that keloid tissues are relatively hypoxic tissues compared to normoxic tissues and that hypoxia induces a pro-fibrotic state in dermal fibroblasts via the TGF-β1/SMAD3 pathway [60]. *Periostin* is an extracellular matrix (ECM) protein, which was initially identified in osteoblasts, periodontal ligaments, and the periosteum [61] and is also expressed in the basement membrane, the dermis, and hair follicles [62]. *Periostin*, induced by TGF in human dermal fibroblasts, increases in the days after injury, reaching a peak amount after about 7 days post injury, before decreasing afterwards [63, 64]. *Periostin* induces angiogenesis, fibroblast proliferation, and *myofibroblast* persistence; thus, it has an important role in *wound healing* and scar pathogenesis. *Periostin* is shown to be elevated in hypertrophic scars and keloids compared to normal tissues [62, 65-68].

MicroRNAs (miRNAs) are a group of short non-coding RNAs that are thought to be de-regulated in many skin diseases, such as malignant skin diseases and keloids [69-71]. Moreover, miRNA expression has been reported to be upregulated or downregulated in keloid tissues compared to normal tissues [72, 73]. Since hypoxia, periostin, and miRNAs induce fibrotic activity, they may also play a role in *contracture* development.

Another factor affecting the development of the *contracture* is the depth of the initial wound. The healing of a wound may result either in restitution (complete regeneration) or substitution. If the injury is limited to stratum papillare, and all the specialized cells of the organ are preserved, complete regeneration occurs. The epithelial appendages, such as pilosebaceous units and sweat glands, extend into the deep dermis and survive partial-thickness injuries. The epithelial cells are derived from these epithelial appendages in the central portion, and from wound edges at the periphery. Cellular detachment, migration, proliferation, and differentiation lead to re-epithelization. However, if the injury is deeper, the defect is covered by substitutive, unspecialized connective tissue. This results in a smaller or more extensive formation of the cicatrix. In situations with full-thickness loss of skin, wound contraction and re-epithelization occurs from the margins, which leads to *contracture*s [5].

Contraction provides a decrease in the area of skin loss in an open wound and concentric reduction in the size of the wound. As the size of the wound gets smaller, connective tissue deposition and the amount of re-epithelialization also decrease. Fibroblasts, myofibroblasts, and collagen deposition comprise wound contraction. Contraction is effective if the tissue loss is small, in a noncritical area, and surrounded by loose skin. The final, improper, result of excessive contraction is scar *contracture* [5].

In the *wound healing* process, contraction can help to heal the original wound and reduce the surface area. However, the continuation of contraction after wound healing can result in high clinical morbidity of joint *contracture*s, functional loss, delayed return to work, and poor cosmetic results [5].

*Contracture*s after injuries, particularly burns, may be multiple, severe, and diffuse [5]. Pain and pruritus are common complaints in cases of *contracture*s, as well as proliferative scar formation. These symptoms are unpleasant for the patient. Although the exact pathophysiological mechanism of the symptoms is as yet unclarified, histamine or kinin formation and activation of C-fiber nociceptors are thought to be responsible for the symptoms [4].

The Vancouver Scar Scale (VSS), which is a method used to objectively evaluate scars, attributes scar *contracture*s to poor outcomes of scar development [74]. Therefore, it is important to prevent and treat *contracture*s. The application of grafts to fresh wounds or over healthy granulating areas may inhibit contraction. Thicker grafts are believed to be more effective in the inhibition of *contracture*s. Delayed grafting is thought to be insufficient in preventing *contracture*s compared with immediate grafting [5].

The treatment of *contracture*s can be differently planned according to the area of the body. The eyelids, neck, dorsum of the hand, and popliteal fossa are areas where *contracture*s should be immediately released, since the delayed intervention might result in functional and vital morbidities [5]. Localization and the characteristics of the *contracture* are important factors when determining the treatment; they include its laxity, whether it is linear or a plaque, and whether the surrounding skin is normal or scarred. Areas that can limit the patient's airway, such as the neck, or the tissues surrounding the mouth, are additional factors that may help to ascertain the correct treatment.

Contractures at the axilla, and those generally located at the proximal areas require early interventions since they may lead to debilitating loss of function of the joints [75]. Splintage and physiotherapy have been shown to be for the prevention of *contractures* in the early stages [76, 77]. Massaging the wound improves the pliability of the scar, particularly if the scar is dry. The management of scar *contractures*, through means such as surgical intervention, drugs, silicon materials, pressure therapy, splinting, lasers, and radiation, is used to control scar formation and *contracture*, but an optimum therapy has not yet been achieved [78]. Medical and surgical treatment options are also available, and these will be discussed later.

2.3. Scar Malignancies

Ultraviolet radiation (UVR) exposure is known as the most important environmental cause of skin cancer, but cutaneous malignancies have also been reported to develop from scars caused by vaccinations, burns, and other injuries [79, 80]. Furthermore, in non-white skin types, scar tissue is thought to have a greater influence in skin carcinogenesis than UVR exposure [81]. Although proportions may vary in each ethnicity, the most common types of skin cancers are basal cell carcinoma (BCC) (~70%), followed by squamous cell carcinoma (SCC) (~15%), and cutaneous melanomas (~10%) [82]. However, SCCs are reported to be the most common *malignancy* arising in scars. The typical form is known to present as *Marjolin's ulcers*, which are the chronic ulcers in burn scars [86].

The majority of scar malignancies consist of burn scar carcinomas, including several types, such as Kangri, Kang, and Kairo cancers, associated with various cultural practices related to self-warming and heating methods [84]. Among the malignancies arising in scars, SCC has been reported to be equal in men and women, while BCC is more common in men and melanoma is more common in women. The majority of the patients with skin cancer arising in burn scars have been reported to have experienced the burn injury during childhood. Among the post-burn skin cancers, BCC has been demonstrated to have the shortest latency period of development in patients who are significantly older when burnt, in comparison to patients developing other scar cancers who were burnt when they were younger [85].

The mean latent period between injury causing scar tissue and skin cancer development has been reported to range from 23 to 48 years [86-89]. An inverse relationship has been identified between the age of the patient and the latency period from initial insult to SCC formation; no such relationship has been observed for BCC [89].

Although the exact mechanism of cancer occurrence in scars is not yet clearly understood, the most accepted hypotheses include prolonged proliferation due to chronic inflammation and irritation of tissue, ongoing exposure of tissues to toxins and co-carcinogens after the injury, and poor vascularization of the scar tissue resulting in impaired immunological defense [83, 90]. Genetic factors, such as mutations in the p53 [91] and Fas [92] genes in patients with burn scar carcinoma, are also thought to be responsible in scar carcinogenesis.

In the literature, most of the data on scar neoplasms are related to patients with burn scars; thus, the potential carcinogenicity of scars of other etiologies remains unquantified. The incidence of skin cancer in burn scars is thought to be higher than in other scars, but this has not yet been elucidated [85].

Although the malignant potential of burn scars has been described, the possible mechanisms are still unclarified. Burn scar tissue has been suggested to increase tumor progression in which cancer is already initiated rather than increasing the rate of the cancer. But this explanation is limited, since in temperate climates, this would only apply to adults [85, 93].

The link between inflammation and skin cancer has been shown in *Marjolin's ulcer* and other nonhealing wounds, including those associated with lupus erythematosus and osteomyelitis, in which the malignant transformation occurs in association with the prolonged cell proliferation of chronic inflammation [94]. SCCs arising in the areas of scarring from discoid lupus erythematosus [95], in the sinus tracts of patients with chronic osteomyelitis [96], and in the acral skin of patients with epidermolysis bullosa [97] have been reported.

Cytokines and growth factors play a major role in epidermal *wound healing*, of which interleukin (IL)-1α, and transforming growth factor betas (*TGF-β*)1, -β2, and -β3 are the most important in initiating keratinocyte proliferation and tissue repair [98]. In addition to normal *wound healing*, IL-6 and TGF-β1, -β2, and -β3 are also found to be associated with in vitro tumorigenesis [99, 100]. Moreover, an imbalance of cytokines and growth factors is thought to be related to tumorigenesis [98]. Several mechanisms have been proposed in the development of *scar malignancies*. It has been suggested that scars are immunologically privileged sites; since scar tissue is poorly vascularized, a decrease in lymphocyte penetration occurs, resulting in decreased immune surveillance of tumor growth [101]. Immunologic isolation has also been suggested in the development of scar carcinogenesis, as lymphatic channel obliteration at the site of injury decreases the delivery of antigens or specially stimulated antigen presenting cells to the regional lymph nodes from that site. As a result, antigenically-foreign tumor cells that initially arise by spontaneous mutation or develop under the influence of viral or chemical carcinogens can proliferate and progress without immunologic interruption. The delayed tumor antigen recognition may then allow the tumors to reach critical size, and by this point immune mechanisms are no longer sufficient to prevent continued neoplastic progression [102].

Continuous irritation has also been defined as another mechanism resulting in a repetitive healing process and eventual tumorigenesis. Tight or thickened scars can repeatedly become ulcerated when subjected to constant stretching, and the continuous process of skin breakdown and healing creates an environment for mitotic errors to occur [102].

One interesting finding is that *TGF-β*1 and -β2 are observed in adult *wound healing* processes with scarring, while TGF-β3 is associated with scar-free embryonic *wound healing* [99, 100]. Investigations have not yet been concluded into the possible role of cytokines, which are involved in *wound healing,* in tumor progression, as opposed to in tumor initiation [85].

Although the malignant transformation of scar tissue has been extensively described on a case-by-case basis, it has not been well investigated at the population level yet. Epidemiological investigations to determine the risk of skin cancer arising in scars other than burn scars are lacking.

Conclusion

The development of scar complications can result in disfigurement and cause loss of function, limited mobility, pruritus, and pain. Cosmetic disfigurement impairs the quality of life of patients and has both psychosocial and social effects. It is important to establish the mechanisms of scar complications in order to develop effective strategies to prevent the morbidities related to these complications. Emerging therapies for wounds, which control the factors inhibiting the healing process, will lead to fast re-epithelization and fewer complications. Wounds that are effectively treated should be expected to heal without causing serious scar complications like scar cancers.

References

[1] Oosterwijk, Anouk M., and Leonara J Mouton, Hennie Schouten, Laurien M. Disseldorp, Cees P. van der Schans, Marianne K. Nieuwenhuis. 2017. "Prevalence of scar contractures after burn: A systematic review." *Burns* 43:41–9.

[2] Martin, Paul. 1997. "Wound healing-aiming for perfect skin regeneration." *Science* 276:75–81.

[3] Heng, Madalene C.Y. 2011. "Wound healing in adult skin: aiming for perfect regeneration."*International Journal of Dermatology* 50:1058–66.

[4] Hertz, Marshall I., and Linda S. Snyder, Keith R. Hamon, Peter B. Bitterman. 1992. "Acute lung injury." In *Wound Healing: Biochemical and clinical aspects,* edited by I. Kelman Cohen, Robert F. Diegelmann and William J. Lindblad, 416-432. Philidelphia: W.B Saunders Company.

[5] Goel, Arun, and Prabhat Shrivastava. 2010. "Post burn scars and contractures." *Indian Journal of Plastic Surgery* 43:S63-S71.

[6] Meaume, Sylvie. 2002. "Chronic wound scars." *Wound Repair and Regeneration* 10:103-6.

[7] Profyris, Christos, and Christos Tziotzios, Isabel Do Vale. 2012. "Cutaneous scarring: pathophysiology, molecular mechanisms, and scar reduction therapeutics Part I. The molecular basis of scar formation." *Journal of American Academy of Dermatology* 66:1–10. doi: 10.1016/j.jaad.2011.05.055.

[8] Bayat, Ardeshir, and Duncan A. McGrouther, Mark W.J. Ferguson. 2003. "Skin scarring." *British Medical Journal* 326:88–92.

[9] Sherris, David A., and Wayne F. Larrabee, Craig S. Murakami. 1995. "Management of scar contractures, hypertrophic scars, and keloids." *Otolaryngologic Clinics of North America* 28:1057–68.

[10] Brissett, Anthony E., and David A. Sherris. 2001. "Scar Contractures, Hypertrophic Scars, and Keloids." *Facial Plastic Surgery* 17:263-72.

[11] Esselman, Peter C., and Brett D. Thombs, Gina Magyar-Russell, James A. Fauerbach. 2006. "Burn rehabilitation: state of the science." *American Journal of PhysicalMedication and Rehabilation* 85:383–413.

[12] Leblebici, Berrin, and Mehmet Adam, Selda Bagis, Akın M. Tarim, Turgut Noyan, Mahmut N. Akman, Mehmet A. Haberal. 2006. "Quality of life after burn injury: the impact of joint contracture." *Journal of Burn Care and Research* 27:864–8.

[13] Desmouliere, Alexis, and Christin Chaponnier, Giulio Gabbiani. 2005. "Tissue repair, contraction, and the myofibroblast." *Wound Repair and Regeneration* 13:7–12.

[14] Ehrlich, H. Paul, and Alexis Desmoulière, Robert F. Diegelmann, I. Kelman Cohen, Carolyn C. Compton, Warren L. Garner, Yusuf Kapanci, Guilio Gabbiani. 1994. "Morphological and immunochemical differences between keloid and hypertrophic scar." *American Journal of Pathology* 145:105–13.

[15] Lawrence, W. Thomas. 1998. "Physiology of the acute wound." *Clinics in Plastic Surgery* 25:321–40.

[16] Monaco, Joan L., and W. Thomas Lawrence. 2003. "Acute wound healing an overview." *Clinics in Plastic Surgery* 30:1–12.

[17] Dietch, Edwin A., and Timothy M. Wheelahan, M. Paige Rose, Jill Clothier, John Cotter. 1983. "Hypertrophic burn scars: analysis of variables." *Journal of Trauma* 77;744-51.

[18] Junker, Johan P.E., and Camilla Kratz, Anna Tollback, Gunnar Kratz. 2008. "Mechanical tension stimulates the transdifferentiation of fibroblasts into myofibroblasts in human burn scars." *Burns* 34:942–6.

[19] Nedelec, Bernadette, and Aziz Ghahary, Paul G. Scott, Edward E. Tredget. 2000. "Control of wound contraction. Basic and clinical features." *Hand Clinics* 16:289–302.

[20] Derderian, Christopher A., and Nicholas Bastidas, Oren Z. Lerman, Kirit A. Bhatt, Shin E. Lin, Jeremy Voss, Jeffrey W. Holmes, Jaime P. Levine, Geoffrey C. Gurtner. 2005. "Mechanical strain alters gene expression in an in vitro model of hypertrophic scarring." *Annals of Plastic Surgery* 55:69–75.

[21] Shin, Dongmin, and Kyung W. Minn. 2004. "The effect of myofibroblast on contracture of hypertrophic scar." *Plastic and Reconstructive Surgery* 113:633–40.

[22] Kwan, Peter, and Keijiro Hori, Jie Ding, Edward E. Tredget. 2009. "Scar and contracture: biological principles." *Hand Clinics* 25:511–28.

[23] Tan, Jianglin, and Xu Peng, Gaoxing Luo, Bing Ma, Chuan Cao, Weifeng He, Shunzong Yuan, Shirong Li, John A. Wilkins, Jun Wu. 2010. "Investigating the role of P311 in the hypertrophic scar." *PLoS One* 5:e9995. doi: 10.1371/journal.pone.0009995.

[24] Yao, Zhihui, and Sisi Yang, Weifeng He, Lian Li, Rui Xu, Xiaorong Zhang, Haisheng Li, Rixing Zhan, Wei Sun, Jianglin Tan, Junyi Zhou, Gaoxing Luo, Jun Wu. 2015. "P311 promotes renal fibrosis via TGFbeta1/Smad signaling." *Scientific Reports* 5:17032. doi: 10.1038/srep17032.

[25] Nedelec, Bernadette, and Heather Shankowsky, Paul G. Scott, Aziz Ghahary, Edward E. Tredget. 2001. "Myofibroblasts and apoptosis in human hypertrophic scars: the effect of interferon-alpha2b." *Surgery* 130:798–808.

[26] Werner, Sabine, and Richard Grose. 2003. "Regulation of wound healing by growth factors and cytokines." *Physiological Reviews* 83:835–70.

[27] Gurtner, Geoffrey C. 2007. "Wound healing: normal and abnormal" In *Grabb and Smith's Plastic Surgery*, edited by Charles H. Thorne, 15-22. Philadelphia: Lippincott Williams and Wilkins.

[28] Bochaton-Piallat, Marie-L., and Giulio Gabbiani, Boris Hinz. 2016. "The myofibroblast in wound healing and fibrosis: answered and unanswered questions." *F1000 Research* 5:1-8. doi: 10.12688/f1000research.8190.1.

[29] Tan, Jianglin, and Jun Wu. 2017. "Current progress in understanding the molecular pathogenesis of burn scar contracture." *Burns and Trauma* 5:14. doi: 10.1186/s41038-017-0080-1.

[30] Gabbiani, Guilio. 2003. "The myofibroblast in wound healing and fibrocontractive diseases." *Journal of Pathology* 200:500–3.

[31] Gokcinar Yagci, Beyza, and Duygu Uckan Cetinkaya, Betül Celebi Saltik. 2015. "Pericytes: properties, functions and applications in tissue engineering." *Stem Cells Reviews and Reports* 11:549–59.

[32] Hinz, Boris. 2016. "Myofibroblasts." *Experimental Eye Research* 142:56–70.

[33] Sun, Yu B. Y., and Xinli Qu, Georgina Caruana, Jinhua Li. 2016. "The origin of renal fibroblasts/myofibroblasts and the signals that trigger fibrosis." *Differentiation* 92:102–7. doi: 10.1016/j.diff.2016.05.008.

[34] Yan, Chunli, and Wesley A. Grimm, Warren L. Garner, Lan Qin, Taryn Travis, Neiman Tan, Yuan P. Han. 2010. "Epithelial to mesenchymal transition in human skin wound healing is induced by tumor necrosis factor-alpha through bone morphogenic protein-2." *The American Journal of Pathology* 176:2247–58. doi: 10.2353/ajpath.2010.090048.

[35] Li, Haisheng, and Zhihui Yao, Weifeng He, Hongyan Gao, Yang Bai, Sisi Yang, Lu Zhang, Rixing Zhan, Jianglin Tan, Junyi Zhou, Masao Takata, Jun Wu, Gaoxing Luo. 2016. "P311 induces the transdifferentiation of epidermal stem cells to myofibroblast-like cells by stimulating transforming growth factor beta1 expression." *Stem Cell Reearch and Therapy* 7:175. Doi: 10.1186/s13287-016-0421-1

[36] Yao, Zhihui, and Haisheng Li, Weifeng He, Sisi Yang, Xiaorong Zhang, Rixing Zhan, Rui Xu, Jianglin Tan, Junyi Zhou, Jun Wu, Gaoxing Luo. 2017. "P311 accelerates skin wound reepithelialization by promoting epidermal stem cell migration through Rho A and Rac1 activation." *Stem Cells and Development* 26:451–60. doi: 10.1089/scd.2016.0249.

[37] Markeson, Daniel, and Jonathan M. Pleat, Justin R. Sharpe, Adrian L. Harris, Alexander M. Seifalian, Suzanne M. Watt. 2015. "Scarring, stem cells, scaffolds and skin repair." *Journal of Tissue Engineering and Regenerative Medicine* 9:649–68. doi: 10.1002/term.1841.

[38] Meng, Xiao-M., and David J. Nikolic-Paterson, Hui Y. Lan. 2016. "TGF-beta: the master regulator of fibrosis." *Nature Reviews Nephrology* 12:325–38. doi: 10.1038/nrneph.2016.48.

[39] Robert, Sacha, and Thomas Gicquel, Aude Bodin, Vincent Lagente, Elisabeth Boichot. 2016. "Characterization of the MMP/TIMP imbalance and collagen production induced by IL-1beta or TNF-alpha release from human hepatic stellate cells." *PLoS One* 11:e0153118. doi: 10.1371/journal.pone.0153118.

[40] Bowley, Erin, and David B. O'Gorman, Bing S. Gan. 2007. "Beta-catenin signaling in fibroproliferative disease." *Journal of Surgical Research* 138:141–50.

[41] Pan, Desi, and Xiaoning Zhe, Sandhya Jakkaraju, Gregory A. Taylor, Lucia Schuger. 2002. "P311 induces a TGF-beta1 independent, nonfibrogenic myofibroblast phenotype." The *Journal of Clinical Investigation* 110:1349–58.

[42] Peng, Xu, and Shunzong Yuan, Jianglin Tan, Bing Ma, Xiuwu Bian, Chengping Xu, Weifeng He, Hongwei Cao, Zhenggen Huang, Yanyan Cui, Chengjun Gan, Xiaojuan Wang, Junyi Zhou, Jie Hu, Sisi Yang, Gaoxing Luo, Jun Wu. 2012. "Identification of ITGB4BP as a new interaction protein of P311." *Life Sciences* 90:585–90. doi: 10.1016/j.lfs.2012.02.008.

[43] Yang, Si-si, and Jiang-lin Tan, Dai-song Liu, Fabrizio Loreni, Xu Peng, Qing-qing Yang, Wei-feng He, Zhi-hui Yao, Xiao-rong Zhang, Ilaria D. Prà, Gao-xing Luo, Jun Wu. 2015. "Eukaryotic initiation factor 6 modulates myofibroblast differentiation at transforming growth factor-beta1 transcription level via H2A.Z occupancy and Sp1 recruitment." *Journal of Cell Sciences* 128:3977–89. doi: 10.1242/jcs.174870.

[44] Lian, Naqi, and Taiping Li. 2016. "Growth factor pathways in hypertrophic scars: molecular pathogenesis and therapeutic implications." *Biomedicine and Pharmacotherapy* 84:42–50. doi: 10.1016/j.biopha.2016.09.010.

[45] Mattyasovszky, Stefan G., and Jochen Wollstadter, Anne Martin, Ulrike Ritz, Andreas Baranowski, Christian Ossendorf, Pol M. Rommens, Alexander Hofmann. 2016. "Inhibition of contractile function in human joint capsule myofibroblasts by targeting the TGF-beta1 and PDGF pathways." *PLoS One* 11:e0145948. doi: 10.1371/journal.pone.0145948.

[46] Shintani, Yasushi, and Ayako Fujiwara, Toru Kimura, Tomohiro Kawamura, Soichiro Funaki, Masato Minami, Meinoshin Okumura. 2016. "IL-6 secreted from cancer-associated fibroblasts mediates chemoresistance in NSCLC by increasing epithelial-mesenchymal transition signaling." *Journal of Thoracic Oncology* 11:1482–92. doi: 10.1016/j.jtho.2016.05.025.

[47] Clement, Sophie, and Stephanie Pascarella, Stephanie Conzelmann, Carmen Gonelle-Gispert, Kevin Guilloux, Francesco Negro. 2010. "The hepatitis C virus core protein indirectly induces alpha-smooth muscle actin expression in hepatic stellate cells via interleukin-8." *Journal of Hepatology* 52:635–43.

[48] Yorifuji, Makiko, and Yasunobu Sawaji, Kenji Endo, Taiichi Kosaka, Kengo Yamamoto. 2016. "Limited efficacy of COX- 2 inhibitors on nerve growth factor and metalloproteinases expressions in human synovial fibroblasts." *Journal of Orthopaedic Science* 21:381–8. doi: 10.1016/j.jos.2016.01.004.

[49] Kiya, Koichiro, and Tateki Kubo, Kenichiro Kawai, Shinsuke Matsuzaki, Rieko Muramatsu, Daisuke Maeda, Toshihiro Fujiwara, Akimitsu Nishibayashi, Shigeyuki Kanazawa, Kenji Yano, Genki Amano, Taiichi Katayama, Ko Hosokawa. 2017. "Endothelial cell-derived endothelin-1 is involved in abnormal scar formation by dermal fibroblasts through RhoA/Rho-kinase pathway." *Experimental Dermatology* 26:705-12. doi: 10.1111/exd.13264.

[50] Park, Joon S., and Jeum Y. Kim, Jae Y. Cho, Jin S. Kang, Young H. Yu. 2000. "Epidermal growth factor (EGF) antagonizes transforming growth factor (TGF)-beta1-induced collagen lattice contraction by human skin fibroblasts." *Biological and Pharmaceutical Bulletin* 23:1517–20.

[51] Shi, Jihong, and Jun Li, Hao Guan, Weixia Cai, Xiaozhi Bai, Xiaobing Fang, Xiaolong Hu, Yaojun Wang, Hongtao Wang, Zhao Zheng, Linlin Su, Dahai Hu, Xiongxiang Zhu. 2014. "Anti-fibrotic actions of interleukin-10 against

hypertrophic scarring by activation of PI3K/AKT and STAT3 signaling pathways in scar-forming fibroblasts." *PLoS One* 9:e98228. doi: 10.1371/journal.pone.0098228.

[52] Wang, Jiaxu, and Ron Zohar, Christopher A. McCulloch. 2006. "Multiple roles of alpha-smooth muscle actin in mechanotransduction." *Experimental Cell Research* 312:205–14.

[53] Gates, Douglas H., and Jin S. Lee, C. Scott Hultman, Bruce A. Cairns. 2007. "Inhibition of rho-kinase impairs fibroblast stress fiber formation, confluence, and contractility in vitro." *Journal of Burn Care and Research* 28:507–13.

[54] Sandbo, Nathan, and Andrew Lau, Jacob Kach, Caitlyn Ngam, Douglas Yau, Nickolai O. Dulin. 2011. "Delayed stress fiber formation mediates pulmonary myofibroblast differentiation in response to TGF-beta." *American Journal of Physiology Lung Cellular and Molecular Physiology* 301:L656–66. doi: 10.1152/ajplung.00166.2011.

[55] Abe, Masatoshi, and Yoko Sogabe, Tomoko Syuto, Yoko Yokoyama, Osamu Ishikawa. 2007. "Evidence that PI3K, Rac, Rho, and Rho kinase are involved in basic fibroblast growth factor-stimulated fibroblast-collagen matrix contraction." *Journal of Cellular Biochemistry* 102:1290–9.

[56] Dai, Xiaoming, and Peilu She, Fangtao Chi, Ying Feng, Huan Liu, Daqing Jin, Yiqiang Zhao, Xiaocan Guo, Dandan Jiang, Kun-Liang Guan, Tao P. Zhong, Bin Zhao. 2013. "Phosphorylation of angiomotin by Lats1/2 kinases inhibits F-actin binding, cell migration, and angiogenesis." *Journal of Biological Chemistry* 288:34041–51. doi: 10.1074/jbc.M113.518019.

[57] DiPersio, C. Micheal, and Rui Zheng, James Kenney, Livingstone Van De Water. 2016. "Integrin-mediated regulation of epidermal wound functions." *Cell Tissue Research* 365:467–82. doi: 10.1007/s00441-016-2446-2.

[58] Chen, Ruim, and Zhiliang Zhang, Zhujia Xue, Lin Wang, Mingang Fu, Yi Lu, Ling Bai, Dongqing Zhang, Zhihong Fan. 2014. "Focal adhesion kinase (FAK) siRNA inhibits human hypertrophic scar by suppressing integrin alpha, TGF-beta and alpha-SMA." *Cell Biology International* 38:803–8. doi: 10.1002/cbin.10265.

[59] Hu, Xialong, and Na Li, Ke Tao, Xiaobing Fang, Jiaqi Liu, Yaojun Wang, Hongtao Wang, Jihong Shi, Yunchuan Wang, Peng Ji, Weixia Cai, Xiaozhi Bai, Xiongxiang Zhu, Juntao Han, Dahai Hu. 2014. "Effects of integrin alphanubeta3 on differentiation and collagen synthesis induced by connective tissue growth factor in human hypertrophic scar fibroblasts." *International Journal of Molecular Medicine* 34:1323–34. doi: 10.3892/ijmm.2014.1912.

[60] Zhao,Bin, and Hao Guan, Jia-Qi Liu, Zhao Zheng, Qin Zhou, Jian Zhang, Lin-Lin Su, Da-Hai Hu. 2017. "Hypoxia drives the transition of human dermal fibroblasts to a myofibroblast-like phenotype via the TGF-β1/Smad3 pathway." *International Journal of Molecular Medicine* 39:153–9. doi: 10.3892/ijmm.2016.2816.

[61] Horiuchi, Keisuke, and Norio Amizuka, Sunao Takeshita, Hiroyuki Takamatsu, Mieko Katsuura, Hidehiro Ozawa, Yoshiyaki Toyama, Lynda F. Bonewald, Akira Kudo. 1999. "Identification and characterization of a novel protein, periostin, with restricted expression to periosteum and periodontal ligament and increased expression by transforming growth factor." *Journal of Bone and Mineral Research* 14:1239–49.

[62] Zhou, Hong-Ming, and Jian Wang, Christopher Elliott, Weiyan Wen, Douglas W. Hamilton, Simon J. Conway. 2010. "Spatiotemporal expression of periostin during skin development and incisional wound healing: Lessons for human fibrotic scar formation." *Journal of Cell Communication and Signalling* 4:99–107. doi: 10.1007/s12079-010-0090-2.

[63] Conway, Simon J., and Kenji Izuhara, Yasusei Kudo, Judith Litvin, Roger Markwald, Gaoliang Ouyang, Joseph R. Arron, Cecile T.J. Holweg, Akira Kudo. 2014. "The role of periostin in tissue remodeling across health and disease." *Cellular and Molecular Life Sciences* 71:1279–88. doi: 10.1007/s00018-013-1494-y.

[64] Boeters, Linda J., and Weiyan Wen, Douglas W. Hamilton. 2009. "Periostin localizes to cells in normal skin, but is associated with the extracellular matrix during wound repair." *Journal of Cell Communication and Signalling* 3:125–33. doi: 10.1007/s12079-009-0057-3.

[65] Crawford, Justin, and Karen Nygard, Bing S. Gan, David B. O'Gorman. 2015. "Periostin induces fibroblast proliferation and myofibroblast persistence in hypertrophic scarring." *Experimental Dermatology* 24:120–6. doi: 10.1111/exd.12601.

[66] Elliott, Christopher G., and Jian Wang, Xiaolei Guo, Shi-wen Xu, Mark Eastwood, Jianjun Guan, Andrew Leask, Simon J. Conway, Douglas W. Hamilton. 2012. "Periostin modulates myofibroblast differentiation during full-thickness cutaneous wound repair." *Journal of Cell Science* 125:121–32. doi: 10.1242/jcs.087841.

[67] Zhang, Zhe, and Fangfei Nie, Chunfu Kang, Bin Chen, Zelian Qin, Jianxun Ma, Yongguang Ma, Xia Zhao. 2014. "Increased periostin expression affects the proliferation, collagen synthesis, migration and invasion of keloid fibroblasts under hypoxic conditions." *International Journal of Molecular Medicine* 34:253–61. doi: 10.3892/ijmm.2014.1760.

[68] Zhang, Zhe, and Fangfei Nie, Xinlei Chen, Zelian Qin, Chunfu Kang, Bin Chen, Jianxun Ma, Bolin Pan, Yongguang Ma. 2015. "Upregulated periostin promotes angiogenesis in keloids through activation of the ERK 1/2 and focal adhesion kinase pathways, as well as the upregulated expression of VEGF and angiopoietin1." *Molecular Medicine Reports* 11:857–64. doi: 10.3892/mmr.2014.2827.

[69] Kashiyama, Kazuya, and Norisato Mitsutake, Michiko Matsuse, Tomoo Ogi, Vladimir A. Saenko, Kenta Ujifuku, Atsushi Utani, Akiyoshi Hirano, Shunichi Yamashita. 2012. "miR-196a downregulation increases the expression of type I and III collagens in keloid fibroblasts." *Journal of Investigative Dermatology* 132:1597–604. doi: 10.1038/jid.2012.22.

[70] Liu, Ying, and Daping Yang, Zhibo Xiao, Miaobo Zhang. 2012. "miRNA expression profiles in keloid tissue and corresponding normal skin tissue." *Aesthetic Plastic Surgery* 36:193–201. doi: 10.1007/s00266-011-9773-1.

[71] Lovendorf, Marianne B., and Love Skov. 2015. "miRNAs in inflammatory skin diseases and their clinical implications." *Expert Review of Clinical Immunology* 11:467–77. doi: 10.1586/1744666X.2015.1020301.

[72] Luan, Yang, and Yun Liu, Chun-yun Liu, Qingfang Lin, Fuchu He, Xuelin Dong, Zewen Xiao. 2016. "Serum miRNAs Signature Plays an Important Role in Keloid Disease." *Current Molecular Medicine* 16:504–14.

[73] Yao, Xiadong, and Xiaomei Cui, Xiaoyan Wu, Pan Xu, Wenyan Zhu, Xiaodong Chen, Tianlan Zhao. 2018. "Tumor suppressive role of miR-1224-5p in keloid proliferation, apoptosis and invasion via the TGF-β1/Smad3 signaling pathway." *Biochemical and Biophysical Research Communications* 495:713-20. doi: 10.1016/j.bbrc.2017.10.070.

[74] Cubison, Tania, and Sarah A. Pape, Nicholas Parkhouse. 2006. "Evidence for the link between healing time and the development of hypertrophic scars (HTS) in paediatric burns due to scald." *Burns* 32:992-9.

[75] Hudson, Donald A., and Anthony Renshaw. 2006. "An algorithm for the release of burn contractures of the extremities." *Burns* 32:663-8.

[76] Walsh, Karl, and Dariush Nikkhah, Baljit Dheansa. 2013. "Burn scar contractures & their management." *Plastic and Reconstructive Surgery* 3:25-31.

[77] Procter, Fiona. 2010. "Rehabilitation of the burn patient." *Indian Journal of Plastic Surgery* 43:101-13.

[78] Berman, Brian, and Martha H. Viera, Sadegh Amini, Ran Huo, Isaac S. Jones. 2008. "Prevention and management of hypertrophic scars and keloids after burns in children." The *Journal of Craniofacial Surgery* 19:989–1006.

[79] Lang, Pearon G., and John C. Maize. 2011. "Basal cell carcinoma." In *Cancer of the Skin,* edited by Darrell R. June, Robinson Merrick, Ross Robert, Friedman Clay, Cockerell Henry, Lim J. Kirkwood, 101-32. Sydney: Elsevier Inc.

[80] Nguyen, Tri H., and Jaeyoung Yoon. 2011. "Squamous cell carcinoma." In *Cancer of the Skin,* edited by Darrell R. June, Robinson Merrick, Ross Robert, Friedman Clay, Cockerell Henry, Lim J. Kirkwood, 133-50. Sydney: Elsevier Inc.

[81] Lai, Vivien, and William Cranwell, Rodney Sinclair. 2018. "Epidemiology of skin cancer in the mature patient." *Clinics in Dermatology* 36:167-76. doi: 10.1016/j.clindermatol.2017.10.008.

[82] Holterhues, Cynthia, and Esther de Vries, Marieke W. Louwman, Senada Koljenović, Tamar Nijsten. 2010. "Incidence and trends of cutaneous malignancies in the Netherlands, 1989-2005." *Journal of Investigative Dermatology* 130:1807–12. doi: 10.1038/jid.2010.58.

[83] Kowal-Vern, Areta, and Bryan K. Criswell. 2005. "Burn scar neoplasms: a literature review and statistical analysis." *Burns* 31:403–13.

[84] Suryanarayan, Col C.R. 1973. "Kangri cancer in Kashmir Valley: preliminary study." *Journal of Surgical Oncology* 5:327–33.

[85] Wallingford, Sarah C., and Catherine M. Olsen, Elsemieke Plasmeijer, Adele C. Green. 2011. "Skin Cancer Arising in Scars: A Systematic Review." *Dermatologic Surgery* 37:1239–44. doi: 10.1111/j.1524-4725.2011.02060.x.

[86] Nthumba, Peter M. 2010. "Marjolin's ulcers in sub-Saharan Africa." *World Journal of Surg*ery 34:2272–7.

[87] Edwards, Michael J., and Rose M. Hirsch, J. Ralph Broadwater, David T. Netscher, Frederick C. Ames. 1989. "Squamous cell carcinoma arising in previously burned or irradiated skin." *Archieves of Surgery* 124:115–7.

[88] Atzeni, Matteo, and Francesco Serratore, Francesco Zaccheddu, Marcella Buosia, Sonia Nemolato, Diego Ribuffo. 2009. "Multiple melanoma arising on a burn scar and extensive sunburn: a case report and a review of the literature." *Melanoma Research* 19:195–8. doi: 10.1097/CMR.0b013e32832ccd3f.

[89] Husein-ElAhmed, Husein. 2012. "Multiple basal cell carcinomas arising in a surgical scar after radiotherapy." *Annals of the Academy of Medicine, Singapore* 41:536–7.

[90] O'Byrne, Kenneth, and Angus G. Dalgleish. 2001. "Chronic immune activation and inflammation as the cause of malignancy." *British Journal of Cancer* 85:473–83.

[91] Hayashi, Masahiro, and Gen Tamura, Noriko Kato, Shin-ichi Ansai, Shigeo Kondo, Teiichi Motoyama. 2003. "Genetic analysis of cutaneous squamous cell carcinomas arising from different areas." *Pathology International* 53:602–7.

[92] Lee, Sug H., and Min S. Shin, Hong S. Kim, Won S. Park, Su Y. Kim, Ja J. Jang, Kyung J. Rhim, Jin Jang, Hun K. Lee, Jik Y. Park, Ro R. Oh, Seo Y. Han, Jong H. Lee, Jung Y. Lee, Nam J. Yoo. 2000. "Somatic mutations of Fas (Apo-1/CD95) gene in cutaneous squamous cell carcinoma arising from a burn scar." The *Journal of Investigative Dermatology* 114:122–6.

[93] Mellemkjaer, Lene, and Lisbet R. Holmich, Gloria Gridley, Charles Rabkin, Jorgen H. Olsen. 2006. "Risks for skin and other cancers up to 25 years after burn injuries." *Epidemiology* 17:668–73.

[94] Kaplan, Richard P. 1987. "Cancer complicating chronic ulcerative and scarifying mucocutaneous disorders." *Advances in Dermatology* 2:19–46.

[95] Harper, James G., and Mary F. Pilcher, Sarah Szlam, David S. Lind. 2010. "Squamous cell carcinoma in an African American with discoid lupus erythematosus: a case report and review of the literature." *Southern Medical Journal* 103:256–9.

[96] Laffosse, J.M., and H. Bensafi, F. Accadbled, F. Fabie, J.L. Tricoire, J. Puget. 2007. "Squamous-cell carcinoma and osteomyelitis: three cases and a review of the literature." *Revue De Chirurgie Orthopedique et Traumatologique* 93:72–7.

[97] Mallipeddi, Raj. 2002. "Epidermolysis bullosa and cancer." *Clinical and Experimental Dermatology* 27:616–23.

[98] Mueller, Margareta M. 2006. "Inflammation in epithelial skin tumours: old stories and new ideas." *European Journal of Cancer* 42:735–44.

[99] Lederle, Wiltruid, and Sofia Depner, Sabine Schnur, Eva Obermueler, Nicola Catone, Alexandra Just, Norbert E. Fusenig, Margareta M. Mueller. 2011. "IL-6 promotes malignant growth of skin SCCs by regulating a network of autocrine and paracrine cytokines." *International Journal of Cancer* 128:2803–14. doi: 10.1002/ijc.25621.

[100] Laverty, Hugh G., and Lalage M. Wakefield, Nick L. Occleston, Sharon O'Kane, Mark W.J. Ferguson. 2009. "TGF-[beta]3 and cancer: a review." *Cytokine and Growth Factor Reviews* 20:305–17. doi: 10.1016/j.cytogfr.2009.07.002.

[101] Noodleman, F. Richard, and Sheldon V. Pollack. 1986. "Trauma as a possible etiologic factor in basal cell carcinoma." The *Journal of Dermatologic Surgery and Oncology* 12:841–6.

[102] Ozyazgan, Irfan, and Olgun Kontacs. 1999. "Basal cell carcinoma arising from surgical scars: a case and review of the literature." *Dermatologic Surgery* 25:965–8.

In: Cutaneous Scars: Biology, Clinics and Management ISBN: 978-1-53615-657-7
Editors: Berna Aksoy, Hasan Mete Aksoy et al. © 2019 Nova Science Publishers, Inc.

Chapter 6

MODELS FOR WOUND HEALING AND SCARRING

Berna Aksoy*

Department of Dermatology,
Faculty of Medicine, Bahcesehir University, Istanbul, Turkey

ABSTRACT

Cutaneous wound healing represents a vital response which repairs various types of injury all over the body. Wound healing is designed to restore physiological and anatomical functions. Understanding mechanisms of wound healing and its complications is vital to patient care in all fields of medicine such as trauma, burns, obesity, diabetes and cancer. A variety of wound healing/scarring models have been developed: preclinical models that include *in vitro* cell culture and tissue engineered models; *in vivo* animal models, and clinical human volunteer/patient models. All these models have their own advantages and disadvantages. The *in vitro* and *in vivo* models of wound healing/scarring are intended to study mechanisms of wound healing and its complications, underlying cellular pathways, preventive and therapeutic alternatives. The important factor in choosing the ideal model is to determine which type of wound/scarring and wound healing stage are planned to be investigated.

Keywords: animal model, burns, chronic wounds, *ex vivo* model, human model, *in silico* model, *in vitro* model, *in vivo* model, proliferative scars, scar formation, scar contracture model, scarless healing, scarring, wound healing

1. INTRODUCTION

The burden of wounds and scars; especially chronic wounds, proliferative and atrophic scars has increased over the past 5 decades all over the world in parallel with ever-increasing number of human beings, extension of life expectancy and the increased need of surgical procedures. Accordingly, scientific and medical interest and research increased in these areas. In order to conduct a *wound healing* and/or *scarring* research, a variety of models have been developed: preclinical models that include *in vitro* cell culture and tissue engineered *models; in vivo animal models,* and clinical *human* volunteer/patient *models* [1, 2]. All of them have their own advantages and disadvantages [1]. All these models have made it possible to study on different aspects of *wound healing, chronic wounds* and normal and abnormal *scar formation,* and to test available therapeutic agents or methods [1, 2]. In laboratory scientists have shifted from conventional monolayer cell culture models to tissue engineered 3D models and from *animal models* even to humanized *animal models* (human skin transplanted onto the animals) [3]. The important factor in choosing the ideal model is to determine which type of wound/*scarring* or *wound healing* stage (granulation tissue formation, contraction, re-epithelization and remodeling) is intended to be investigated [2].

Initial screening of potential therapeutics for *chronic wounds* and *burns* is usually done by *in vitro* tests. Before being applied in the clinic, promising therapeutic agents should be tested *in vivo* by using immunocompetent animals to prove efficacy, to reveal advantages and/or disadvantages of the agent and to provide information on safety issues [4].

2. Laboratory Based Models

Laboratory based *in vitro models* are used regularly to investigate etio-pathogenetic mechanisms and efficacy of various therapeutics in *wound healing* and *proliferative scars* [1]. These models include *in silico, in vitro* and *ex vivo models* to study wound repair mechanisms and processes in humans [2]. Table 1 summarizes the *wound healing* assays and models that can be studied by these laboratory models. Different *wound healing* models have been compared and 57% concordance was found between humans and *in vitro model* studies [5]. Laboratory based models lack various types of cells that participate in *in vivo wound healing* process as these cell types could not be incorporated in cell culture models [2].

An emerging novel model is the organ-on-a-chip or skin-on-a-chip that involves engineered tissues similar to their *in vivo* equivalents. They consist of multiple different cell types interacting with each other under closely controlled conditions of microfluidic chip. These controlled conditions make it possible to mimic the natural environment of the skin (oxygen levels, humidity, temperature, pH), the elasticity of the skin, complex cellular interactions within and between different cell types and complex structures of the skin [2].

Table 1. Laboratory models to study wound healing and scarring

Method	Models	Assays
In vitro	Single cell Co-culture Organotypic	Proliferation Migration Invasion Senescence
Ex vivo	Normal skin Pathological skin	Proliferation Apoptosis Re-epithelization Fibrosis Angiogenesis
In silico	Agent based Hybrid Differential equations Deterministic Finite element	Epidermal healing Dermal repair Contraction Angiogenesis

2.1. *In Vitro* Models

"Physiologically relevant" *in vitro* cell culture *models* have provided valuable information and had a significant role in the study of *wound healing* and *scarring* [6]. *In vitro models* provide valuable information regarding one or a few components of the skin, *wound healing or scarring* at a time. However they do not correlate with *in vivo models* as they lack complexity of skin *wound healing*. These cultures are used to answer basic questions related to specific mechanistic issues, cell signaling, cellular cycling and behavior during *wound healing* and *scarring*. They allow direct quantitative evaluation of a particular effect on specific cell types alone without incorporation of other tissue components, and that limits their utility. These *in vitro models* have a significant role in the study of biomarkers, role and activity of keratinocytes and fibroblasts and effects of various therapeutics/stimuli in *wound healing* and *scar formation* [2]. Traditionally the investigation of *proliferative scars* has been based on studying respective scar cells grown in two dimensional cell culture conditions [6]. An adverse scar is generated by a complex cascade of cellular and molecular interactions starting at the time of injury and that could not be simulated in human cell culture methods [3].

In vitro models can be categorized as single cell culture, co-culture including more than one cell line or organotypic cultures [2]:

- Single cell culture models are produced by the relevant cells (mostly keratinocytes and fibroblasts) being grown and cells are traumatized by scraping the dish surface with a rubber device or tip of the pipette to create a wound. Later on, the rate at which these cells proliferate and migrate into this scratch wound area is determined by microscopic evaluation. The processes analyzed are viability, gene expression, protein synthesis and secretion, proliferation, differentiation and migration. Scratch assays are usually used to evaluate proliferation and migration of cells. This model can be used to analyze various agents used for the enhancement of re-epithelization and fibroblast migration [2].

- Co-culture of keratinocytes and fibroblasts in monolayers enabled the study of keratinocyte - fibroblast interactions [2].
- It is very difficult to study biology of three dimensional (3D) macroscopic wound or scar tissue by using only monolayer cell cultures. To overcome this limitation of monolayer cell culture models several three-dimensional *in vitro models* have been utilized. These models include fibroblasts seeded in a collagen lattice or collagen construct enabling analysis of cell contraction or migration [2]. A skin like 3D organotypic culture is created when keratinocytes are cultured separately and then placed on top of the extracellular matrix containing fibroblasts [2, 6]. This model allows for studying interactions of these two cell types in a 3D manner and this is important for investigating scar pathogenesis, especially that of *proliferative scars* [2]. The evolution of this 3D model has yielded improvements in the study of inflammatory response to scar formation and this has provided better simulation of the *in vivo* response to scar [6].

There are various *in vitro* assays to investigate *wound healing* as:

- Cell proliferation assay: It has been developed to test if the number of cells in a test culture is increasing with the presence/absence of a test substance (a chemical, a material, etc.) [1].
- Cell cytotoxicity assay: It has been developed to test if cells are killed by the presence of a test substance (a chemical, a material, etc.) [1].
- Cell viability assay: It has been developed to test if cells maintain their viability (staying alive) when they are exposed to a test substance (a chemical, a material, etc.) [1].
- Cell migration and chemotaxis assay [2],
- Endothelial cell *in vitro* tube formation assay [2],
- Transwell migration assay can be used for many different cell types including fibroblasts and keratinocytes to study cell to cell interactions [2].

Researchers are able to test a large number of test substances quickly and under controlled conditions by using these laboratory assay models. These assay methods provide laboratory data on how these test substances affect cells [1]. The results should be interpreted with caution with regard to:

- the relevance of these *in vitro* assays to the clinical situation [1],
- the representation of the conglomerate of molecular and cellular synergies of *wound healing, scarring* or *proliferative scars* in human skin [6], and human cell culture models are still limited in this respect as a result of their extreme simplicity [3],
- the accuracy of representation of mode of action of a therapeutic as it would take place in a patient [1],
- the usefulness of the results in decision-making [1].

The majority of cell culture models employ serum, which is an inflammatory fluid compared to plasma and interstitial fluid (that resting cells are exposed in body), to support and enhance the growth of cells *in vitro*. Hence any observation made in cells grown in a serum environment should be cautiously compared to normal cellular function and behavior in the human body [2].

It is generally accepted that *in vitro* tests are not good indicators of how the substances being tested will affect biological processes in a patient. This is due to the fact that these assays could not reconstitute the interaction of the wound/scar and peri-wound/scar tissue with any therapeutic substance occurring in a patient [1].

2.2. *Ex Vivo* Models

Ex vivo human skin tissue *models* use whole normal or pathological (stretch marks, scar, hypertrophic scar or keloid scar) skin biopsies maintained in organ culture. These *ex vivo models* provide immediate and short term evaluation of cells and their surrounding tissue components, hence they are appropriate for certain types of research. They allow studying the effects of individual agents and formulations in an environment more closely mimicking the normal skin, understanding human skin pathophysiology and evaluating novel therapeutics. Different wound types (partial or full thickness) can be studied in these studies by using different skin (normal and pathological) biopsies. There is a wide range of different culture conditions, various support and growth mediums used [2]. Keloid scar biopsies can remain viable in culture up to 6 weeks without tissue deterioration encountered in long term *in vitro* studies [3]. Angiogenesis, apoptosis, cell proliferation, fibrosis and the rate of epithelization assays can be successfully performed in *ex vivo models*. Despite promising results, they lack standardization and comparable simulation of *in vivo wound healing* and scar environment [2].

2.3. *In Silico* Models

The complexity of the biophysical and biochemical processes involved in tissue repair highlighted the need for computational models to understand cell growth, migration, organization, access to nutrients, extracellular matrix deposition, and to design tissue substitutes and efficient scaffolds [2]. *In silico models* are summarized in Table 1. *In silico models* are advantageous as a first virtual screening tool to predict the effects of a drug/stimulus on cells/tissues and they help to plan future experimental researches or clinical studies. These *in silico models* can be useful theoretically but lack validation and human skin biophysical characteristics [2].

3. Animal Models

Various aspects of *wound healing* and *scarring* can be investigated by using *animal models* in a controlled and reproducible environment [1]. Animal skin structure, *wound healing* and *scarring* can never be the same as and a true and accurate reflection of human skin structure, *wound healing* and *scarring* with their clinical challenges [1, 2, 6]. No animal model has been shown to be an exact replica of the human clinical *wound healing* but the best current *animal model* in terms of dermal structure and underlying mechanisms is considered to be the pig models [2].

There are several specific advantages of the use of domestic pig as an animal for *wound healing* studies that can be summarized as follows;

- Human and pig skin have great overall similarity, similar dermal architecture and lack of panniculus carnosus,
- Several therapeutics can be compared in the same animal due to the large size of the animals that reduces the variability [4].

There are also several disadvantages related to the use of domestic pig as an animal for *wound healing* studies and these can be summarized as follows;

- Pigs are expensive to buy and care for,
- Treatments with systemic effects are difficult to study in pigs as they cannot be tested in the same animal. Pig studies involve small number of animals while small animal (rat and mice) studies involve great number of animals,
- In immunohistochemistry, cross-reactivity is lacking among monoclonal antibodies against human or rodent antigens, and specific antibodies are required for porcine tissues,
- *Animal models* lack humanoid clinical complexity in general [4].

These *in vivo animal models* can provide tools to investigate basic research and development regarding *wound healing*, *chronic wounds* and *proliferative scars* [1, 2]. Animal studies have been proposed to overcome problems confronted by patient studies such as ethical issues [3]. The potential cost, ethical and moral issues associated with the use of laboratory animals can be challenging and problematic [2]. *Animal models* are not excellent substitute for studying human *wound healing* and adverse *scar formation* as animal skin and immune system are very different from humans and the pivotal factors responsible for differences between normo-trophic, hypertrophic and keloid *scar formation* are not identifiable. Additionally genetic predisposition factors of humans (except extreme burn trauma that nearly always results in hypertrophic scarring) can not be taken into account by using *animal models* to study *proliferative scars* [3].

Rodents like mice and rats represent an excellent preclinical *animal model* for studying *wound healing* as they are readily available, of low cost and easily handled [1,7]. Additionally various experimental reagents like monoclonal antibodies, knockout and transgenic breeds are readily available [7]. Aged rodents display delayed cutaneous *wound healing* compared to younger ones and this should be taken into account when planning experiments [8]. Disadvantages of rodent models include a predominant *wound healing* phenotype of contraction due to a well-developed contractile panniculus carnosus muscle layer. Additionally rodent skin contains much higher density of epidermal appendages with hair follicles that differ from human hair follicles. Furthermore murine skin is only of 50 μm in thickness and this makes it difficult to create partial thickness skin wounds. However mice have been extensively used to study various aspects of wound healing including incisional and excisional wounds, diabetic wounds, *scarring* and *burns* [7].

Guinea pigs and rabbits show basically similar *wound healing* characteristics as of rodents. However, their *wound healing* also fundamentally differs from that of humans [1]. This is especially because of the fact that guinea pigs and rabbits are like mice and rats, and have panniculus carnosus layer which helps *wound healing* to take place primarily by providing contraction as opposed to granulation tissue formation and re-epithelization seen in humans [1, 9].

Porcine skin is more similar to human skin anatomically and physiologically [1, 7]. Similarities between pig and human skin make pig an appropriate animal model of cutaneous *wound healing*. Pig skin, like human skin, is adherent to underlying structures unlike those of rodents and rabbits which are loose and slide over subcutaneous fascia. The turnover time is also approximately 30 days in pig epidermis like human epidermis. Pig hair is also sparse but coarser than human hair. Pigs have a relatively thick epidermis, distinct rete pegs, dermal papillae and dense elastic fibers in dermis like humans. Additionally histopathological localization of epidermal keratins 10 and 16, dermal collagen IV, vimentin and fibronectin is also similar between pigs and humans. Porcine collagen has a similar biochemical structure to human collagen. Immune cells including dendritic cells in pig skin are similar to those present in human skin. However, human and pig skins also have important differences: The pig hair follicles and dermis are less vascular and the endothelium of cutaneous vascular structures does not produce alkaline phosphatase. Pilosebaceous system also differs. Pig skin has only apocrine sweat glands and eccrine sweat glands are located only in snout, lips and carpal organ (located between the two hind toes). On the other hand, humans have eccrine sweat glands distributed all over the entire body surface and they provide essential sources of keratinocytes during re-epithelization. There are several disadvantages of using pig models over other animal models; pigs are more expensive to get and feed, their large size makes them more difficult to manage and house, anesthesia administration is more difficult and requires a skilled veterinarian, and some research reagents like antibodies of PCR arrays are less readily available. Many of the molecular mechanisms of *wound healing* have been elucidated by using small-animal models but they remain unexplored in pigs and transgenic pigs because these mechanisms are more difficult to be produced in pig models [7].

Recently adult zebrafish was introduced as a model system for cutaneous *wound healing* research. Full-thickness wounds were created on the flank of adult zebrafish and shown to exert all steps of adult mammalian wound repair process [10].

Basic characteristics of comparative cutaneous *wound healing* are summarized in Table 2. Different *wound healing animal models* have been compared; pig models have been found to be 78% concordant with human *wound healing*, other small *animal models* were only 53% concordant with humans [5, 11]. Despite the presence of some differences, porcine cutaneous *wound healing* model has been determined to have major advantages over other *animal models* with respect to simulation of human cutaneous *wound healing* by the Wound Healing society. But rodents and *in vitro* models are used frequently in the published literature and this leads to low concordance rate between research findings and real life clinical situations [1]. Nonetheless, many aspects of *wound healing* process and therapeutic agents can be studied in *animal models* provided that the limitations of these models are kept in mind [4].

To execute a *wound healing/scarring* study in an *animal model,* first a researcher must evaluate human wound/scar tissue samples to generate a hypothesis. Once a hypothesis is formulated and confirmed by using human tissue samples, the planning of a research involving *animal models* to search for the same mechanisms is an eligible approach. So it is strongly encouraged that researchers should validate their preclinical *in vitro* and *in vivo animal model* findings by using human wound/scar tissue to make them more translational and clinically significant [1].

Table 2. Basic characteristics of comparative wound healing (adapted from [9])

Species	Skin type	Inflammation	Granulation tissue formation	2° healing mode	Area reduction of 2cm² square excisional wound
Rodents, guinea pig and rabbits	Loose	Intense, peaks 4-7 days post-wounding	Good	Contraction	Mice: ≥ 50% contraction in 3-7 days
Pigs	Tight	Intense at 7 days post-wounding	Good (hypertrophic scar in Red duroc pigs)	Re-epithelization	20% at 11 days post-wounding
Humans	Tight	Intense, 48-72 hours	Good	Re-epithelization	20-40% by contraction, re-epithelization complete in 10-12 days

3.1. Wound Healing Models

Wound healing studies in humans are limited by a paucity of experimental models and the questionable practice of taking serial biopsies of human wounds that are painful and this practice may cause infection or *scarring* and ethical issues [7]. Adult animal skin *wound healing* is basically similar to that of human skin *wound healing* [12]. However, the anatomy and physiology of the skin significantly affect the healing process as various fundamental phenotypic variabilities exist between rodent, pig and human skin and also with regard to wound healing [1, 7]. An accurate model of human *wound healing* must use an animal with similar skin and *wound healing* characteristics [7].

3.1.1. Acute Wound Healing Models

Acute *wound healing* includes incisional, partial-thickness and full-thickness excisional models [7]. They are the simplest to replicate and study by using *in vivo animal models* [1]. Each of these wounding categories includes wounds of varying depths and different etiologies of injury [7]. These models can be used to evaluate *wound healing* processes, effects of various therapeutics and surgical interventions on *wound healing* and resulting scars can be analyzed or used for further scar research.

Rodents are widely used to study acute *wound healing* and *scar formation.* It is recommended to use male rodents in order to eliminate the influence of female hormones on *wound healing* and *scarring.* Additionally animals should be housed singly in cages (1 week pre-wounding and entire period of post-wounding) in order to prevent lesions and interference from fighting males. The number and size of incisional and/or excisional wounds may be varied according to study protocol, appropriate ethical and regulatory approval. The wounds are advised to be located on the dorsal surface of the animal, on either side of the midline, in order to minimize differences in the wound gape, interference from the cage environment or normal behavior of the animal (grooming or scratching). As rodents do not have tethered skin, pigs with fixed skin more closely resembling human tissue can be used to study *wound healing*. Pigs are also advantageous because they can tolerate a greater number of wounds, and therapeutics. Different dose ranges of therapeutics can be studied in one animal. When planning experiments and deciding on which animal to be used it is important to remember that a greater number of immune-cytochemical antibodies are available for mice than rats [12]. Additionally rats are more aggressive animals than mice.

The sites of the wounds should be marked before the operation and all surgical and wound care procedures should be performed under general anesthesia. Incisional wounds can be performed by taking the skin of the rodent between index finger and thumb of one hand and cutting the tissue and the incision is made along the predetermined line penetrating the epidermis, dermis and panniculus carnosus [12]. Incisional wounds can be created with a blade which causes minimal tissue damage with more bleeding or an electrocautery or laser surgical device which causes minimal bleeding with more tissue damage. Incisional wound models are appropriate to study the biomechanical properties of the wound and re-epithelization (epithelial migration) but they provide little wound or scar tissue for analysis [7].

Excisional wounds can be superficial, partial-thickness or full-thickness. Superficial excisional wounds can be created by repeated tape stripping that removes only the stratum corneum and granulosum. This model is an excellent one to study the absorption of pharmaceutical products through compromised skin. Partial-thickness excisional wounds include removal of the epidermis and variable amounts of dermis, but the deepest parts of sebaceous glands and hair follicles are usually left intact. Partial-thickness excisions are frequently made by using a dermatome; they closely resemble partial-thickness burns or donor sites following partial-thickness skin grafting [7]. Full-thickness excisional wounds can be produced by using a biopsy punch, scalpel or multiple passes of a dermatome and in this procedure the epidermis, entire dermis and panniculus carnosus down to the subcutaneous tissue or fascia are removed [7, 12]. By using a biopsy punch, a circular piece of skin is removed. Excisional wounds can also be produced by creating round or square excisional wounds with a scalpel [12]. These wounds are optimal for inducing and studying hypertrophic scarring. Excisional wounds provide more wound and scar tissue for analysis [7].

Wound depth is a critical variable in planning excisional *wound healing* studies. Re-epithelization time of pig back skin excisional wounds has been found to be 2-4 days for superficial partial-thickness wounds (300-600 μm), and 3-5 days for deep partial-thickness wounds (700-900 μm). After 5 days, all partial-thickness wounds were completely re-epithelialized but none of full-thickness wounds were re-epithelialized [7].

Type of chronic wound	Injury	Animal	Advantages	Limitations
Chronic Ischemic Wounds	Bi-pedicle flap creation followed by full-thickness excisional wounding	Pig	The skin of the flaps has decreased skin perfusion Wounds created in flaps have delayed macrophage infiltration	Requires advanced surgical skills to produce an ischemic skin flap
Chronic Non-Ischemic Wounds	Radiation exposure followed by full-thickness excisional wounding	Pig	Wounds created in irradiated tissue have delayed formation of granulation tissue, angiogenesis and re-epithelization	Effects of radiation could not be generalized to other causes of chronic wounds Healing rate returns to normal 2 weeks following wounding
	Uni/bilateral extremity nerve root transection followed by tissue compression	Pig	Full-thickness ulcers develop	Requires advanced surgical skills to transect nerve roots Wounds resolve within 3 weeks Denervated limb develop muscle atrophy
	Panniculus carnosus excision followed by third degree burn injury	Rabbit	Wounds heal slower in average of 43.2 days Scars are broader and more irregular Simple, economic and effective	Need to surgically excise panniculus carnosus and waiting 3 weeks prior to creation of chronic wounds, Limited clinical relevance to human chronic wounds
Diabetic Wounds	Streptozocin injection followed by full-thickness excisional/burn wounding	Pig	Animals experience persistent hyperglycemia Delayed re-epithelization	Wounds heal after 18 days Wounds were inflicted 14 days after induction of diabetes so do not evaluate long term effects of diabetes
Diabetic Wound Infections	Streptozocin injection followed by full-thickness excisional wounding and wound inoculation with *S. aureus*	Pig	Sustained tissue infection Delayed re-epithelization	Substantial epithelization after 12 days Wounds were inflicted 14 days after induction of diabetes so do not evaluate long term effects of diabetes

Incisional and excisional wounds can also be created on the same animal approach allows direct comparison of healing of different wound types. The wc allowed to heal without further operational procedures. In both techniques u muscle may be visible. There should be very little or no bleeding from the w prevent mortality [12]. It should also be kept in mind during planning the ex that incisional wounds heal with less apparent *scarring* than excisional wounds optimal method to deliver therapeutic agents to incisional and excisional intradermal injection [12].

3.1.2. Chronic Wound Healing Models

The pathophysiology of *chronic wounds* is complex but the major causa include venous insufficiency, diabetes, ischemia, foreign bodies, prolong pressure and radiation [7]. *In vivo models* of chronic *wound healing* are However there is no perfect model that can adequately mimic the cellular an changes of human chronic non-healing wounds like venous ulcers [12].

Chronic animal wound healing models can be created as chronic ische ischemic wounds, diabetic wounds or inoculation of bacteria to diabetic w model has their own advantages and limitations (Table 3) [7].

Chronic slowly healing wounds can be created in small animal model with panniculus carnosus excision followed by full-thickness burn injury. heal slowly and produce more irregular scars compared to non-excision carnosus (Figure 1) [14]. This model can be used to study effect of variou on healing of chronic wounds and resulting scars can be used to evaluat therapies.

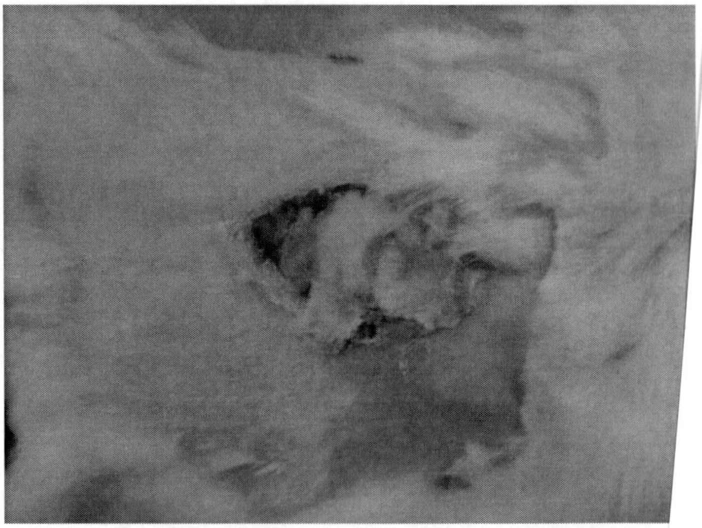

Figure 1. Chronic wound model is developed by excision of panniculus carnosus fc thickness burn injury in rabbits. The appearance of the wound at 3rd week postburn

Table 3. Chronic wound healing models

Diabetes is induced by administering streptozocin to animals like rodents and pigs. Streptozocin is a chemotherapeutic agent that is toxic to insulin secreting pancreatic β-cells. Persistent hyperglycemia with blood glucose levels greater than 350 mg/dl develops 22 hours after streptozocin administration. Full-thickness excisional/burn wounds were created on the backs of animals 14 days after streptozocin administration. Wound fluid can be collected in a wound chamber and analyzed for glucose, cytokines and growth factors. *Wound healing* properties and potential therapeutics can be studied. Full-thickness diabetic wounds can be inoculated with bacteria to investigate the effects of bacterial infection on diabetic *wound healing* [7].

3.1.3. Burn Models

A burn wound is a dynamic wound that can become deeper and wider in time, thus increasing the total amount of tissue damage and the risk of complications like hypertrophic scarring which may develop after healing process. A well-known reason for deepening of a burn wound is wound infection [4]. *Burns* also cause an area of central tissue necrosis and a surrounding area of ischemia which can progress to necrosis [7]. The reason for this is the fact that different types of *burns* may lead to different levels of vascular damage that determine the eventual level of tissue damage [4]. There are three zones of vascular damage in a burn site;

- A peripheral hyperemic zone with increased capillary bleeding that is produced by superficial burn damage,
- An intermediate ischemic stasis zone with retarded capillary filling,
- A central coagulation zone with no capillary refill [4].

Depending on the type of burn treatment the ischemic stasis zone may convert to coagulation zone by desiccation [4]. The main goal of burn wound care is to prevent progression of this ischemia zone to necrosis [7].

Burn models can be designed to create partial-thickness or full-thickness injuries. They can be used to study burn *wound healing* mechanisms, various burn wound therapeutics and surgical burn wound interventions like excision and grafting of deep *burns*. They represent a specific type of *wound healing* models because they create more necrosis and generate a greater inflammatory response than other types of injury. A contact burn can be made by directly applying a heated metal bar, comb or a container filled with hot water to the skin (Figure 2). Contact *burns* produce a small surface area of burn, so the results may not apply to large *burns* [7]. Placing a heated (100-170ºC) brass block on the porcine dorsal skin for 10 sec creates a superficial contact burn and for 20 sec creates a deep partial thickness burn [4, 14]. An aluminum bar pre-heated in hot water (70-80ºC) and applied for 20-30 sec produces mid-dermal partial-thickness *burns* [15, 16] and if it is preheated to 100ºC and applied for 30 sec than it produces full-thickness contact *burns* in domestic porcine skin [17]. Cylindrical aluminum templates (3.76 cm diameter, 500 g) were pre-heated in a water-bath for 2 hour to 75°C and applied for 5 sec to moistened, clipped and depilated dorsal skin of guinea pigs to create deep partial skin thickness *burns* [18]. Contact burn created with a brass comb represents an excellent model of zone of ischemia. The unburned tissue between the prongs of the comb has been shown to progress to full thickness necrosis over a period of 7 days. This model is ideal to evaluate processes that convert ischemic zones to coagulated or hyperemic zones [7]. Brass, aluminum plate or comb models are used in both pigs and small animals [15].

Alternative models include scalding or flame burn mechanisms [7]. Scalds were made by pouring hot water (80°C) into a PVC cylinder positioned on the back of the animal for 10-40 sec [4]. Deep dermal burns were created by pouring 300 ml of heated water at 92°C from a kettle into a bottomless mug in large white pigs. The base of the mug is fitted with a latex membrane and the base of the jug is kept in contact with the flank skin for 20 sec. Radiant heater at 400°C applied for 20 sec can be used to create *burns* in pigs and rats. Burn models based on immersing animal in hot water is the commonest protocol used in small animals [15].

In burn models it is difficult to create a consistent wound depth in comparison with excisional wounding models [7]. A novel burn device to create tailored and repeatable depths of *burns,* independent of user, is described including an electrically heated burn stylus, a temperature control feedback loop using an electronic microstat and a digital pressure monitoring scale which measures downward force. This kind of device provides a uniform starting burn injury for the study of anti-scar and other *wound healing* therapies [19].

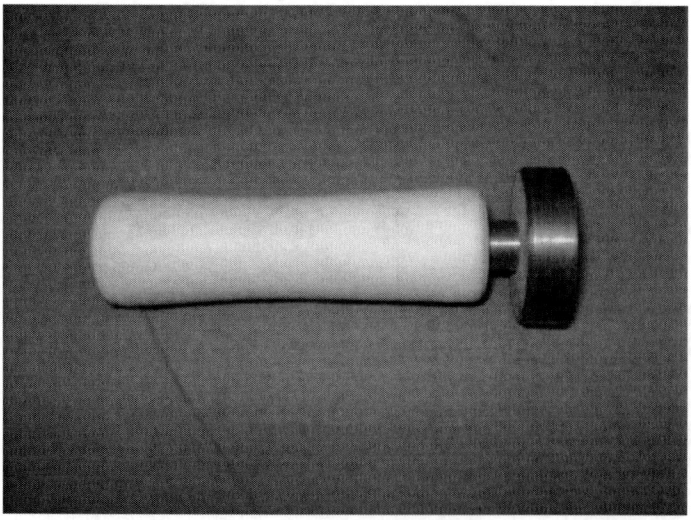

Figure 2. Brass plate with a handle, having 3.5 cm diameter and weighing 500 gr, used to inflict contact burn injury.

Burn wounds can be inoculated with *S. aureus* to create a burn wound infection model. The inoculated wounds have deep tissue infection and destruction but the wound chambers used in this model do not reflect the actual clinical wound environment [7].

Mice are frequently used as a model for burn wounding but they can only tolerate 30% total body surface area *burns* and *burns* of this size do not provoke the hypermetabolic response seen following large human *burns* [7]. Another limitation of these mice and other small *animal models* is the relatively higher rate of mortality caused by anesthetic overdose or burn injury compared to pigs. Additionally, rodent skin and *wound healing* are different from the human skin and wound healing, and hence proliferative scars do not develop [15]. Also small animals differ substantially in their innate and adaptive immune response systems in comparison to humans [7]. It was shown that mice models poorly mimic the human inflammatory events to burn wound trauma in general [3]. These observations have reinforced the need to develop burn *wound healing* models that more closely resemble human burn injury pathophysiology [7]. Pigs seem to represent a better model for burn *wound healing* research. Domestic pigs are most commonly used in burn studies because of their low cost [15]. However the site of burn is important in healing in pigs as caudal burns heal significantly better than cranial burns, displaying earlier closure of wounds, less scar formation and better cosmetic results. It is recommended to create symmetrical burns to compare burn *wound healing* processes and potential therapeutic agents [20]. The disadvantages of porcine models are their cost, difficulty to house and handle. This is why small animals like rodents have been widely used in a variety of studies [15].

Humanized murine burn models are developed due to the limitations of rodent burn models. These models include grafting human skin onto the backs of nude mice and creation of burn injury one month after grafting [15].

Usually an hourglass contracted scar or sometimes proliferative scars develop after burn injury in laboratory animals [15]. In animal burn models wound healing mechanisms, re-epithelialization, wound contraction and various therapeutics can be studied.

3.1.4. Scarless Healing Models

All species respond to injury by *wound healing* mechanisms to restore homeostasis and tissue function and these mechanisms result in either regeneration/*scarless healing* or repair [21, 22]. Regeneration results in restoration of complete tissue architecture and function similar to pre-wounding state in teleost fish and urodele amphibians when their fin or limb has been amputated. However, repair process causes scar formation in mammals. Among vertebrates two types of regeneration have been detected: epimorphic (true) regeneration and compensatory re-growth. Epimorphic regeneration is based on the formation of a blastema structure that is composed of progenitor/stem cells formed underneath the epithelial apical cap which covers the post-amputated region. During true regeneration blastema cells differentiate into cells that regenerate the amputated parts of the body. The blastema structure has been analyzed and detected during limb regeneration in axolotls, fin regeneration in zebrafish and during re-growth of punch holes in rabbit ears, nude and spiny mice [21]. Compensatory re-growth is observed in liver tissue or bone or mucosal membranes characterized by proliferation of differentiated/mature cells to replace damaged tissues [21, 22].

3.1.4.1. Lower Vertebrate Models

Zebrafish and urodele amphibians are well known models to study regeneration. Amputated fins, the tip of the heart and jaws in zebrafish regenerate resulting in full functional reconstruction of lost/damaged tissues [21]. Skin *wound healing* was studied by performing full-thickness skin wounds in zebrafish and they displayed *scarless healing* in less than 24 hours [21, 22]. Zebrafish skin and fin regenerative models have proven to be useful for studying signaling mechanisms of regenerative healing [22]. Limbs of salamander and tails of adult reptiles, in particular lizards, also regenerate similarly [21, 22]. Scarless skin wound healing was also observed in both aquatic and terrestrial axolotls and in both limbs and tails (regenerative structures) and dorsal flank [21].

3.1.4.2. Mammalian Models

Mammalian fetuses (including marsupials, mice, rats, sheep, pigs, rabbits and humans) have the ability for *scarless healing* up to late gestational periods. As a general rule, mammalian fetuses heal their skin wounds by regeneration during the first two trimesters of gestation [21]. This period is up to day 18.5 of 19 days long total gestation period in mice, day 16 of 22 days long total gestation period in rats, 75 of 165 days long total gestation period in Rhesus monkeys and 24 weeks of total gestation period in humans. There are distinct differences in inflammation (decreased) and extracellular matrix composition (collagen type III, collagen deposited in fine reticular patterns, increased hyaluronic acid, differences in MMP expression and activity) in fetal *scarless healing* [22].

A xenograft model of *scarless healing* has been described by transplanting human fetal skin grafts into subcutaneous pockets created under the murine panniculus carnosus or onto the skin of athymic mice. Wound healing of subcutaneous grafts displayed *scarless healing* whereas cutaneous grafts healed with scarring [23].

Another xenograft model uses fetal mouse skin (gestational day 16.5 out of 20 days) grafted onto the chorioallantoic membrane of chichen embriyos (12 day old) and culturing for up to 7 days. Circular laser wounds were created at 48 hours post-engraftment and wound healing properties were evaluated by visual inspection and histopathologically [24].

FOXN1 deficient nude mice lack T lymphocytes and heal their skin injuries better than their wild type controls. Punch holes measuring 2 mm in diameter made in their external ears reveal epimorphic regeneration, develop blastema structure and display dermal, cartilage and muscle re-growth. Nude mice also display features of scarless incisional skin wound healing. Skin healing in nude mice is characterized by extracellular matrix characteristics of rapid establishment of collagen content and remodeling, high levels of hyaluronic acid, higher expression of matrix metalloproteinases, lower levels of TIMPs (tissue inhibitors of matrix metalloproteinases) and intrinsic differences in fibroblasts [21].

African spiny mice are able to shed up to 60% of the total dorsal surface area of their skin as an escape behavior to predator attack. Following this their wounds heal unexpectedly in a short period of time in a scarless manner with rapid re-growth of hair. African spiny mice are the only wild type adult mammal capable of healing severe skin wounds in a regenerative manner. This provides the evidence that even adult mammals have the molecular machinery for regenerative *scarless healing*. The regenerative ability of African spiny mice can be evaluated by creating 4 mm diameter punch holes in their external ears. These punch holes close in a regenerative manner [21].

Both of extreme time points of life are characterized by *scarless healing* with reduced levels of TGF-beta. Older mammals including humans exhibit skin *wound healing* with features of regeneration. It has been reported that acute wounds in old humans and animals heal in a scarless manner resembling healing in fetuses. Elderly *wound healing* is characterized by a prolonged inflammatory phase, reduced macrophage numbers and function, decreased proliferation and migration of cells, decreased collagen and growth factor synthesis resulting in delayed epithelization and wound closure with changes in tissue remodeling (increased MMP and decreased TIMP) [21].

All these *scarless healing* models of fetuses, older mammals and nude mice display lack of or reduced FOXN1 expression. Healing with a scar formation in mammals is related to differential expression profiles of cytokines and MMPs, development of immune system and the phenomenon of bioelectricity in living organisms [21].

3.2. Proliferative Scar Models

Scar models are required to investigate the pathogenesis of adverse scar formation, identify new drug targets and to test new therapeutic agents [3]. The incidence of keloids after deep dermal injury ranges from 4-16% in the black and Hispanic populations. The incidence of hypertrophic scarring is certainly greater [5]. Nowadays various *animal models* are used along with *in vitro* cell culture and tissue-engineered models with varying degrees of success to simulate human *proliferative scars* [3]. As a rule, pathophysiological mechanisms are better studied in tissue cultures whereas therapeutic testing is more appropriately studied in *animal models.* A cell culture can be used to verify the action mechanism of a new therapeutic agent and to establish a safe dose range for human use. However an animal model study is still needed to assess the safety of a therapeutic agent before use in humans [5]. Despite the growing knowledge of *wound healing* and *scarring,* we could only demonstrate the fibrotic nature of *proliferative scars* but could not elucidate how and why these proliferative scarring occurs in certain populations or why they develop in response to certain types of injury [6]. There exist a large number of studies describing mice, rabbits, pigs and other laboratory animals to investigate proliferative scarring, but the basic skin physiology, immunology and wound healing processes are markedly different within these models and hence animals do not develop scars completely comparable to human proliferative scars [3]. *Proliferative scar* research is also challenging in that rodents do not naturally develop *proliferative scars* and burn size, location and depth cannot be controlled in human studies [25]. Most studies used keloid and hypertrophic scarring terms interchangeably. But here it is intended to differentiate hypertrophic scar and keloid models from each other.

3.2.1. Hypertrophic Scar Models

Hypertrophic scars are elevated, red and rigid scars that are confined within the boundaries of the original wound unlike keloids [7]. The exact incidence of hypertrophic scarring is unknown but it may affect up to 58% of adult and 88% of children human burn victims [7, 15]. The pathophysiology of hypertrophic scarring is poorly understood due in part to the lack of a robust *animal model* [26]. Additionally appropriate *animal models* addressing the hypertrophic scar as an endpoint following *burns* are also lacking. Lower species like rodents heal mainly by contraction of panniculus carnosus and hence without development of a proliferative scar [27]. Rodent skin is very thin with poor collagen content and heals mainly by contraction because of the underlying panniculus carnosus layer that prevents hypertrophic scarring [15]. Higher species like pigs, heal more similarly to humans, with *proliferative scars* in some instances; but are associated with high cost, poor manageability, longer duration for scar development and challenges in quantifying scar hypertrophy [27].

Over the past 20 years, several investigative teams found that genetic variation differences in animals led to development of hypertrophic scar models in nonhuman species [9]. The female Red Duroc pig has emerged as a promising *in vivo* hypertrophic scar *animal model* after deep dermal injury [5, 26]. The model was first described in 1972 but not widely used till 2000s [5]. Hypertrophic scars only occur in deep dermal excisional wounds with residual dermis and these wounds are difficult to create in Red Duroc pigs. The model has been validated against wounds in humans and Yorkshire pigs [7]. The scars look similar to that of human hypertrophic scars; thick, firm, hairless and hypo- or hyper-pigmented, but not identical; less erythematous and raised [7, 15]. The scars also have disorganized collagen bundles in a whorl-like pattern, similar to human hypertrophic scars [7]. The hypertrophic scars were shown to persist up to 46 weeks after injury and demonstration of comparable results to human hypertrophic scars has confirmed the value of this model for the study of human hypertrophic scarring [5, 15]. Both human hypertrophic scars and Red Duroc scars have a high number of myofibroblasts and mast cells. The Red Duroc scars also have similar immunolocation and expression of epidermal keratins, cytokines and extracellular matrix proteoglycans [7]. The dermal fibroblasts of Red Duroc pig display pro-fibrotic gene and protein expression profile, enhanced collagen contraction, impaired migration and increased adhesion complex formation compared to those of Yorkshire dermal fibroblasts at baseline. Red Duroc fibroblasts also over-express TGF-β1 and respond less to exogenous TGF-β1. So Red Duroc dermal fibroblasts are supposed to have inherent myofibroblastic differentiation that accounts for pathologic scarring capacity in these animals and these fibroblasts can be cultured *in vitro* to study fibroproliferative scarring [26]. Cones are skin structures that contain epidermal appendages and a fat dome which is adipose tissue extending up into the dermis and continuous with the underlying subcutaneous tissue. Cones are shown in the regions to be affected by hypertrophic scarring in humans; earlobe, cheek, neck, back, chest, abdomen, and extremities [5]. Cones are found in the skin of Red Duroc female pigs but not in mouse or rabbit skin (traditionally proliferative scar free animals) [5, 28]. Recently burn injury created by stainless steel custom burn device, that is heated to 200±10ºC and applied to the dorsal skin for 40 sec, has been described as a new mode of injury to produce hypertrophic scarring in Red Duroc pigs. Burn scars were found to be hairless, had mixed pigmentation, more erythematous, less elastic, less pliable and weaker than scars resulting from excisional injuries and they were analyzed over 150 days. This burn injury induced Red Duroc pig hypertrophic scar model was proposed to have more similarity to human burn hypertrophic scarring and this model is valuable to be used in studies evaluating pathophysiology and therapeutics of burn hypertrophic scars [25]. The large size, housing difficulty and high cost of Red Duroc pigs are the major limitations to their use [26]. They have a life-span of only 6-8 years [7]. Scars also remodel and regress over time [15].

Another porcine model of hypertrophic scarring relies on wounding mechanisms (burn) in juvenile Large White pigs rather than a unique breed [7, 29]. Large burn wound (50 cm2) was created with tissue damage down to the base of the hair follicles but sparing enough dermal cells for repair. Complete re-epithelialization occurred over 3-5 weeks. The burn injury is created by a modified glass bottle filled with water heated to 92ºC, bottom of the bottle is replaced with a plastic wrap and it is applied for 15 sec. Most wounds developed contracted, purple and hypertrophic scars. Burn scar tissue is 1.8 times thicker at week 6 than control skin; approximately 2.2 times thicker than control skin and requires 10 times less force to break after 99 days. Immunohistochemistry and electron microscopy findings are similar to human hypertrophic scars [30]. Interestingly Large White pigs also have skin cones that are important for hypertrophic scarring [5].

This model has the advantage of simulating burn wounds that have multiple zones of injury in the same area but this is also a disadvantage as it creates variability within the model [7]. Scars remodel and regress over time [15]. Additionally the collagen is organized in a parallel pattern, rather than the characteristic nodules and whorls of human and Red Duroc pig hypertrophic scars [7].

Domestic pigs have also been used to develop burn hypertrophic scar model recently. Thermal contact burns were created on dorsal skin by the use of a branding iron at 170 ºF for 20 sec yielding deep partial-thickness *burns*. Overall stiffness increased and elasticity decreased in the scars from the initial burn to 8 weeks in comparison to normal skin. Scars were found to be thicker, more erythematous and uniform in the caudal dorsal skin [30].

To overcome the heavy and cumbersome nature of Red Duroc pigs, recently lightweight Clawn miniature pig hypertrophic scarring model was described. Skin wounds measuring 7.5 x 7.5 cm with a depth of 0.15 cm were created, scar thickness was increased and peaked on day 90 after injury, then gradually decreased [31].

Rabbits are other animal species that are used to develop hypertrophic scar models. Full thickness 6 mm excisions including perichondrium performed on the ventral surface of rabbit ears were shown to heal by elevated hypertrophic scars. The scars were evaluated over 9 months and total area of scar and hypertrophic index were used to evaluate hypertrophy [32]. This model is extensively used in the literature for proliferative scar studies including molecular mechanisms involved in hypertrophic scarring, treatment with cytokines or blockage of cytokine pathways by antibodies or retroviral injections. Rabbit ear hypertrophic scar model is also valuable that older animals display decreased hypertrophic scarring as in humans [5]. But this model lacks the usability in hypertrophic scarring studies caused by *burns*. To overcome this Friedrich et al. developed thermal injury hypertrophic scar model in rabbit ear by creating burn wounds via application of dry-heated brass rod for 20 sec at 90ºC in the rabbit ear. They showed burn wounds exhibited progression of wounds in the first 3 days and there was development of larger hypertrophic scars in comparison to excisional wounds [27].

A brief (one week) augmented mechanical stress applied during the early proliferative phase of *wound healing* in mice results in hypertrophic scars that are identical to human hypertrophic scars and persist for more than 6 months. The authors have concluded that mechanical loading results in scar hypertrophy by inhibiting cellular apoptosis [33].

Guinea pigs are also used to develop a chemically induced *proliferative scar* model. Circular skin excisions in combination with panniculectomies were performed in Guinea pigs. Starting from postoperative one week, coal tar applied to the surgical sites two times weekly. This model yielded hourglass shaped hypertrophic scarring in one third of animals. But the model needs improvements to induce hypertrophic scarring in more animals and to decrease the high mortality associated with coal tar application [34].

Twenty eight days of subcutaneous infusion of bleomycin to dorsal murine skin induces hypertrophic scarring similar to those observed in humans at 28 (developing hypertrophic scar) and 56 (mature hypertrophic scar) days postoperatively [35]. These models are appropriate for testing therapies directed at dampening the inflammatory response that drives fibroproliferation (28 days model) and therapies intended to increase the scar remodeling (56 days model) [36].

Full thickness human skin grafts implanted on the back of nude mice develop morphologically and histologically similar hypertrophic scars to those of humans and they persist even 6 months after transplantation [37]. Humanized murine burn models include grafting human skin onto the backs of nude mice and creation of burn injury one month after grafting. Hypertrophic scar developed in normal human skin and contracture developed in meshed normal human skin grafts. The hypertrophic scars are similar to those in humans and persisted up to 8 months after transplantation [38]. In this model the unburned parts of grafted human epidermis and upper portions of dermis shed and mechanism of this shedding may involve rejection of the graft. This raises the possibility that the hypertrophic scarring may not be because of the burn injury itself but rather it may be the result of failure of the transplant [15].

Pieces of human hypertrophic scars taken from burn patients can be implanted onto or into subcutaneous pockets of the backs of nude mice [15, 38]. Human hypertrophic skin explants are shown to survive more than a year and allow additional experiments to be done in these scars. Microvascular anastomoses occur between nude mice and the implant within the first several days and remodeling of the edges of the implant occur very early [15]. Another similar model involves explantation of human proliferative scars on flaps based on isolated vascular pedicles in nude mice. Explanted scar specimens retain both fibroblastic and epithelial histological characteristics of original human scar specimens for up to 12 months. The microvasculature of these scar explants demonstrate a double basement membrane suggesting that host vessels grow into ghost vessels of human donor scar [39].

Animal *in vivo* hypertrophic scar models are summarized in Table 4.

3.2.2. Scar Contracture Models

Vertical progression porcine burn model is a validated *scar contracture model* that includes creation of partial-thickness burn wound and removal of necrotic epidermis by scrapping and resulting wound was later covered with a polyurethane occlusive dressing. Porcine skin contact *burns* were created on the backs and flanks by using a 150 gr aluminum bar preheated to 80ºC and applied for 30 sec and these burns lead to contracted scars in 75% of wounds. Burn wounds created by aluminum bar preheated to 90ºC and applied for 20 sec lead to contracted scars in 100% of the wounds [40].

Table 4. Animal *in vivo* hypertrophic scar models: advantages and disadvantages

Model definition	Wound model	Advantage	Disadvantage
Full-thickness dermal wounds in pigs	Deep partial-thickness excisional wounds in Red Duroc pig	Formation of thick scars Increased collagen deposition in scars Aberrant expression of TGF-β1, IGF-1, decorin and versican similar to human hypertrophic scars	Large animals, expensive and difficult to house, handle and anesthetize, Wounds are created by an excision rather than a burn (hypertrophic scars develop mostly following burns in humans) Scars are less erythematous and raised than human hypertrophic scars
	Deep dermal burn wounding in juvenile Large White pigs	Simulates burn wounds and hypertrophic scars Ki-67 and cytokeratin 16 immunolocations are similar to human hypertrophic scars	Large animals, expensive and difficult to house, handle and anesthetize, Variability and multiple zones of injury Collagen organized in parallel pattern so lack of nodules and whorls
Specific anatomic sites	Rabbit ear hypertrophic scar model (excisional)	Easy to handle, cheap, widespread availability	Need excision of perichondrium and resulting scar is also related to response of chondrocytes to wounding in excisional model.
Chemical application to full-thickness wound	Guinea pig dorsal skin, excisional injury with panniculectomy and coal tar application	Easy to handle, cheap	Not all animals develop hypertrophic scarring, high mortality
Chemically induced	Subcutaneous bleomycin infusion in mice	Similar to human hypertrophic scars, Mice are readily available, cheap and easy to handle	Only fibroproliferative process can be evaluated
Heterologous hypertrophic scarring in immune privileged site	Hamster cheek pouch	Not need for specialized laboratory conditions	Need surgical experience Need human hypertrophic scar donation
Heterologous hypertrophic scarring in immunodeficient animals	Athymic mice	Similar wound healing mechanisms as in humans, similar histological and morphological findings, Persist for 135 days	Expensive, need special laboratory conditions, high morbidity and mortality rates, Need human skin donation

Another hypertrophic *scar contracture model* was developed in immune-competent murine skin by creating a third degree burn on the dorsal skin and excising the tissue 3 days post-burn followed by grafting with ear skin of green fluorescent protein mice. Grafts were shown to contract approximately 45% of their original size by day 14 and maintained their size later. Hair follicles were shown to disappear after grafting and regenerated in ear skin configuration by day 30 [41].

3.2.3. Keloid Models

Keloid scarring has been known to occur only in humans and no other animal species naturally develop scar tissue comparable to that of human keloids [42]. One of the major limitations in keloid research is the lack of a naturally occurring keloid animal model that can mimic human keloidal scarring. This limits investigative efforts on studying cellular interactions and biochemical processes that occur normally in *in vivo* keloid scar [43].

In vitro models (tissue cultures) are appropriate to study pathophysiological steps in keloid formation or a treatment's mechanism of action or to establish a dose range for a therapeutic. Tissue cultures from a donated keloid tissue are less expensive than animal models. But a tissue culture including only fibroblasts cannot entirely reproduce the complex nature of human keloids and thus it cannot be used to evaluate prophylactic treatments or the efficacy of a treatment in humans [44].

Fibrosis can be searched in genetic models of fibrosis (tight skin mouse), trauma induced animal models of fibrosis (Red Duroc pig, rabbit ear models and horse exuberant granulation tissue "proud flesh") and chemically induced fibrosis models (bleomycin model, reactive oxygen species models) [42]. All these models are a kind of fibrosis model and not specific to keloid scarring.

Instead of inducing keloid scarring in animals, grafting human keloid tissue to an animal has proved to be more successful in creating a keloid animal model [44]. About 30 years ago human keloid tissue implanted subcutaneously in athymic mice was described as a model of keloid scarring. Histological evaluation yielded preservation of histological characteristics at 60 days and grafts were shown to be still alive at 246 days post implantation [5]. Angiographic studies have yielded that peripheral vascularization of implant begins within 8 days and host-graft anastomoses occur at about the 16-postimplant day [5, 44]. The experiments are advised to be performed at day 16 in this model [5]. Oral or systemic acting therapeutics can only be studied in athymic mice models as keloid tissue vasculature is not isolated from the host. Athymic mice models are extensively characterized but small sized keloids can be implanted and the length of the experiment is limited (up to 60 days) [44].

About 10 years later an analogous model was described in athymic rats. Histological features were stable for 12 months but levels of procollagen peptide III were equivalent to surgical samples for only 6 months. Also capacity of fibroblast proliferation was decreased in comparison to human samples [5]. Keloid tissue vasculature is isolated from the host so systemic acting therapeutics cannot be studied in athymic rat xenograft models. Larger keloid tissue sample can be implanted in athymic rats, serial biopsies can be done and length of the experiment can be much longer (up to 12 months) [44].

These subcutaneous heterologous implantation models have made some progress. These models enabled researchers to study specific signaling pathways and test various therapeutics in-vivo. The advantages of these models are; it is comparable to studying the specific human tissue in an *in vivo* environment while limiting the impact of environmental factors; it keeps the tissue as a whole thus preserving the complex human cell-cell interactions in both the epidermis and dermis in some models; fibroblasts continue to thrive in a 3-dimensional organotypic environment and so not one cell type is studied in culture [42]. These xenograft models are valuable in studying pathophysiology, pharmacological agents, safety of treatments, and establishing dose ranges [44]. Keloid xenografts can maintain viability for several months after transplantation with evidence of continued collagen production and angiogenesis. However, after several months, most xenografts lose weight and matrix synthesis decreases. Athymic nude mouse is not completely immunodeficient, there are still functioning innate and humoral adaptive immune systems and additionally resident immune cells in graft tissue may also result in graft rejection affecting graft viability [42]. Moreover, the subcutaneous position of most of the grafts prevents the study of epidermis-dermis interactions and efficacy of topical agents cannot be evaluated. Additionally there is a constant need for donation of human keloid scar in these models. The human keloid tissue is isolated from its *in vivo* environment and this may prove to be misleading as a result of differences in rodent and human *wound healing* processes. Although aseptic conditions are obeyed, specific laboratory technology is used for creating, maintaining and handling these athymic animals. They are fragile and have a high degree of morbidity and mortality because of their own immunodeficiency states [5]. Prophylactic therapies cannot be tested in athymic rodent models [44]. Although xenograft keloid models have demonstrated success in short term; limited longevity, potential for rejection and decrease of fibroblast functioning over time limit the use of these models [5, 42].

Another attempt to develop *in vivo* keloid models was made by culturing and growing donor derived keloid cells in 3-dimensional scaffolding materials and implanting them into immunocompromised mice. Use of these tissue engineered models to study keloid pathogenesis is a relatively recent effort and entirely dependent upon fibroblasts which are expected to maintain their cellular phenotype in culture after being removed from their native environment [42].

Clinically active human keloid tissue was implanted in sub-epithelial cheek pouches of hamsters. The grafts were evaluated up to 168 days after implantation and displayed similar histological findings compatible with human keloids. This model represents an easier to handle and more economic model than athymic rodent models [5].

Horses develop exuberant granulation tissue that is accepted as naturally occurring fibroproliferative keloid-like process following dermal trauma [44, 45]. However equine exuberant granulation tissue possesses markedly increased myofibroblasts, small vessels and acute inflammatory reaction in comparison to human keloids [45]. Additionally, histological analysis demonstrated that the equine exuberant granulation tissue is more closely resembled granulation tissue and these lesions spontaneously regress [44].

3.3. Xenograft Models

Nude mice have greatly reduced numbers of T cells and this reduces the chance of graft rejection. As a result, the immune component of wound healing and scar formation is severely compromised in these models. The only human immune cells present are those which are derived from the transplanted tissue itself, and human circulating immune cells from the blood are absent [3]. Models relying on the implantation of excised human skin should theoretically be more relevant to the clinical situation and represent the standard for *in vivo* experiments. However, their use is limited by the availability of human skin tissue and variability among patients donating the skin in terms of age, gender, race or anatomical site of the tissue sample [15]. Additionally, these nude mice models still fall short of the profound immunologic and inflammatory derangements of human physiologic response to wound healing and scarring. The major limitations are the compulsory human subject involvement and the lack of sufficient specimens [6].

There are hypertrophic scar models in which healthy human split-thickness skin graft is transplanted onto the back of a nude mouse and develops hypertrophic scarring. Similarly keloid skin (full thickness keloid skin or dermis only) has been directly transplanted onto nude mouse [3]. *Proliferative scars* especially keloid tissue explants transplanted into/onto nude mouse models demonstrate scientific potential by allowing the cells of interest to stay in their pathologic state and this is important in studies [6].

Genetically modified skin-humanized mice model is based on the regeneration of a cultured bioengineered skin equivalent (a retroviral vector encoding enhanced green fluorescent protein is used to genetically modify human keratinocytes). Nine to 12 weeks after grafting, wounding recapitulated native skin wound healing features during the first 15 days in this model [5].

4. Human Models

Using humans to investigate acute *wound healing* enables researchers to generate identical pathology and physiology of healing (in acute wounds) and all these processes are identical to those found in the patient [1]. Studies can be performed by using volunteers or patients [1, 2]. Patient models can include all types of wounds and scars but volunteer models are unable to create abnormal wound or pathological scar types (ie. *chronic wounds*, keloid scars) [2].

There are various acute *wound healing* models described in humans (volunteers or patients) (Table 5). Volunteer models include scratch, blister, tape stripping, incisional and excisional wounds and burns; patient models include surgical wound, donor site wounds, incisional and excisional wounds. Despite clear advantages, there is a lack of standardization and conformity in design, evaluation and follow-up for all (acute and chronic) wounds and scars. Many of these models have a limited duration of days or weeks whereas human scars develop over a period of months or years including wound contraction and remodeling. Hence human acute *wound healing* models can only reflect early stages of wound healing [2].

4.1. Partial Thickness Wound Models

It is limited to epidermis and superficial dermis; there is no damage to the dermal blood vessels and adnexa [1].

4.1.1. Tape Stripping Model

It is limited to removal of only stratum corneum. This results in the temporary compromise of permeability of the skin. Epidermal compartment is generally left intact. Wound depth is variable and depends on various methodological factors such as adhesiveness of the tape, pressure applied onto the skin, direction and velocity of tape removal and the number of repeat tape strip applications [1].

It is mainly used to evaluate skin barrier function and the effect of topical wound healing therapeutics or dressings on skin barrier function. The advantages of this model are; it is quick and simple to use, and relatively painless; it allows evaluation of re-epithelization component of *wound healing*. The disadvantages of this model are; it allows only a limited component of *wound healing* to be evaluated; and it is not relevant to deeper *wound healing* processes [1].

4.1.2. Blister Model

It is limited to removal of epidermis from dermis by forming a blister between lamina lucida and lamina densa of the epidermal basement membrane. The blister cavity is filled with interstitial fluid. The blister can be formed by mechanical forces, chemical or biological vesicants or thermal (heat) damage. The suction blister model was developed by induction of a blister by constant application of 300 mmHg negative pressure for 3-4 hours on the skin with the use of various forms of mechanical suction devices. Later the blister roof is excised leaving a clean wound that heals without *scarring* [1].

This model can be used to measure drug concentrations in various parts of the skin and for the evaluation of *wound healing* (re-epithelization; keratinocyte migration, proliferation, differentiation kinetics), for the assessment of treatments for impaired healing and for investigating skin barrier function. Suction blister wounds offer advantages over uncontrolled patient conditions in that they are controlled and well standardized for clinical acute *wound healing* studies [1].

4.1.3. Abrasive Wound Model

This model removes only epidermis and hence basal membrane stays intact. It involves superficial standardized abrasion formation by repeatedly abrading skin with a surgical brush until the first signs of punctate bleeding and uniform glistening develop. This model creates a wound depth that is comparable to suction blister model but the basal membrane stays intact and heals without *scarring*. However the removal of epidermal layer is not as clean and as complete as with the suction blister method [1].

Uniform and identical standardized wounds could be created by using abrasive wound model and they can be used to evaluate superficial *wound healing* and various wound dressings. The advantage of this model is that it is faster and very similar to real-life conditions of superficial minor wounds [1].

4.1.4. Laser and Microdermabrasion Induced Wound Models

CO2 and Er:YAG lasers and microdermabrasion devices can be effectively used to create experimental wounds. Er:YAG laser at a total fluence of 15 J/cm^2 and a pulse length of 250 microsec can be used to induce 1x1 cm^2 wounds that are shown to be more superficial than suction blister wounds. These various devices can be used to create wounds of various depths in a highly reproducible way. Healing time is comparable between laser - induced wounds and suction blister wounds. The disadvantage of this model is the cost of these devices and this may limit their more widespread use [1].

4.1.5. Split-thickness Wounds

Split thickness injury generally involves the use of a dermatome that cuts parallel to the skin surface at a predefined depth of 100-1500 μm thick layer of epidermis with/without superficial dermis. The remaining reticular dermis contains intact lower portions of epidermal appendageal structures and the resulting wound heals with re-epithelization [1].

This model can be used to evaluate *wound healing* process and various treatment methods for acute (or chronic) superficial wounds located at various depths of the skin [1].

Table 5. Human wound healing models (Adapted from [1])

Wound Model	Depth into skin	Advantage	Disadvantage	Wound healing process	Scarring
Skin stripping by adhesive tape	Stratum corneum	Simple, quick, painless, less damaging to epidermis	Time consuming	Re-epithelization	-
Suction blister	Epidermis (split in basal membrane)	Standardized clean epidermal wound	Time consuming	Re-epithelization	-
Abrasive wound	Epidermis (basal membrane intact)	Standardized wounds with high similarity to real world superficial wounds	Epidermal removal not clean and not complete as of suction blister model	Re-epithelization	-
Laser wounds	Variable depth (depending on laser type and energy)	Flexibility in wound depth, Great reproducibility	High cost	Re-epithelization	+/-
Microdermabrasion	Variable depth	Less expensive than lasers	Require high investigator skills	Re-epithelization	+/-
Dermatome	Split thickness wounds (epidermis + upper dermis)	Time-honored technique, Various depths available	Require high investigator skills	Re-epithelization	+
Excisional wounds	Full thickness (various techniques)	Healing involving all dermal and epidermal components	Greater susceptibility to infection, More extensive bleeding and fluid loss	Granulation tissue formation, Re-epithelization (secondary healing)	+
Incisional wounds	Variable	Can be accurately reproduced and used for multiple investigations	Inability to study secondary healing	Primary healing	+
Burns	Partial thickness	Standardized burn wound can be inflicted by using thermaprobe	Susceptibility to infection	Granulation tissue formation, Re-epithelization	+/-

4.2. Full-thickness Wound Models

These models involve the complete removal of epidermis and dermis down to the depth of subcutaneous fat or fascial planes and are associated with disruption of dermal blood vessels. Excisional wound healing involves granulation tissue formation and re-epithelization. These models involve usage of various devices like punch biopsy instrument, scalpel, dermatome or laser to inflict a full thickness wound in a standardized fashion [1].

This model has the advantage of evaluating *wound healing* involving all dermal and epidermal components (granulation tissue formation and re-epithelization). Healing rate can be measured macroscopically; biopsies can be obtained to analyze chemistry, histology, cellular components, angiogenesis and biochemical content of the healing tissue. Punch biopsy wounds are widely used in both *animal models* and human volunteer studies to study *wound healing* and investigate the effects of new treatments on wound healing. The disadvantages of this model are the greater risk of infection and more extensive bleeding and fluid loss [1].

4.3 Patient Models

Patient studies remain essential part of *wound healing* and scar studies and are always necessary to validate potential novel therapies identified in other wound and scar models [2, 3]. Patient models are useful and any acute wound type can be assessed but chronic wound studies have limitations due to the heterogeneity of the patient population and lack of uniformity of wounds. Patients with various types of scars (stretch marks, normal scar, hypertrophic scar) can be used to explore the pathogenesis and therapy of scar formation. However keloid formers are seldom included in such studies [2]. Patients are rarely used to evaluate the pathogenesis of adverse scar formation probably due to patient variation with regard to extent and duration of inciting trauma, logistical problems and most importantly ethical issues [3].

5. Overview of Methods for the *In Vivo* Evaluation of Wound Healing/Scar Models

Evaluation methods that are currently used for the clinical evaluation of *wound healing in vivo* can be divided into noninvasive and invasive methods [46]. Noninvasive methods can be further subdivided into subjective and objective methods to assess specific scar features:

5.1. Noninvasive Macroscopic Evaluation Methods

These methods aim to evaluate *wound healing* and *scarring in vivo* by subjective and objective methods.

5.1.1. Subjective Methods

These methods predominantly include scar assessment methods developed for easy and quick evaluation of a scar. Most are filled out by the Observer (O) and some are additionally by the Patient (P). There are various types of scar scales reviewed in part 3 - chapter 4 that can be used in clinical studies. POSAS scale can be used routinely in scar evaluation but in animal studies only Observer part is filled out. Additionally signs of granulation tissue or epithelization and the absence of signs of infection/inflammation or necrosis, appearance of healing wounds in time and observation of specified areas (granulation tissue and neo-epithelium) can be macroscopically evaluated in healing wounds [46].

A proposed standard checklist for performing studies includes usage of a subjective scar assessment tool (ie: OSAS which contains 1-10 scale to score vascularity, pigmentation, thickness, relief, pliability and surface area) and evaluation of wound contraction and re-epithelization subjectively [46].

5.1.2. Objective Methods

Objective evaluation methods use specialized tools to measure;

- color (like DermaSpectrometer, Mexameter, Labscan XE…),
- thickness (like DermascanC, Tissue Ultrasound Palpation System -TUPS, Vivid 900),
- relief (like Optical or Mechanical or Laser profilometry…),
- mechanical properties (like Cutometer, Dermal torque meter, Tonometry…),
- planimetry (like transparent acetate wound perimeter tracing, computer assisted planimetry, Stereophotogrammetry…),
- epidermal barrier functions (like evaluating surface hydration by Raman spectroscopy, corneometer; transepidermal water loss evaluation by vapometer, evaporimeter…),

in normal skin, surgical and burn scars, hypertrophic and keloid scars and wounds [46].

Proposed standard for studies includes evaluation of wound contraction and re-epithelization by planimetry. For objective evaluation of wound area and contraction; a caliper can be used manually, photographs can be taken (a ruler must be included in photographs), transparent papers can be used to trace wound edges and a software can be used to calculate wound area. However, most studies do not correct for the growth of the animals during the study. So, in evaluation of contraction a larger square outside of the original wound and the original wound margins must be marked by tattoo to calculate contraction as a percentage of the unaffected square with time. Re-epithelization can be examined by tracing epidermal edges on transparent papers but the presence of crust covering the newly formed epithelium makes it problematic and the presence of synchronous contraction complicates the re-epithelization rate calculations [46].

5.2. Invasive Evaluation Methods

Tissue specimens are obtained at different time points during *wound healing/scarring* to explore the effects of a specific treatment or to identify the sequential events in time. Since this gives inconvenience to the patients, these invasive methods are mainly confined to laboratory animal studies. In humans, sampling is mostly limited to the scenario that a scar surgically corrected. Cells may be isolated from these samples and cultured. Tissue samples are usually evaluated by histological and molecular techniques. Invasive evaluation methods are usually performed directly, but cells may also be isolated from tissue samples and cultured for special research purposes [46].

The time of harvesting tissue specimens in *in vivo* post-wounding studies depends on the parameter to be evaluated. Inflammatory response can be evaluated in wounds from 1 hour to 14 days post-wounding. Following wounding, typical time course of obtaining specimens to evaluate inflammatory response may be 1, 6, 12, 24 and 48 hours and 3, 5, 7, 10 and 14 days. Re-epithelization can be evaluated from immediately post-wounding up to 7 days. Vascularization can be assessed from 1 to 7 days. Scar quality can be assessed up to at least post-wounding 70 days in mice and 80 days in rats. Wound image analysis and wound breaking strength measurement can be done at all mentioned time points. The tissue specimens should be taken after photographs are taken. In *animal models* the wound/scar should be excised together with 3-4 mm unwounded surrounding tissue and underlying muscle layer [12].

5.2.1. Histopathology and Immunohistochemistry

The most important issues for reliable histopathological and immunohistochemical evaluation are correct sampling and processing of these tissue samples. Different histological staining methods can be used depending on the structures of interest. Tissue sections may be stained by standard histopathological staining techniques [such as hematoxylin-eosin (H&E) staining] to evaluate tissue cellularity, cellular type and morphology, presence and thickness of granulation tissue, vascularization, re-epithelization or epithelial gap, epidermal differentiation, presence of normal skin structures (rete ridges, appendages) and architectural aspects of the tissue like dermal and epidermal thickness, and collagen bundle orientation. Alternative dyes can be used for further distinguishing between different tissue components like Elastic-van Gieson dye, Trichrome-Goldner staining, Mallory's trichrome staining, orcein dye or periodic acid-Schiff (PAS) (glycogen) staining. They are used to evaluate elastic and collagen fibers or basement membrane formation. Architecture of collagen fibers can also be evaluated by polarized microscopy with the help of special staining techniques like picrosirius red staining, and phase-contrast microscopy on H&E stained sections [46].

Quantification of histopathological data can be done by a semiquantitative 1-5 scale to score inflammation severity, total area of granulation tissue; counting blood vessels; using softwares like Image Based Analysis System (IBAS) or ImageJ to quantify contraction, epithelization, volume fractions of different cells, and vascularization [46]. The distance across the healing surface from the junction between normal and proliferating epidermis on one side of the wound to the similar junction on the opposite wound margin can be measured histopathologically either by calculating manually on micrographs or by using image analysis software [12].

The proposed standard for histopathological evaluation includes search for presence or absence of key players of wound healing (keratinocytes, fibroblasts, macrophages, blood vessels) and quantification of the area occupied by certain cells/structures or total number of cells [46].

Immunohistochemical techniques are used to evaluate presence, expression level and localization of specific cells and proteins in the tissue specimens. One or more antibodies can be used to evaluate proliferation and differentiation of the epidermis, dermal-epidermal basement membrane components, blood vessels, proteins of specific dermal structures and cells, markers for cell proliferation, differentiation and migration. The standard panel of antibodies recommended cover most important structural aspects of the skin: keratin 14 (basal keratinocytes), involucrin (corneocytes), type IV collagen (epidermal basement membrane and blood vessels), CD31 (blood vessel endothelium) and α-smooth muscle actin (myofibroblasts and mature blood vessels) [45]. Antibodies to CD31 can be used to evaluate the angiogenic response from existing blood vessels and CD34 to evaluate vasculogenesis from precursor cells [12].

Visual analog scale can be used to score wound/scarring; wound/scar width at the epidermis, mid-wound/mid-scar and at the level of panniculus carnosus; wound/scar perimeter; size and orientation of collagen bundles, spacing between fibers; overall score [12].

5.2.2. Molecular Biological Methods

The main interest of molecular biological methods is the expression of mRNA and proteins in cells isolated from tissue specimens [46].

5.2.2.1. mRNA Expression

Two common methods are used to evaluate mRNA expression levels of corresponding proteins: microarrays and real-time quantitative reversed transcription polymerase chain reaction (qRT-PCR). Even the expression profile of the whole genome can be studied. Microarrays are appropriate to explore differentially expressed genes in different RNA populations. qRT-PCR is usually used to confirm the differences detected with microarrays. In qRT-PCR the expression levels of target genes are determined relative to a reference gene, hence validation of these reference genes is important. Following identification of differentially expressed genes with previous methods, mRNA expression can also be localized by using in situ hybridization techniques [46].

5.2.2.2. Protein Expression

It is the resulting protein that plays a role in *wound healing* and *scarring* process and many processes are involved in translation. Hence it is important to figure out whether the differences found at the mRNA level are also present at the active protein level. Proteins, proteolytic enzymes, cytokines and growth factors can be evaluated by western blot or enzyme linked immunosorbent assay (ELISA) to analyze levels, to differentiate types, activity or inactivity and to study localization. Specific ELISA techniques like Azocoll assay or zymography were developed to analyze activity and in situ zymography was developed to study the localization of proteolytic enzymes [46].

5.2.2.3. Cellular Viability

Cells isolated from a proliferative scar can be investigated to assess the balance between cell proliferative capacity and apoptosis. The techniques involve DNA fragmentation assay using agarose gel electrophoresis, MTT assay for cell viability, and propidium iodide staining for apoptotic cells [46].

5.2.3. Electron Microscopy

Transmission electron microscopy (TEM) and scanning electron microscopy (SEM) can be used to examine individual epidermal components, basement membrane components, dermal elastic fiber, collagen, fibroblast and myofibroblasts in detail. As small samples can be used in electron microscopy evaluations, these methods are most suitable to answer specific research questions at a detailed level but not appropriate in general wound/scar evaluation [46].

5.3. Transillumination to Observe Vascularization

The explanted skin from laboratory animals can be evaluated by transillumination method to observe blood vessels. Removed skin is placed over a transilluminator and digital pictures are taken; vessel area and length can be calculated afterwards by semi-automated systems [46].

5.4. *In Situ*/*In Vivo* Imaging

Optical coherence tomography (OCT) can be used to evaluate *wound healing* and scarring *in vivo* and it can be combined with conventional H&E staining in obtained tissue sections. Images obtained by OCT can go down to a maximum depth of 0.5 mm, reaching upper part of the subcutaneous fat layer [46].

Fluorescently labeled cells can be evaluated for survival and distribution by using *in vivo* imaging methods [46].

5.5. Mechanical Properties

Tissue strength is closely related to its functional performance. Mechanical strength of explanted skin strips can be evaluated in terms of ultimate tensile strength, elasticity, stiffness and failure strength by using special tools (like Instron tester). The limitation of this method is the requirement of relatively large skin samples [46]. However, nowadays the breaking strength can be assessed by applying stress to wounds *in vivo*. Multi-axial stress can be applied to wounds in an anesthetized animal [12].

5.6. Microbiological Sampling

Signs of infection can be scored macroscopically or microscopically or by culture. However it can sometimes be problematic to differentiate between colonization, contamination and tissue infection. Quantitative microbiology of tissue samples is the only reliable method to prove tissue infection [46].

5.7. Recommended Standard Work-Out for Comparable Evaluation of Wound Healing/Scarring

The studies are recommended to include both macroscopic and microscopic methods to make studies comparable to each other (Table 6). Minimum set of evaluation methods should include observation of behavior of animals to get an idea about adverse effects like itching or pain, subjective scar assessment method (OSAS), measurement of wound area (planimetry), histopathological examination of H&E stained sections and immunohistochemistry examination of stained sections if it is available [46].

Table 6. Proposed standard assessment methods (Adapted from [46])

Characterization of method		Method	Wound/scar feature
Noninvasive	Subjective	OSAS	Vascularity, pigmentation, thickness, relief, pliability, surface area
	Objective	Planimetry	Re-epithelization Contraction
Invasive	Histopathology	H&E staining	Number and distribution of cells / blood vessels, architecture of epidermal/ dermal structures
	Immunohistochemistry	Keratin 14, involucrin, α-smooth muscle actin, type IV collagen, CD31	Keratinocyte differentiation, myofibroblasts, (mature) blood vessels

Conclusion

Understanding the basic mechanisms and pathophysiology of how wounds heal and scars form is mandatory to develop optimal therapeutics/strategies in the future to prevent pathologic/delayed wound healing and abnormal scar formation. Although there is a growing knowledge of the wound healing and scarring, we have neither created *an in vitro/in vivo* laboratory model that demonstrates the complex nature of human wound healing/scar formation and immunologic responses in these processes nor discovered the ways to prevent and perfectly treat the proliferative scars (hypertrophic scars and keloids).

Additionally wound healing/scar models have a limited duration of time (weeks to months) while human adverse wound healing/scarring develops over longer time periods (months to years). Hence wound healing/scar models can only provide data on early processes of wound healing/scarring. Additionally, we should clarify in the future the answers to questions like: Why does an adverse scar forms instead of a normotrophic scar? What causes a scar to become a hypertrophic scar instead of becoming a keloid scar? Ideal wound healing/scar models should mimic cells, structure, elasticity, cellular and molecular interactions and immunologic responses of all wound/scar types in human skin. The future may bring the skin-on-a-chip or even scar-on-a-chip model into reality to study wound healing/scarring and this development will be a valuable one.

REFERENCES

[1] Wilhelm, Klaus P., and D. Wilhelm, S. Bielfeldt. 2017. "Models of wound healing: an emphasis on clinical studies." *Skin Research and Technology* 23:3-12. doi: 10.1111/srt.12317.

[2] Ud-Din, Sara, and Ardeshir Bayat. 2017. "Non-animal models of wound healing in cutaneous repair: *In silico, in vitro, ex vivo*, and *in vivo* models of wounds and scars in human skin." *Wound Repair and Regeneration* 25:164-76. doi: 10.1111/wrr.12513.

[3] van den Broek, Lenie J., and Grace C. Limandjaja, Frank B. Niessen, Susan Gibbs. 2014. "Human hypertrophic and keloid scar models: principles, limitations and future challenges from a tissue engineering perspective." *Experimental Dermatology* 23:382-6. doi: 10.1111/exd.12419.

[4] Middelkoop, E., and A. J. van den Bogaerdt, E. N. Lamme, M. J. Hoekstra, K. Brandsma, M. M. Ulrich. 2004. "Porcine wound models for skin substitution and burn treatment." *Biomaterials* 25:1559-67.

[5] Ramos, Maria L. C., and Alfredo Gragnani, Lydia M. Ferreira. 2008. "Is there an ideal animal model to study hypertrophic scarring? *Journal of Burn Care & Research* 29:363-8. doi: 10.1097/BCR.0b013e3181667557.

[6] Williams, Felicia N., and David N. Herndon, Ludwik K. Branski. 2014. "Where we stand with human hypertrophic and keloid scar models." *Experimental Dermatology* 23:811-2. doi: 10.1111/exd.12506.

[7] Seaton, Max, and Anne Hocking, Nicole S. Gibran. 2015. "Porcine models of cutaneous wound healing." *ILAR Journal* 56:127-38. doi: 10.1093/ilar/ilv016.

[8] Soybir, Onur C., and Sibel O. Gurdal, Ebru S. Oran, Feti Tulubas, Meral Yuksel, Aysenur I. Akyıldız, Ayhan Bilir, Gursel R. Soybir. 2012. "Delayed cutaneous wound healing in aged rats compared to younger ones". *International Wound Journal* 9:478-87. doi: 10.1111/j.1742-481X.2011.00897.x.

[9] Volk, Susan W., and Mark W. Bohling. 2013. "Comparative wound healing--are the small animal veterinarian's clinical patients an improved translational model for human wound healing research?" *Wound Repair and Regeneration* 21:372-81. doi: 10.1111/wrr.12049.

[10] Richardson, Rebecca, and Krasimir Slanchev, Christopher Kraus, Philipp Knyphausen, Sabine Eming, Matthias Hammerschmidt. 2013. "Adult zebrafish as a model system for cutaneous wound-healing research." *Journal of Investigative Dermatology* 133:1655-65. doi: 10.1038/jid.2013.16.

[11] Sullivan, T. P., and W. H. Eaglstein, S. C. Davis, P. Mertz. 2001. "The pig as a model for human wound healing." *Wound Repair and Regeneration* 9:66-76.

[12] Mary Birch, Annette T., and Mark W. J. Ferguson. 2005. "Animal Models for Adult Dermal Wound Healing" In *Methods in Molecular Medicine, Vol. 117:*

Fibrosis Research: Methods and Protocols edited by Varga, John, and David A. Brenner, Sem H. Phan, 223-35. Totowa, NJ: Humana Press Inc.

[13] Singer, Adam J., and Steve A McClain. 2006. "Development of a porcine incisional wound model and novel scarring scales." *Wound Repair and Regeneration* 14:492-7. doi: 10.1111/j.1743-6109.2006.00149.x.

[14] Aksoy, Berna, and H. Mete Aksoy, Ekrem Civas, Huseyin Ustun, Nilgun Atakan. 2009. "A new experimental delayed wound healing model in rabbits." *European Journal of Dermatology* 19:565-9. doi: 10.1684/ejd.2009.0788.

[15] Domergue, Sophie, and Christian Jorgensen, Daniele Noël. 2015. "Advances in Research in Animal Models of Burn-Related Hypertrophic Scarring." *Journal of Burn Care & Research* 36:e259-66. doi: 10.1097/BCR.0000000000000167.

[16] Macri, L. K., and A. J. Singer, S. A. McClain, L. Crawford, A. Prasad, J. Kohn, R. A. Clark. 2016. "Immediate tangential excision accelerates wound closure but does not reduce scarring of mid-dermal porcine burns." *Annals of Burns and Fire Disasters* 29:54-61.

[17] Carlsson, Anders H., and Lloyd F. Rose, John L. Fletcher, Jesse C. Wu, Kai P. Leung, Rodney K. Chan. 2017. "Antecedent thermal injury worsens split-thickness skin graft quality: A clinically relevant porcine model of full-thickness burn, excision and grafting." *Burns* 43:223-31. doi: 10.1016/j.burns.2016.08.006.

[18] Kaufman, T., and S. N. Lusthaus, U. Sagher, M. R. Wexler. 1990. "Deep partial skin thickness burns: a reproducible animal model to study burn wound healing." *Burns* 16:13-6.

[19] Kim, J. Y., and D. M. Dunham, D. M. Supp, C. K. Sen, H. M. Powell. 2016. "Novel burn device for rapid, reproducible burn wound generation." *Burns* 42:384-91. doi: 10.1016/j.burns.2015.08.027.

[20] Wang, Xue-Qing, and Pei-Yun Liu, Margit Kempf, Leila Cuttle, Allen H.-E. Chang, Michael Wong, Olena Kravchuk, Julie Mill, Roy M. Kimble. 2009. "Burn healing is dependent on burn site: a quantitative analysis from a porcine burn model." *Burns* 35:264-9. doi: 10.1016/j.burns.2008.05.030.

[21] Gawronska-Kozak, Barbara, and Anna Grabowska, Marta Kopcewicz, Anna Kur. 2014. "Animal models of skin regeneration." *Reproductive Biology* 14:61-7. doi: 10.1016/j.repbio.2014.01.004.

[22] Ud-Din, Sara, and Susan W. Volk, Ardeshir Bayat. 2014. "Regenerative healing, scar-free healing and scar formation across the species: current concepts and future perspectives." *Experimental Dermatology* 23:615-9. doi: 10.1111/exd.12457.

[23] Lorenz, H. Peter, and Michael T. Longaker, Luke A. Perkocha, Russell W. Jennings, Michael R. Harrison, N. Scott Adzick. 1992. "Scarless wound repair: a human fetal skin model." *Development* 114:253-9.

[24] Carre, Antoine L., and Barrett J. Larson, Joseph A. Knowles, Kenichiro Kawai, Michael T. Longaker, H. Peter Lorenz. 2012. "Fetal mouse skin heals scarlessly in

a chick chorioallantoic membrane model system." *Annals of Plastic Surgery* 69:85-90. doi: 10.1097/SAP.0b013e31822128a9.

[25] Blackstone, Britani N., and Jayne Y. Kim, Kevin L. McFarland, Chandan K. Sen, Dorothy M. Supp, J. Kevin Bailey Heather M., Powell. 2017. "Scar formation following excisional and burn injuries in a red Duroc pig model. *Wound Repair and Regeneration* 25:618-31. doi: 10.1111/wrr.12562.

[26] Sood, Rafi F., and Lara A. Muffley, Max E. Seaton, Maricar Ga, Pornthep Sirimahachaiyakul, Anne M. Hocking, Nicole S. Gibran. 2015. "Dermal Fibroblasts from the Red Duroc Pig Have an Inherently Fibrogenic Phenotype: An *In Vitro* Model of Fibroproliferative Scarring." *Plastic and Reconstructive Surgery* 136:990-1000. doi: 10.1097/PRS.0000000000001704.

[27] Friedrich, Emily E., and Solmaz Niknam-Bienia, Ping Xie, Sheng-Xian Jia, Seok J. Hong, Thomas A. Mustoe, Robert D. Galiano. 2017. "Thermal injury model in the rabbit ear with quantifiable burn progression and hypertrophic scar." *Wound Repair and Regeneration* 25:327-37. doi: 10.1111/wrr.12518.

[28] Zhu, Kathy Q., and Loren H. Engrav, Nicole S. Gibran, Jana K. Cole, Hajime Matsumura, Michael Piepkorn, F. Frank Isik, Gretchen J. Carrougher, Paul M. Muangman, Murad Y. Yunusov, Tai-Mei Yang. 2003. "The female, red Duroc pig as an animal model of hypertrophic scarring and the potential role of the cones of skin. *Burns* 29:649-64.

[29] Cuttle, Leila, and Margit Kempf, Gael E. Phillips, Julie Mill, Mark T. Hayes, John F. Fraser, Xue-Qing Wang, Roy M. Kimble. 2006. "A porcine deep dermal partial thickness burn model with hypertrophic scarring." *Burns* 32:806-20.

[30] Rapp, Scott J., and Aaron Rumberg, Marty Visscher, David A. Billmire, Ann S. Schwentker, Brian S. Pan. 2015. "Establishing a Reproducible Hypertrophic Scar following Thermal Injury: A Porcine Model." *Plastic and Reconstructive Surgery Global Open* 3:e309. doi: 10.1097/GOX.0000000000000277.

[31] Jimi, Shotaro, and Hajime Matsumura. 2017. "Effect of chymase activity on skin thickness in the Clawn miniature pig hypertrophic scarring model." *Journal of Plastic Surgery and Hand Surgery* 51:446-52. doi: 10.1080/2000656X.2017.1310733.

[32] Morris, D. E., and L. Wu, L. L. Zhao, L. Bolton, S. I. Roth, D. A. Ladin, T. A. Mustoe. 1997. "Acute and chronic animal models for excessive dermal scarring: quantitative studies." *Plastic and Reconstructive Surgery* 100:674-81.

[33] Aarabi, Shahram, and Kirit A. Bhatt, Yubin Shi, Josemaria Paterno, Edward I. Chang, Shang A. Loh, Jeffrey W. Holmes, Michael T. Longaker, Herman Yee, Geoffrey C. Gurtner. 2007. "Mechanical load initiates hypertrophic scar formation through decreased cellular apoptosis." *The FASEB Journal* 21:3250-61.

[34] Aksoy, H. Mete, and Ibrahim Vargel, H. Ibrahim Canter, Yucel Erk, Mustafa Sargon, Asli Pinar, G. Guler Tezel. 2002. "A new experimental hypertrophic scar model in guinea pigs." *Aesthetic Plastic Surgery* 26:388-96.

[35] Cameron, Alexander M., and Damian H. Adams, John E. Greenwood, Peter J. Anderson, Allison J. Cowin. 2014. "A novel murine model of hypertrophic scarring using subcutaneous infusion of bleomycin." *Plastic and Reconstructrive Surgery* 133:69-78. doi: 10.1097/01.prs.0000436821.26709.a7.

[36] Cameron, Alexander M. 2014. "Reply: a novel murine model of hypertrophic scarring using subcutaneous infusion of bleomycin. *Plastic and Reconstructive Surgery* 134:164e. doi: 10.1097/PRS.0000000000000257.

[37] Yang, Dong Y., and Shi R. Li, Ju L. Wu, Yan Q. Chen, Gang Li, Sheng Bi, Xia Dai. 2007. "Establishment of a hypertrophic scar model by transplanting full-thickness human skin grafts onto the backs of nude mice." *Plastic and Reconstructive Surgery* 119:104-9.

[38] Robb, Edward C., and J. Paul Waymack, Glenn D. Warden, Paul Nathan, J. Wesley Alexander. 1987. "A new model for studying the development of human hypertrophic burn scar formation." *The Journal of Burn Care & Rehabilitation* 8:371-5.

[39] Polo, Max, and Young-Jin Kim, Ahmet Kucukcelebi, Peter G. Hayward, Francis Ko, Martin C. Robson. 1998. "An *in vivo* model of human proliferative scar." *Journal of Surgical Research* 74:187-95.

[40] Singer, Adam J., and Douglas Hirth, Steve A. McClain, Laurie Crawford, Fubao Lin, Richard A. Clark. 2011. "Validation of a vertical progression porcine burn model." *Journal of Burn Care and Research* 32:638-46. doi: 10.1097/BCR.0b013e31822dc439.

[41] Ibrahim, Mohamed M., and Jennifer Bond, Andrew Bergeron, Kyle J. Miller, Tosan Ehanire, Carlos Quiles, Elizabeth R. Lorden, Manuel A. Medina, Mark Fisher, Bruce Klitzman, M. Angelica Selim, Kam W. Leong, Howard Levinson. 2014. "A novel immune competent murine hypertrophic scar contracture model: a tool to elucidate disease mechanism and develop new therapies." *Wound Repair and Regeneration* 22:755-64. doi: 10.1111/wrr.12238.

[42] Marttala, Jaana, and Jonathan P. Andrews, Joel Rosenbloom, Jouni Uitto. 2016. "Keloids: Animal models and pathologic equivalents to study tissue fibrosis." *Matrix Biology* 51:47-54. doi: 10.1016/j.matbio.2016.01.014.

[43] Duong, Hai S., and Qunzhou Zhang, Abraham Kobi, Anh Le, Diana V. Messadi. 2005. "Assessment of morphological and immunohistological alterations in long-term keloid skin explants." *Cells Tissues Organs* 181:89-102.

[44] Hillmer, M. P., and S. M. MacLeod. 2002. "Experimental keloid scar models: a review of methodological issues." *Journal of Cutaneous Medicine and Surgery* 6:354-9.

[45] Theoret, Christine L., and Oluyinka O. Olutoye, Laura K.S. Parnell, John Hicks. 2013. "Equine exuberant granulation tissue and human keloids: a comparative histopathologic study." *Veterinary Surgery* 42:783-9. doi: 10.1111/j.1532-950X.2013.12055.x.

[46] Lammers, Gerven, and Pauline D. H. M. Verhaegen, Magda M. W. Ulrich, Joost Schalkwijk, Esther Middelkoop, Daniela Weiland, Suzan T. M. Nillesen, Toin H. Van Kuppevelt, Willeke F. Daamen. 2011. "An overview of methods for the *in vivo* evaluation of tissue-engineered skin constructs." *Tissue Engineering: Part B Review* 17:33-55. doi: 10.1089/ten.TEB.2010.0473.

In: Cutaneous Scars: Biology, Clinics and Management ISBN: 978-1-53615-657-7
Editors: Berna Aksoy, Hasan Mete Aksoy et al. © 2019 Nova Science Publishers, Inc.

Chapter 7

HISTOPATHOLOGY OF CUTANEOUS SCARS

Duru Onan*

Department of Dermatology, University of Health Sciences,
Ankara Numune Training and Research Hospital, Ankara, Turkey

ABSTRACT

Skin wound healing is a complex process, the interruption of which gives rise to development of pathological scars. Scarring mainly arises from external trauma or skin disorders. Dermal damage results in persistent scarring, whereas damage confined to epidermis or papillary dermis can heal in a scarless manner. The distinction between normal scars and pathological scars may be so obscure that histopathologic examination might be necessary in some circumstances. Awareness of the specific histological features in different scar types might guide the physician to make an appropriate diagnosis.

Keywords: atrophic scar, cicatricial alopecia, Marjolin's ulcer, proliferative scars, scar, scar contracture, unstable scar

1. INTRODUCTION

The cutaneous scar is the consequence of a healed injury of the skin [1]. The interruption of the skin wound healing process with conditions that are significant enough

*Corresponding Author's Email: t_duru@hotmail.com.

to cause permanent loss or alteration of the collagen fiber architecture might lead to scar formation [2, 3]. Scarring may result from external trauma as well as from a skin disease (connective tissue disease, diseases of the pilosebaceous unit such as acne, infections of the skin or adnexal structures) or other organic diseases (Crohn's disease) [1]. Dermal damage is more permanent and results in a gain or loss of tissue. However, damage limited to the epidermis or papillary dermis can heal without scarring [4].

Scars normally pass through the stages of the wound-healing process: inflammation, proliferation, and remodeling [4]. The inflammatory stage limits the injury and prevents infection. The proliferative stage is characterized by granulation tissue composed of endothelial cells, fibroblasts, and epithelial cells. The remodeling stage involves extracellular matrix (ECM) reorganization at the site of injury [5]. The role of epidermis is important in the control of scarring. Elastic fibers and collagen are the main components of ECM which are closely related to the process of scar formation [6].

The structure of the skin is histologically changed in cutaneous scars [2]. Keratinocytes in scarring epidermis are more proliferative than in normal skin and the collagen bundles in scars are arranged in a more parallel manner [2, 7].

2. Normal Scar

After injury, a complex physiologic tissue repair process takes place up till scar formation; in which damaged dermis and other tissues are substituted with fibrosis. Normal scars appear initially erythematous, later skin-colored, hyper- or hypopigmented; may be elevated or depressed but they are usually flat. They have a smooth, firm quality and do not significantly displace the underlying subcutis or adnexal structures [3, 8].

In the early stage normal scars reveal an acanthotic epidermis with a fibromyxoid stroma consisting of loose fine collagen fibers; increased fibroblasts, myofibroblasts, and capillaries, and presence of a mixed infiltrate. In the chronic stage; an increased collagen fiber deposition in which the fibers are oriented parallel to each other as well as to the overlying atrophic epidermal surface can be observed. The capillaries are oriented perpendicular to the collagen fibers and epidermal surface. The fibroblasts are increased in number, and there is a predominantly lymphocytic infiltrate [3, 8].

Most of the normal scars have thinner epidermis with attenuation or loss of the rete ridge pattern and thinner elastic fibers compared to normal skin [3, 6]. The obviously thicker collagen underneath the basal membrane zone and partly disrupted collagen in deep dermis complicates the distinction between the papillary and the reticular dermis [6].

3. Proliferative Scars

Proliferative scars are a variation of the physiologic wound healing process [9]. Keloids and hypertrophic scars are two forms of excessive cutaneous scarring; characterized by local fibroblast proliferation and excessive amounts of collagen production in response to cutaneous injury [10, 11]. Superficial injuries that do not reach to the level of reticular dermis never cause keloidal and hypertrophic scarring; so these pathological scars develop due to injury to reticular dermis with subsequent development of chronic inflammation composed of inflammatory cells, numerous fibroblasts, newly formed blood vessels, and collagen deposits [12].

Proliferative scars have different clinical and histopathologic features [11]. Keloids have been defined as painful or pruritic, raised cutaneous scars that grow beyond the borders of the initial trauma, and hypertrophic scars have been defined as raised scars that remain within the margins of the original wound [9]. In addition to increased number of fibroblasts producing much more collagen compared to normal scars; keloids and hypertrophic scars have a distinct pattern of vascularization with higher number of vessels in papillary and reticular dermis [13]. The distribution pattern of fibrillin-1 and elastin also differs in proliferative scars compared to normal scars [10].

3.1. Keloid Scar

Unique to humans, keloids represent benign fibroproliferative tumors characterized by an excessive deposition of extracellular matrix (ECM) components, especially collagen, in the dermis and subcutis that extends beyond the boundaries of the original wound and infiltrating into the adjacent healthy skin [1, 14, 15]. The pathogenesis of keloid formation is proposed to be related to an increased formation of connective tissue together with a change in the crosslinking of the collagen fibers due to an absence of differentiation of myofibroblasts from fibroblasts [1]. Keloids continue to grow over the years and spontaneous regression is rare [15]. Young age, black skin and localization at the sternum are the main predisposing factors regarding keloid formation [1].

Early keloids show abundant fibroblasts and fibrillary collagen within the reticular dermis but elastic fibers are largely absent [1, 9]. In the late stage the picture is entirely dominated by characteristic thick sclerotic collagen strands, however in longstanding lesions, there may be a return to the earlier fibrillary pattern [1, 11].

The overlying epidermis may be unchanged or moderately thin, and underneath it there are often some telangiectatic capillaries. A sparse, perivascular chronic inflammatory cell infiltrate may be observed [1, 9]. In the papillary dermis an advancing edge that resembles invasive tumour growth can be observed. Whorls and nodules of randomly arranged, strikingly thick, brightly eosinophilic collagen bundles composed of densely packed fibrils dominate the dermis with obliteration of the papillary-reticular border along with displacement and ultimate destruction of skin appendages [1, 11, 14]. The orientation of numerous fibroblasts and accompanying collagen bundles is similar (Figure 1) [9].

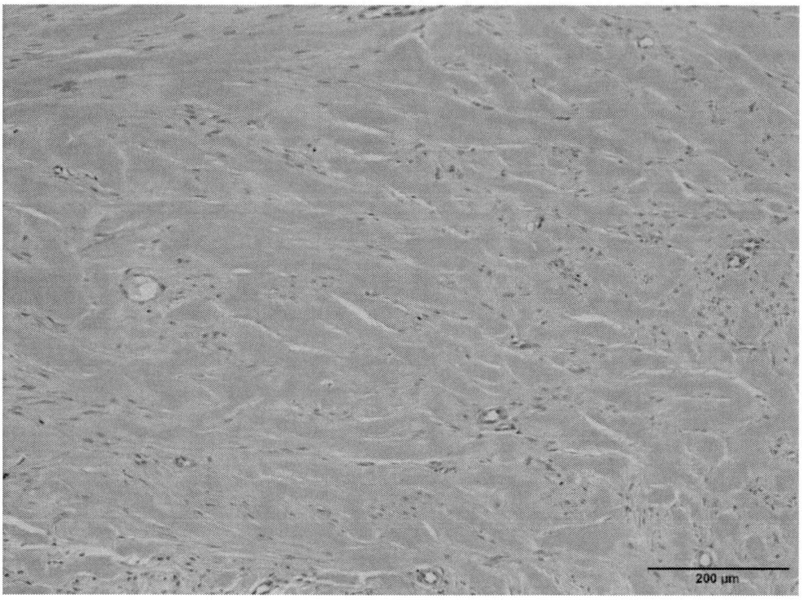

Figure 1. Keloid scar - randomly arranged, markedly broad, sclerotic, and brightly eosinophilic collagen bundles admixed with numerous fibroblasts (H.&E. x100).

3.2. Hypertrophic Scars

Clinically hypertrophic scars are mildly elevated above the perilesional skin, but do not extend beyond the margins of the initial trauma [3, 9]. These scars are most common within the first couple of months postinjury, and then, contrary to keloids, tend to normally mature with occasional spontaneous regression [4]. In the histologic pattern, below the moderately thin epidermis, a nodular proliferation of randomly oriented fascicles composed of collagen fibers that maintain a parallel array with one another. The fascicles are demarcated by small, thin-walled blood vessels [1, 3]. Densely packed collagen bundles and the fibroblasts are typically oriented parallel to the skin surface, but they are less organized compared to regular and well-defined orientation seen in normal skin tissues [9, 16]. These collagen bundles which are markedly increased in number, contain distinctly more cellular nuclei than the keloid. Hyalinization is less marked. Capillaries are usually oriented vertical to the skin surface, and chronic perivascular sparse inflammatory infiltrates are often noticeable within the scar. A decrease or loss of elastic tissue can be noted (Figure 2) [1, 9].

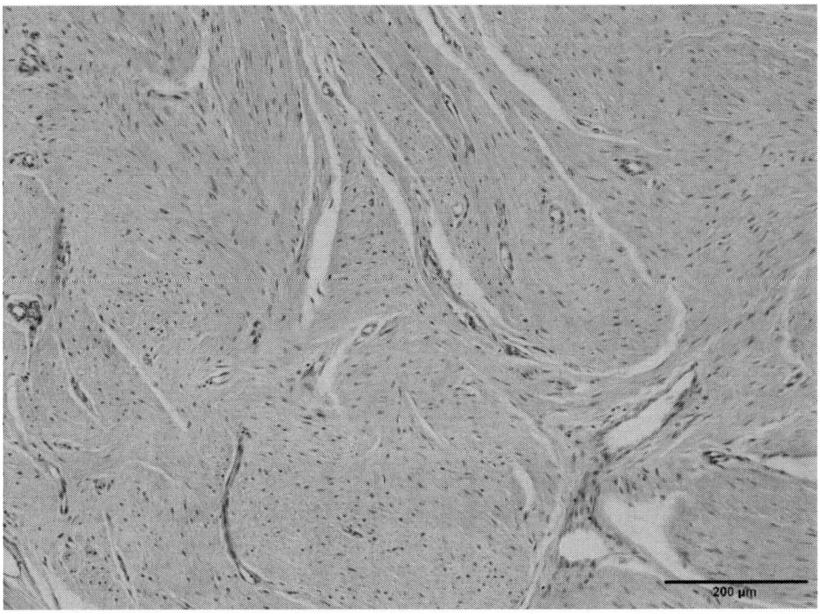

Figure 2. Hypertrophic scar - whorls of thickened collagen and fibroblasts, randomly oriented fascicles demarcated by small, thin-walled blood vessels (H&Ex100).

Distinguishing between a keloid and a hypertrophic scar histopathologically is not always easy because thickened hyalinized collagen fibers that are typically situated in the centers of the fibrotic nodules (keloidal collagen, so-called "red crayons"), are not always detectable in keloids and alpha -smooth muscle actin (α -SMA), a differentiating marker of HS, is variably expressed by myofibroblasts in both forms of scar [3, 11, 17]. Expression of cyclooxygenase (COX)-1 favors but does not specifically identify keloids, since it can also be seen in hypertrophic scars. However, a study investigated additional distinguishing features between keloid and HS in scars with no detectable keloidal collagen. No flattening of the epidermis, a lack of fibrosis within the papillary dermis, presence of a tongue-like extending edge, presence of a horizontal cellular fibrous zone in the upper reticular dermis forming a sharp demarcation from the normal-appearing dermis, and presence of prominent fascia-like fibrous bands in the deeper portion of the scar were reported as the features favoring the diagnosis of keloid [11, 17].

3.3. Differential Diagnosis of Proliferative Scars

Histopathologically, some dermal or subcutaneous neoplasms may resemble keloids or hypertrophic scars. Dermatofibroma, dermatofibrosarcoma protuberans, desmoplastic melanoma, scar-like variant of squamous cell carcinoma (SCC) and the fibrotic stroma of cutaneous endometriosis are the most prominent conditions that must be differentiated from proliferative scars [3, 11]. Keloidal collagen fibers can occasionally be observed focally in lesions of morphea, dermatofibroma, and basal cell carcinoma [3, 9]. These conditions can often be differentiated by clinical data or by selected histopathologic features [9]. However, in some circumstances immunohistochemical studies may be required to arrive at a specific diagnosis [3]. Immunostaining for CD34 and factor XIIIa, which is usually positive in dermatofibrosarcoma protuberans and dermatofibroma respectively, is negative in keloids and hypertrophic scars. Desmoplastic melanomas generally exhibit strong expression of S100 protein, however minimal immunostaining for this marker can also be encountered in cutaneous scars [11]. Care needs to be taken on these conditions in order not to overdiagnose them as desmoplastic melanomas. In contrast, desmoplastic melanomas can also be confused with scars [9].

4. Atrophic Scars

An atrophic scar is an incomplete replacement of necrotic connective tissue by cicatricial tissue. These scars are more or less below skin level and can be perceived as an indentation. Although the involved skin areas are covered by epidermis, dermal structures are largely absent [1].

4.1. Post-Acne Scars

Acne scars result from an altered wound healing response to cutaneous inflammation. Abnormal production and degradation of collagen during the healing process leads to various types of acne scars; thus, the result of inflammation and scarring is either an atrophic scar or a hyperplastic response. Atrophic scars that result in the loss of tissue due to a net destruction of collagen in the dermis, are much more common than thickened scars (hypertrophic or keloid scars) where there is a net gain of collagen [18, 19].

As the inflammation is started under the epidermis in the lower part of the pilosebaceous unit, the resultant scarring often involves deeper structures instead of just the surface. As the scars mature and contract they pull these surface layers down by fibrous anchoring of the dermis to the subcutis, leading to the appearance of atrophy to the overlying skin [19, 20]. Besides, the enzymatic activity and inflammatory mediators make contribution to the development of atrophic scarring by destroying the deeper structures [19]. Atrophic acne scars are categorized as icepick, boxcar, and rolling scars. Icepick scars are narrow, deep, sharply marginated epithelial tracts that extend vertically to the deep dermis or subcutaneous tissue [4, 20]. Boxcar scars have a small orifice with sharp edges and a wide atrophic base surrounded by almost vertical walls [4]. Rolling scars develop from dermal tethering of otherwise relatively normal-appearing skin [20].

4.2. Striae Distensae

Striae distensae (SD) are linear bands of atrophic skin that develop following excessive dermal stretching. SD often shows scar-like features because early striae (striae rubrae) appear erythematous and late striae (striae albae) show hypopigmentation and dermal fibrosis [21]. The process of elastolysis of the mid-dermis, followed by reorganization of collagen and fibrillin is proposed to be involved in its pathogenesis [22].

Histopathology of early striae exhibits excessive fine elastic fibers that are split up in the papillary dermis with thicker tortuous fibers in the periphery, accompanying perivascular lymphocytes, dilated dermal vessels and edema. Elastin and fibrillin fibers are reduced in number and reorganized. Additionally, there are structural changes in collagen fibers, which are thicker and densely packed horizontally [22]. Histopathology of late striae reveals epidermal atrophy, loss of rete ridges, less vascularity, and densely packed, fine collagen bundles arranged in parallel lines [21, 22]. While elastic fibers are completely absent in the center, in the periphery there are glomerular or dilated elastic fibers mixed with hardly stainable fibrils [1]. They appear similar to mature atrophic scars [22].

5. Cicatricial Alopecias

The hair follicles are destructed and replaced by fibrous scar tissue leading to irreversible hair loss in scarring alopecias. Although there are many causes of secondary scarring alopecia (infiltrative conditions, trauma and infections), the term cicatricial alopecia is used mainly to imply primary cicatricial alopecias, a group of disorders in which the hair follicle is the major target of the inflammatory process [23].

5.1. Histopathologic Features of Primary Scarring Alopecias

5.1.1. Chronic Cutaneous Lupus Erythematosus (CCLE)

Parakeratosis, epidermal atrophy, vacuolar interface dermatitis, keratinocyte apoptosis along the follicular basal layer and sometimes at the dermo-epidermal junction between follicles, thickening of PAS-positive epidermal and follicular basal membrane zone, folliculocentric lymphocytic inflammatory infiltrate, hyperkeratosis of the infundibulum with ostial obstruction, destruction of peri- and interfollicular elastic fibers, papillary dermal fibrosis, deep dermal mucin and uneven spacing of scars due to interfollicular dermal inflammation are present on histopathologic examination. Direct immunofluorescence findigs are IgG and C3 deposits along the cutaneous and follicular dermo-epidermal junction [23-25].

5.1.2. Lichen Planopilaris (LPP)

A band-like mononuclear infiltrate concealing the interface between the follicular epithelium and the dermis is typical. Folliculocentric lymphocytic inflammatory infiltrate involves the upper part of the follicle most severely, however, the inflammation may extend all the way along the follicle [23, 24]. Wedge shaped hypergranulosis at the follicular ostia is a useful clue [25]. In later stages perifollicular concentric lamellar fibrosis may be seen. Finally, sebaceous glands and then follicles are damaged and replaced by columns of sclerotic collagen (cradle cap scars). Such scars can be emphasized with elastic tissue stains due to destruction of elastic fibers. In LPP, the abundant Civatte bodies (necrotic keratinocytes) are positive for IgM and they are mainly located in the follicular epithelium of the infundibulum and the isthmus. Civatte bodies formed by aggregates of the basal membrane, can also be observed in CCLE [23, 24].

5.1.3. Pseudopelade of Brocq

Follicular scars and loss of sebaceous glands, with variable amounts of residual chronic inflammation are present. In the absence of typical features of other cicatricial alopecias diagnosis of exclusion is possible for this disorder [23, 24].

5.1.4. Central Centrifugal Cicatricial Alopecia

Premature desquamation of the inner root sheath is the earliest histologic finding. Lamellar fibroplasia around follicular infundibula and a perifollicular lymphocytic inflammation can be observed. Late findings include destruction of the follicular epithelium with residual hair shaft fragments, granulomatous inflammation, fibrous tracts replacing pilosebaceous units, and infrequent infundibular fusion (polytrichia). Thickened elastic fibers can be seen in the dermis [23, 26].

5.1.5. Alopecia Mucinosa

Mucin deposits in the outer root sheath, and lakes of intrafollicular mucin are the main findings. In the end-stage, the pilosebaceous unit is destructed and inflammatory cells surround the residual tracts of mucin [23, 26].

5.1.6. Keratosis Follicularis Spinulosa Decalvans

Compact infundibular hyperkeratosis is the typical finding in this disorder [23].

5.1.7. Primary Neutrophilic Cicatricial Alopecias (Folliculitis Decalvans & Dissecting Cellulitis)

Mixed acute and chronic inflammation with follicular damage is present and this inflammation is most severe in the upper dermis with relative sparing of the deeper dermis. Intra- and perifollicular neutrophilic inflammatory infiltrate, polytrichia (fused infundibula), perifollicular and interstitial fibrosis, and foreign-body type granulomatous reaction to destructed hair shafts are the other findings [23, 26].

5.1.8. Primary Mixed Cicatricial Alopecias

5.1.8.1. Folliculitis Keloidalis

Folliculitis with a granulomatous inflammation (a neutrophilic and lymphocytic infiltrate, rarely with plasma cells) and destruction of sebaceous glands in the early stages are observed [23].

5.1.8.2. Folliculitis Necrotica

Early lesions reveal spongiosis and lymphocytic exocytosis in the follicular epithelium associated with dyskeratosis, with a dense perifollicular and perivascular lymphocytic infiltrate. As the lesions progress, with the coalescence of necrotic keratinocytes overall necrosis of the adjacent follicular epithelium, epidermis, and adventitial dermis develops [23].

5.1.8.3. Erosive Pustular Dermatosis

Marked epidermal thinning with focal erosions and intraepidermal groups of neutrophils (subcorneal pustules) are observed. There is an upper dermal folliculocentric mixed inflammatory infiltrate consisting mainly of neutrophils, lymphocytes, and especially plasma cells and this infiltrate is associated with foreign-body type giant cells [23, 26].

6. Scar Complications

6.1. Scar Contractures

A scar contracture occurs as a result of a contractile wound-healing process in a re-epithelized and adequately healed scar [27]. Scars that cross joints or skin creases at right angles tend to develop shortening or contracture. Scar contractures are usually hypertrophic and they are common after burn injury [28]. The main difference between wounds that ends up with a normal scar and wounds that develop scar contractures may be a lack or late induction of myofibroblast apoptosis. Abnormal extracellular matrix protein production by fibroblasts and myofibroblasts contributes to the formation of an excessive and rigid scar [29].

6.2. Unstable Scar

Non-healing wounds, especially full-thickness ones, may develop hypergranulation in some areas instead of epithelization, whereas some areas that have healed spontaneously may ulcerate or develop hypertrophic scars. The scarring phase of some lesions like large burns may be so unstable that it can go on for months, without reaching completion. Repeated ulcerations of the unstable scar that continue quite a while, can lead to malignant transformation causing an invasive tumor [30].

6.3. Marjolin's Ulcer

Malignant degeneration that typically develops over a period of time in unstable scar areas such as post-burn lesions and any other chronic wound is termed as Marjolin's ulcer. The classic triad of nodule formation, induration, and ulceration on the burn scars necessitates a biopsy to confirm the diagnosis [31]. The first histologic sign of this highly invasive type of malignancy occurs at the edge of the ulcer [30]. Squamous cell carcinoma (SCC) (71%) is the most frequent histological type identified in Marjolin's ulcers; followed by BCC (12%), melanoma (6%), sarcoma (5%), basosquamous cell carcinoma (1%), SCC-melanoma (1%) and other rare neoplasms (4%) [31, 32]. Fibrosarcoma, liposarcoma, dermatofibrosarcoma protuberans, malignant fibrous histiocytoma, eccrine syringofibroadenoma, Merkel cell carcinoma, and keratoacanthoma are the rare types of tumors that may arise in the post-burn wounds and scars [31, 33].

The most significant factor in predicting the prognosis is the grade of the tumor [33]. The grade of the Marjolin's ulcer can be defined as follows; grade I: more than 75% of the cells are differentiated; grade II: 25%-75% of the cells are differentiated; grade III: less than 25% of the cells are differentiated. As the grade increases the incidence of metastasis increases and the prognosis worsens [31].

Conclusion

Cutaneous scars are the inevitable consequences of the wound healing process. Their prevention and treatment are challenging just like their diagnosis. When clinical data is insufficient to make a proper diagnosis, histopathological evaluation enables the physician to make a distinction between various types of pathological scars and to detect their complications. Therefore, a fundamental knowledge of the specific histopathological features of them is necessary.

REFERENCES

[1] Vogt, H. J. 1993-2001. *Scars.* Stuttgart : Hippokrates Verlag GmbH.

[2] Yang, Shao-Wei, and Zhi-Jun Geng, Kui Ma, Xiao-Yan Sun, Xiao-Bing Fu. 2016. 'Comparison of the histological morphology between normal skin and scar tissue.' *Journal of Huazhong University of Science and Technology Medical Sciences.* 36:265-9. doi: 10.1007/s11596-016-1578-7.

[3] Maxwell A. F. 2010. 'Inflammatory Diseases of the Dermis and Epidermis.' In *Dermatopathology*, edited by Busam, K. J., and J. R. Goldblum. 11-78. Philadelphia: Saunders, Elsevier.

[4] Rivera, Albert E. 2008. 'Acne scarring: a review and current treatment modalities.' *Journal of American Academy of Dermatology* 59:659-76. doi: 10.1016/j.jaad.2008.05.029.

[5] Profyris, Christos, and Christos Tziotzios, Isabel Do Vale. 2012. 'Cutaneous scarring: Pathophysiology, molecular mechanisms, and scar reduction therapeutics Part I. The molecular basis of scar formation.' *Journal of American Academy of Dermatology* 66:1-10; doi: 10.1016/j.jaad.2011.05.055.

[6] Zhu, Xiaoqin, and Shuangmu Zhuo, Liqin Zheng, Kecheng Lu, Xingshan Jiang, Jianxin Chen, Bifang Lin. 2010. 'Quantified characterization of human cutaneous normal scar using multiphoton microscopy.' *Journal of Biophotonics* 3:108-16. doi: 10.1002/jbio.200910058.

[7] Verhaegen, Pauline D. H. M, and Paul P. M. van Zuijlen, Noor M. Pennings, Jan van Marle, Frank B. Niessen, Chantal M. A. M. van der Horst, Esther Middelkoop. 2009. 'Differences in collagen architecture between keloid, hypertrophic scar, normotrophic scar, and normal skin: An objective histopathological analysis.' *Wound Repair and Regeneration* 17:649-56. doi: 10.1111/j.1524-475X.2009.00533.x.

[8] Kempf, W., M. Hantschke, H. Kutzner, W. H. C. Burgdorf. 2008. 'Soft tissue proliferations and neoplasms.' In, *Dermatopathology,* 236-59. Germany: Steinkopff Verlag.

[9] Patterson, James W. 2016. 'Disorders of collagen.' In, *Weedon's Skin Pathology*, 11, 347-379.e18. China: Elsevier Limited.

[10] Amadeu, Thais P., and Andre S. Braune, Luis C. Porto, Alexis Desmoulière, Andrea M. A. Costa. 2004. Fibrillin-1 and elastin are differentially expressed in

hypertrophic scars and keloids. *Wound Repair and Regeneration* 12:169-74. Doi : 10.1111/j.1067-1927.2004.012209.x.

[11] Machan, S., and A. M. Molina-Ruiz, L. Requena. 2018. 'Dermal Hypertrophies.' In, *Dermatology*, edited by Bolognia, J. L., and J. V. Schaffer, L. Cerroni, 1712-22. China: Elsevier Limited.

[12] Ogawa, Rei. 2017. 'Keloid and Hypertrophic Scars Are the Result of Chronic Inflammation in the Reticular Dermis.' *International Journal of Molecular Sciences* 18:pii: E606. doi: 10.3390/ijms18030606.

[13] Amadeu, Thais, and Andre Braune, Carlos Mandarim-de-Lacerda, Luis C. Porto, Alexis Desmoulière, Andrea Costa. 2003. 'Vascularization pattern in hypertrophic scars and keloids: a stereological analysis.' *Pathology, Research and Practice* 199:469-73.

[14] Jumper, N., and R. Paus, A. Bayat. 2015. 'Functional histopathology of keloid disease.' *Histology and Histopathology* 30:1033-57. doi: 10.14670/HH-11-624.

[15] Andrews, Jonathan P., and Jaana Marttala, Edward Macarak, Joel Rosenbloom, Jouni Uitto. 2016. 'Keloids: The paradigm of skin fibrosis - Pathomechanisms and treatment.' *Matrix Biology* 51:37-46. doi: 10.1016/j.matbio.2016.01.013.

[16] Chen, G., and J. Chen, S. Zhuo, S. Xiong, H. Zeng, X. Jiang, R. Chen, S. Xie. 2009. 'Nonlinear spectral imaging of human hypertrophic scar based on two-photonexcited fluorescence and second-harmonic generation.' The *British Journal of Dermatology* 161:48-55. doi: 10.1111/j.1365-2133.2009.09094.x.

[17] Lee, Julia Y-Y., and Chao-Cun Yang, Sheau-Chiou Chao, Tak-Wak Wong. 2004. 'Histopathological differential diagnosis of keloid and hypertrophic scar.' The *American Journal of Dermatopathology* 26:379-84.

[18] Connolly, Deirdre, and Ha L. Vu, Kavita Mariwalla, Nazanin Saedi. 2017. 'Acne Scarring-Pathogenesis, Evaluation, and Treatment Options.' The *Journal of Clinical and Aesthetic Dermatology* 10:12-23.

[19] Goodman, G. J. 2000. Postacne scarring: a review of its pathophysiology and treatment. *Dermatologic Surgery* 26:857-71.

[20] Jacob, Carolyn I., and Jeffrey S. Dover, Michael S. Kaminer. 2001. 'Acne scarring: a classification system and review of treatment options.' *Journal of the American Academy of Dermatology* 45(1):109-17.

[21] Ud-Din, Sara, and Ardeshir Bayat. 2014. 'New insights on keloids, hypertrophic scars, and striae.' *Dermatologic Clinics* 32:193-209. doi: 10.1016/j.det.2013.11.002.

[22] Oakley, A. M., and S. S. Bhimji. 2018. *Stretch Marks (Striae).* Treasure Island (FL): StatPearls Publishing LLC.

[23] Bernárdez, C., and A. M. Molina-Ruiz, L. Requena. 2015. 'Histologic features of alopecias: part II: scarring alopecias.' *Actas Dermo-sifiliograficas* 106:260-70. doi: 10.1016/j.ad.2014.06.016.

[24] Bolduc, Chantal, and Leonard C. Sperling, Jerry Shapiro. 2016. 'Primary cicatricial alopecia: Lymphocytic primary cicatricial alopecias, including chronic cutaneous lupus erythematosus, lichen planopilaris, frontal fibrosing alopecia, and Graham-Little syndrome.' *Journal of the American Academy of Dermatology* 75:1081-99. doi: 10.1016/j.jaad.2014.09.058.

[25] Inchara, Y. K., and Rajalakshmi Tirumalae, Reeti Kavdia, Meryl Antony. 2011. 'Histopathology of scarring alopecia in Indian patients.' The *American Journal of Dermatopathology* 33:461-7. doi: 10.1097/DAD.0b013e318201abcd.

[26] Bolduc, Chantal, and Leonard C. Sperling, Jerry Shapiro. 2016. 'Primary cicatricial alopecia: Other lymphocytic primary cicatricial alopecias and neutrophilic and mixed primary cicatricial alopecias.' The *Journal of American Academy of Dermatology* 75:1101-17. doi: 10.1016/j.jaad.2015.01.056.

[27] Brissett, Anthony E., and David A. Sherris. 2001. 'Scar contractures, hypertrophic scars, and keloids.' *Facial Plastic Surgery* 17:263-72. doi: 10.1055/s-2001-18827.

[28] Bayat, Ardeshir, and D. A. McGrouther, M. W. J. Ferguson. 2003. 'Skin scarring.' *BMJ* 326(7380):88-92.

[29] Nedelec, B., and A. Ghahary, P. G. Scott, E. E. Tredget. 2000. 'Control of wound contraction. Basic and clinical features. *Hand Clinics* 16(2):289-302.

[30] Borghese, L, and A. Masellis, M. Masellis. 2018. 'Extremity burn reconstruction. In, *Plastic Surgery: Volume 4: Lower Extremity, Trunk, and Burns,* edited by Song, D., and P. C. Neligan, 424-444. Canada: Elsevier

[31] Saaiq, Mohammad, and Bushra Ashraf. 2014. 'Marjolin's ulcers in the post-burned lesions and scars.' *World Journal of Clinical Cases* 2:507-14. doi: 10.12998/wjcc.v2.i10.507.

[32] Bazaliński, Dariusz, and Joanna Przybek-Mita, Beata Barańska, Pawel Więch. 2017. 'Marjolin's ulcer in chronic wounds - review of available literature.' *Contemporary Oncology (Poznan, Poland)* 21:197-202. doi: 10.5114/wo.2017.70109.

[33] Copcu, Eray. 2009. 'Marjolin's ulcer: a preventable complication of burns?' *Plastic Reconstructive Surgery* 124:156e-64e. doi: 10.1097/PRS.0b013e3181a8082e.

In: Cutaneous Scars: Biology, Clinics and Management ISBN: 978-1-53615-657-7
Editors: Berna Aksoy, Hasan Mete Aksoy et al. © 2019 Nova Science Publishers, Inc.

Chapter 8

SCARLESS HEALING AND FUTURE DIRECTIONS

Nilgun Senturk*
Department of Dermatology,
Faculty of Medicine, Ondokuz Mayis University,
Samsun, Turkey

ABSTRACT

Scarring is a natural consequence of skin injury in which organisation of normal structure is inadequate. Scarless healing can be seen in fetal life along with the development of dermal appendages and it may also be possible in adult life. There is a growing interest in scarless wound healing mechanisms and the progress in this area has improved significantly. Recent advances in stem cell and developmental biology have revealed novel pathways and cell types involved in this area. Targeting components of adult tissue healing, such as inflammation, with molecular therapies offers increased specificity. Combinations of endogenous and exogenous wound healing modulators are more likely to successfully achieve scarless wound healing.

Keywords: regenerative healing, scarless healing, stem cell therapy

1. INTRODUCTION

Scarring is a natural consequence of skin injury in which organisation of scar structure is inadequate. It happens as a result of trauma, wounding, burn injury, and

*Corresponding Author's Email: senturk.nilgun@gmail.com.

inflammatory or infectious processes. Evidence of *scarless healing* can be seen in fetuses of various animals [1, 2]. It has been shown that fetal wounds result in complete regeneration with the development of dermal appendages. It is plausible to think that managing *scarless healing* in postnatal life may be possible [3-6]. If achieved, in pediatric and adult life, scarless wound healing can allow complete functional recovery from different types of traumatic injury. There is a growing interest in scarless wound healing mechanisms and the progress in this area has improved significantly leading to development of promising clinical targets.

2. Scarless Healing in Humans

2.1. Fetal Scarless Healing

In the early gestational period, wounds heal without scar formation resembling regeneration [2, 7]. Fetal environmental factors, such as sterility, amniotic fluid including growth factors, and low oxygen tension are thought to play important roles in decreasing scar formation. In addition, intrinsic fetal factors that is responsible for *scarless healing* were identified especially in animal models [8].

Several histological and chemical differences at the cellular and tissue levels between fetal and adult wound healing are represented in Table 1 [8]. Among these, decreased tensile strength, fewer inflammatory cells and different cytokine microenvironment are the important ones [9].

Fibroblasts may be influenced by different cytokine and growth factors for production of extracellular matrix (ECM) molecules in a regenerative pattern [10]. In fetal wounds hyaluronic acid is present in higher concentrations and fibronectin is deposited more rapidly. These molecules may direct healing process towards a regenerative phenotype [11].

In addition, early remodeling of collagen can be achieved by higher levels of matrix metalloproteinase activity present in fetal wounds [12]. Compared to adult fibroblasts, fetal tissues express higher collagen III and IV and are capable of simultaneous proliferation and deposition of collagen, whereas adult fibroblasts first undergo proliferation then deposit collagen [13]. Fetal cultured fibroblasts' proteome analysis revealed different patterns of protein expression related to *regenerative healing* such as engrailed 1 (En1) which supports the notion that scar formation may be a cell-intrinsic property [14].

Table 1. Features of reperative scar formation and scarless healing

	Scar formation	Scarless healing
Cytokine	TGFβ1↑	TGFβ3↑
ECM	TIMP↑	MMP↑
Collagen	Collagen Type I ↑	Collagen type III ↑
Myofibroblasts	Persist	Apoptosis
Matrix interactions	Wound contraction	ECM remodeling

ECM: extracellular matrix, MMP: matrix metalloproteinase, TGFβ: transforming growth factor beta, TIMP: tissue inhibitor of metalloproteinase.

2.2. Adult Scarless Healing

In adults, *regenerative healing* with decreased scar formation is best represented in oral mucosa. Since oral mucosa is relatively immune privileged, with decreased neutrophil content and attenuated inflammatory environment, negative contibution of inflammation to scar formation is attenuated during wound healing [15, 16]. Also, barrier function provided by salivary mucins protects underlying mucosa from mechanical damage, interaction with pathogens and other insults. This "protected environment" is important but probably not sufficient [17].

Oral mucosa ECM composition characterized by increased fibronectin, its splice variant ED-A, and chondroitin sulfate, may contribute to *scarless healing* [18]. To initiate scar contraction, pro-fibrotic myofibroblast ACTA2 (smooth muscle alpha actin) expression needs interaction of cell surface with ED-A fibronectin and TGFβ1 [19]. On the other hand, higher amount of elastin is present in the skin in comparison to oral mucosa. Oral keratinocytes have higher proliferation rate wheras cutaneous keratinocytes demonstrate increased differentiation [18]. Differantial characteristics of the oral mucosa in comparison to skin may contribute to its ability to heal with minimal scarring.

3. Therapeutic Options for Scarless Healing

3.1. Two- and Three-Dimentional Scaffolds

Scaffolds can be used for refractory chronic wounds and acute burn injuries. Engineered products may be synthetic, natural, two- or three- dimensional (3D), and autologous or non-autologous; transplanted cells may or may not be used. Structural and mechanical support, cellular adhesion, proliferation, and differentiation should be provided by these scaffolds [20]. They can be produced from natural or synthetic polymers, and be composites.

Two-dimensional scaffolds are usually used for debridement, and/or therapeutic material delivery. Three-dimensional scaffolds are used for complicated wounds. These scaffolds have importance in extreme tissue damage, and also in situations where tensile strength preservation is important. In order to create ECM scaffolds natural polymer collagen may be used [21].

Improvements in tissue engineering and biochemistry have provided the discovery of synthetic matrices [21]. HYAFF is a semisynthetic biocompatible and biodegradable material used for matrices and scaffolds. These materials can be tailored according to the therapeutic need, such as drug release, growth factor and cell delivery to injured area [22].

One of the latest developments in this area is siRNA within a silicon bilayer which blocks the TGFβ1-mediated pathway. This approach inhibits scar formation through downregulation of COL1, COL3, and ACTA2 [23].

3D printing technology was used to develop scaffolds composed of adult keratinocytes and fibroblasts to combine stem cell populations with tissue regeneration and *scarless healing* [24, 25].

3.2. Reduction of Mechanical Forces

Extracellular mechanical factors play an important role in healing process by changing mechanosensors, such as dual focal adhesion-tyrosine kinase complex (FAK-SRC), Rho associated coiled-coil containing protein kinase (ROCK), mitogen activated protein kinase 1(MAPK1), and phosphoinositide 3-kinase (PI3K). For that reason the mechanotransduction signaling pathway is an ideal target for the *scarless healing* [26-30]. Inhibiting components of the inflammatory FAK-ERK-MCP-1 pathway, may cause attenuation of scar formation. Based on this mechanism, a device which reduces stress has been developed [31-33].

3.3. Supression of Inflammation

Scar formation is associated with unregulated inflammatory response and supression of inflammation may improve wound healing [13]. Physiological anti-inflammatory molecules may drive regenerative wound healing. In mice, α-melanocyte-stimulating hormone (α-MSH) caused *regenerative healing* with decreased scar formation and better collagen fiber organization [34]. In this model, α-MSH was effective only when it was administered prior to wound creation, so it is possible that prophylactic administration of anti-fibrotic agents may be useful in scar revision surgery.

Fibroblast growth factor 9 (FGF9) may also modulate inflammatory environment. It has been shown that FGF9 promotes monocytes towards M2 macrophage differentiation in cardiac ischemic injury [35]. In cutaneous injury, FGF9 from dermal γδ T cells was shown to facilitate follicle neogenesis. These findings may pave the way to development of new therapies aimed at achieving *regenerative healing* [36].

Administration of interleukin (IL)-10 resulted in restoration of normal skin architecture and attenuation of pro-inflammatory gene expression in mice [37]. Before incision, intradermally injected recombinant human IL-10 showed improved macroscopic scar appearance at 12 months [38].

Antagonism of stromal cell-derived factor 1 (SDF-1) / chemokine receptor type 4 (CXCR-4) results in potent anti-fibrotic and regenerative phenotype. In mice, antagonism of CXCR-4 with CTCE-9908 caused grafts remained flat with limited contraction, contrary to controls with more hypertrophic scars, suggesting the potential role of this agent [39].

3.4. Cellular Targets

Ablation of pro-inflammatory perivascular cells which are activated after acute injury, or destroying the activators of these cells (metalloprotease 12 -ADAM12) have been shown to decrease fibrosis and scarring [40].

Among the heterogenous dermal fibroblast population, those originating from En1-lineage play an important role in cutaneous scarring. Abortion of the En1-fibroblast lineage may be accomplished by the simultaneous expression of CD26 (also known as dipeptidyl peptidase-4, DPP4) surface marker with diprotin A. Treatment with this small molecule reduced cutaneous scarring after full-thickness excisional wounding along with protection of the integrity of the regenerated tissue [14]. Inhibitors of DPP4 supress the fibrogenic capacity of keloid-derived or normal fibroblasts. The underlying mechanism associated with the observed decrease in collagen production and TGF-β1 expression involves the pro-fibrotic pp38 and pERK1/2 pathways [41].

Myofibroblasts and adipocytes are important in normal wound healing and cells having myofibroblast-like characteristics are important in fibrosis development [2, 42]. Myofibroblasts are functionally heterogeneous cell populations. Fibroblasts, mesenchymal stem cells (MSCs), smooth muscle cells, endothelial cells, and fibrocytes are potential precursors for them [43]. Basic fibroblast growth factor (bFGF), when added to myofibroblasts, decrease expression of α-SMA, collagen I, and fibronectin in addition to loss of focal adhesions and stress fibers. These findings suggest that myofibroblast differentiation process is not terminal, and bFGF has a potential to change their phenotype [44].

Usually used for urological or orthopedic purposes, extracorporeal shockwaves (ESW) may also reduce scar formation. ESW treatment led to myofibroblast precursors to differentiate into more fibroblast-like cells with decreased contraction and higher migration potential, concomitantly reducing α-SMA and type I collagen expression [45].

4. Stem Cells in Scarless Healing

4.1. Fetal Stem Cell Therapy

By reducing inflammation, stem cells can modulate the wound environment and improve healing, [46, 47]. However, their contribution to scarring is unclear [48, 49]. Umbilical cord epithelium (UCE), human amniotic epithelial cells, and human foreskin fibroblasts (HFF) are neonatal cell sources for *scarless healing*.

The UCE is structurally similar to the epidermis of the early fetus and surrounded by gelatinous ECM called Warton's Jelly (WJ). Mesenchymal stem cells (MSC) isolated from WJ have been shown to promote wound healing [50, 51].

Another source of *stem cell therapy* is human amniotic epithelial cells, which are capable of forming tissue engineered skin with similar morphology to normal skin [52].

Transfected HFF from newborn males may have a role in *scarless healing*, by increasing expression of TGFβ3 when grafted into wounds [53]. HFF are also used in allogeneic grafting [54]. They can be used with scaffolds or applied directly to wounds to modulate acute or chronic wound healing.

4.2. Adult Stem Cell Therapy

MSCs which have the ability of self-renewal and differentiation are attractive option for many chronic diseases [55]. They accelerate wound closure, reduce inflammation, improve angiogenesis, and positively augment the deposition of the ECM [56].

Conditioned media from umbilical cord (UC)-MSC cultures may have potential benefits. Dermal fibroblasts under the paracrine influence of these cells exhibited characteristics of fetal fibroblasts, with decreased TGF-β1/TGF-β3 ratio, and increased expression of enzymes involved in ECM degradation. Wounds treated with the UC-MSC conditioned media also healed faster with decreased collagen accumulation [57]. Additionally, human amniotic fluid-derived MSC conditioned media inhibit the pro-fibrotic actions of TGF-β1 and reverse the myofibroblast phenotype to a fibroblast-like state. Conditioned media from ASCs produced similar results, but to a lesser extent [58]. These findings suggest that stem cells may promote a *scarless healing* phenotype without the requirement of direct inoculation to the wound bed. Additionally, the use of biological scaffolds in combination with the application of MSCs may allow for improved cellular migration, proliferation, and differentiation [59].

4.3. WNT Signaling

Wnt signaling is a key component of embryological development and involved in wound healing. Of the various subsets, the canonical Wnt pathway is the most relevant to tissue regeneration and repair. The link between TGF-β and the canonical Wnt/β-catenin pathway has been shown in multiple studies [60].

Topical application of Wnt pathway inhibitors (XAV-939, a tankyrase inhibitor, and pyrvinium, a casein kinase activator) caused formation of rete pegs and dermal papillae like intact skin following wound closure and scar formation was inhibited. Wnt activation with lithium chloride (LiCl), reduced regenerative repair [61]. However, in a full thickness excisional wound model in rats, topical LiCl application demonstrated reduction in gross scar appearance without influencing time to wound closure [62]. Furthermore, the activation of epidermal Wnt/β-catenin signaling can cause expansion of the upper dermal fibroblast lineage, which in turn allows hair follicle growth not traditionally observed in physiological wound healing [63, 64]. This observation has led to the notion that upper dermal fibroblasts could be utilized as a means for resolving scar formation and promoting *scarless healing*, with their more abated fibrillary collagen production when compared to the lower dermis lineage [65].

Specific models used to study the role of Wnt in scar formation may differ in part due to the transient mode of action and the different means by which this pathway is manipulated experimentally. It has been shown that long-term Wnt activation limits the efficacy of small molecule Wnt inhibitors [66]. The different outcomes of Wnt stimulation related to target tissues, and partly to the mode of Wnt pathway modulation are likely to account for some of the aforementioned discrepancies concerning upregulation of the canonical pathway which either promotes or inhibits *scarless healing*.

4.4. MicroRNA (miRNA)

MicroRNA (miRNA) therapies are another avenue for potential therapeutic intervention for wound healing. These molecules exert an inhibitory role on mRNA transcription within eukaryotic cells, effectively silencing genes at a post-transcriptional level [67]. Comparison of genome-wide miRNA expression between mid- (E16) and late-gestational (E19) mouse skin showed global repression of these molecules at an earlier time point, which is known to heal without scar formation [68]. In human fetal keratinocytes, the miR-34 family is a potential candidate for *scarless healing*. Expression of these miRNAs was significantly lower in late- as compared to mid-gestational keratinocytes. This family may also heavily suppress genes involved throughout the TGF-β pathway [69]. Numerous tools have been developed to modulate cell and tissue miRNA levels, several of which have been directed towards *regenerative healing*. For example, miR-145, has been found to be three times of normal levels in hypertrophic scars and pro-fibrotic TGF-β1-induced myofibroblasts. Using a commercial inhibitor of miR-145, significant decrease has been shown in type I collagen expression, TGF-β1 secretion, and contractility in skin myofibroblasts [70]. Additionally, miRNAs can be combined with biomimetic scaffolds to enhance wound healing, further supporting their clinical potential [71].

Conclusion

Recent advances in stem cell and developmental biology have revealed novel pathways and cell types involved in scarring and fibrosis. The study of fetal wound healing offers promising insights, with many obvious dissimilarities between fetal and adult wounds. Future studies aimed at assessing therapeutic potential for scarless wound healing would benefit from a more standardized model.

Stem cell therapies may provide a more complex composition of factors to promote scarless wound healing, but there exist many barriers to their utility. Multipotent or pluripotent stem cells carry a potential risk of tumor formation. These cells also exhibit difficulty with survival and engraftment following administration. Targeting some components of adult tissue healing, such as inflammation, takes attention on adult stem cells. Although, molecular therapies offer increased specificity on their targets, they may not be adequate to restore the complex wound healing process towards the regenerative phenotype. Combinations of endogenous and exogenous wound healing modulators are more likely to successfully promote scarless wound healing.

References

[1] Moore, Alessandra L., and Clement D. Marshall, Leandra A. Barnes, Matthew P. Murphy, Ryan C. Ransom, Michael T. Longaker. 2018. "Scarless wound healing: Transitioning from fetal research to regenerative healing." Wiley Interdisciplinary Reviews. *Developmental Biology* 7(2). doi: 10.1002/wdev.309.

[2] Gurtner, Geoffrey C., and Sabine Werner, Yann Barrandon, Michael T. Longaker. 2008. "Wound repair and regeneration." *Nature* 453:314–21. doi: 10.1038/nature07039.

[3] Walmsle, Graham G., and Zeshaan N. Maan, Victor W. Wong, Dominik Duscher, Michael S. Hu, Elizabeth R. Zielins, Taylor Wearda, Ethan Muhonen, Adrian McArdle, Ruth Tevlin, David A. Atashroo, Kshemendra Senarath-Yapa, H. Peter Lorenz, Goeffrey C. Gurtner, Michael T. Longaker. 2015. "Scarless wound healing: Chasing the holy grail." *Plastic and Reconstructive Surgery* 135:907–17. doi: 10.1097/PRS.0000000000000972.

[4] Buchanan, E. P., and M. T. Longaker, H. P. Lorenz. 2009. "Fetal skin wound healing." *Advances in Clinical Chemistry* 48:137–61.

[5] Whyte, Jemima L., and Andrew A. Smith, Bo Liu, Wilfred R. Manzano, Nick D. Evans, Girija R. Dhamdhere, Mark Y. Fang, Howard Y. Chang, Anthony E. Oro, Jill A. Helms. 2013. "Augmenting endogenous Wnt signaling improves skin wound healing." *PLoS One* 8:e76883. doi: 10.1371/journal.pone.0076883.

[6] You, Hi-Jin, and Seung-Kyu Han. 2014. "Cell therapy for wound healing." *Journal of Korean Medical Science* 29:311–9. doi: 10.3346/jkms.2014.29.3.311.

[7] Beanes, Steven R., and Fei-Ya Hu, Chia Soo, Catherine M. H. Dang, Mark Urata, Kang Ting, James B. Atkinson, Prosper Benhaim, Marc H. Hedrick, Peter H. Lorenz. 2002. "Confocal microscopic analysis of scarless repair in the fetal rat: Defining the transition." *Plastic and Reconstructive Surgery* 109:160–70.

[8] Longaker, M. T., and NS Adzick. 1991. "The biology of fetal wound healing: A review." *Plastic and Reconstructive Surgery* 87:788–98.

[9] Longaker, M. T., and D. J. Whitby, N. S. Adzick, T. M. Crombleholme, J. C. Langer, B. W. Duncan, S. M. Bradley, R. Stern, M. W. Ferguson, M. R. Harrison. 1990. "Studies in fetal wound healing, VI. Second and early third trimester fetal wounds demonstrate rapid collagen deposition without scar formation." *Journal of Pediatric Surgery* 25:63–8.

[10] Wang, Zhe, and Xiaoyu Liu, Dianbao Zhang, Xiliang Wang, Feng Zhao, Tao Zhang, Rui Wang, Xuewen Lin, Ping Shi, Xining Pang. 2015. "Phenotypic and functional modulation of 20–30 year old dermal fibroblasts by mid- and late-gestational keratinocytes in vitro." *Burns* 41:1064–75. doi: 10.1016/j.burns.2014.12.013.

[11] Longaker, M. T., and D. J. Whitby, M. W. Ferguson, M. R. Harrison, T. M. Crombleholme, J. C. Langer, K. C. Cochrum, E. D. Verrier, R. Stern. 1989. "Studies in fetal wound healing: III. Early deposition of fibronectin distinguishes fetal from adult wound healing." *Journal of Pediatric Surgery* 24:799–805.

[12] Dang, Catherine M., and Steven R. Beanes, Haofu Lee, Xinli Zhang, Chia Soo, Kang Ting. 2003. "Scarless fetal wounds are associated with an increased matrix

metalloproteinase-to-tissue-derived inhibitor of metalloproteinase ratio." *Plastic and Reconstructive Surgery* 111:2273–85.

[13] Larson, Barrett J., and Michael T. Longaker, H. Peter Lorenz. 2010. "Scarless fetal wound healing: A basic science review." *Plastic and Reconstructive Surgery* 126:1172–80. doi: 10.1097/PRS.0b013e3181eae781.

[14] Rinkevich, Yuval, and Graham G. Walmsley, Michael S. Hu, Zeshaan N. Maan, Aaron M. Newman, Micha Drukker, Michael Januszyk, Geoffrey W. Krampitz, Geoffrey C. Gurtner, H. Peter Lorenz, Irving L. Weissman, Michael T. Longaker. 2015. "Skin fibrosis. Identification and isolation of a dermal lineage with intrinsic fibrogenic potential." *Science* 348:aaa2151. doi: 10.1126/science.aaa2151.

[15] Walraven, Mariella, and Wendy Talhout, Robert H. J. Beelen, Marjolein van Egmond, Magda M. W. Ulrich. 2016. "Healthy human second-trimester fetal skin is deficient in leukocytes and associated homing chemokines." *Wound Repair and Regeneration* 24:533–41. doi: 10.1111/wrr.12421.

[16] Glim, Judith E., and Robert H. J. Beelen, Frank B. Niessen, Vincent Everts, Magda M. W. Ulrich,. 2015. "The number of immune cells is lower in healthy oral mucosa compared to skin and does not increase after scarring." *Archives of Oral Biology* 60:272–81. doi: 10.1016/j.archoralbio.2014.10.008.

[17] Amerongen, A. V. Nieuw, and E. C. I. Veerman. 2002. "Saliva: The defender of the oral cavity." *Oral Diseases* 8:12–22.

[18] Glim, Judith E., and Vincent Everts, Frank B. Niessen, Magda M. W. Ulrich, Robert H. J. Beelen. 2014. "Extracellular matrix components of oral mucosa differ from skin and resemble that of foetal skin." *Archives of Oral Biology* 59:1048–55. doi: 10.1016/j.archoralbio.2014.05.019.

[19] Tomasek, James J., and Giulio Gabbiani, Boris Hinz, Christine Chaponnier, Robert A. Brown. 2002. "Myofibroblasts and mechano-regulation of connective tissue remodelling." *Nature Reviews. Molecular Cell Biology* 3:349–63.

[20] Zhong, S. P., and Y. Z. Zhang, and C. T. Lim. 2010. "Tissue scaffolds for skin wound healing and dermal reconstruction." *Wiley Interdisciplinary Reviews. Nanomedicine and Nanobiotechnology* 2, 510–525. doi: 10.1002/wnan.100.

[21] Benedetti, L., and R. Cortivo, T. Berti, A. Berti, F. Pea, M. Mazzo, M. Moras, G. Abatangelo. 1993. "Biocompatibility and biodegradation of different hyaluronan derivatives (Hyaff) implanted in rats." *Biomaterials* 14:1154–60.

[22] Milella, E., and E. Brescia, C. Massaro, P. A. Ramires, M. R. Miglietta, V. Fiori, P. Aversa. 2002. "Physico-chemical properties and degradability of non-woven hyaluronan benzylic esters as tissue engineering scaffolds." *Biomaterials* 23:1053–63.

[23] Liu, Xing, and Lie Ma, Jun Liang, Bing Zhang, Jianying Teng, Changyou Gao. 2013. "RNAi functionalized collagen-chitosan/silicone membrane bilayer dermal

equivalent for full-thickness skin regeneration with inhibited scarring." *Biomaterials* 34:2038–48. doi: 10.1016/j.biomaterials.2012.11.062.

[24] Abaci, H. E., and Zongyou Guo, Yanne Doucet, J. Jackow, A. Christiano. 2017. "Next generation human skin constructs as advanced tools for drug development." *Experimental Biology and Medicine (Maywood, N.J.)* 242:1657–68. doi: 10.1177/1535370217712690.

[25] Kim, Byoung S., and Jıng-Seob Lee, Ge Gao, Dong- Woo Cho. 2017. "Direct 3D cell-printing of human skin with functional transwell system." *Biofabrication* 9:025034. doi: 10.1088/1758-5090/aa71c8.

[26] Agha, Riaz, and Rei Ogawa, Giorgio Pietramaggiori, Dennis P. Orgill. 2011. "A review of the role of mechanical forces in cutaneous wound healing." *The Journal of Surgical Research* 171:700–8. doi: 10.1016/j.jss.2011.07.007.

[27] Das, Tamal, and Kai Safferling, Sebastian Rausch, Niels Grabe, Heike Boehm, Joachim P. Spatz. 2015. "A molecular mechanotransduction pathway regulates collective migration of epithelial cells." *Nature Cell Biology* 17:276–87. doi: 10.1038/ncb3115.

[28] Januszyk, Michael, and Victor W. Wong, Kirit A. Bhatt, Ivan N. Vial, Josemaria Paterno, Michael T. Longaker, Geoffrey C. Gurtner. 2014. "Mechanical offloading of incisional wounds is associated with transcriptional downregulation of inflammatory pathways in a large animal model." *Organogenesis* 10:186–93. doi: 10.4161/org.28818.

[29] Takada, Hiroya, and Kishio Furuya, Masahiro Sokabe,. 2014. "Mechanosensitive ATP release from hemichannels and Ca(2)(+) influx through TRPC6 accelerate wound closure in keratinocytes." *Journal of Cell Science* 127:4159–71. doi: 10.1242/jcs.147314.

[30] Wang, Jing, and Yifan Zhang, Ning Zhang, Chuandong Wang, Tanja Herrler, Qingfeng Li. 2015. "An updated review of mechanotransduction in skin disorders: Transcriptional regulators, ion channels, and microRNAs." *Cellular and Molecular Life Sciences* 72:2091–106. doi: 10.1007/s00018-015-1853-y.

[31] Wong, Victor W., and Kristine C. Rustad, Satoshi Akaishi, Michael Sorkin, Jason P. Glotzbach, Michael Januszyk, Emily R. Nelson, Kemal Levi, Josemaria Paterno, Ivan N. Vial, Anna A. Kuang, Michael T. Longaker, Geoffrey C. Gurtner. 2012. "Focal adhesion kinase links mechanical force to skin fibrosis via inflammatory signaling." *Nature Medicine* 18:148–52. doi: 10.1038/nm.2574.

[32] Lim, Angeline F., and Jennifer Weintraub, Ernest N. Kaplan, Michael Januszyk, Christy Cowley, Peggy McLaughlin, Bill Beasley, Geoffrey C. Gurtner, Michael T. Longaker. 2014. "The embrace device significantly decreases scarring following scar revision surgery in a randomized controlled trial." *Plastic and Reconstructive Surgery* 133:398–405. doi: 10.1097/01.prs.0000436526.64046.d0.

[33] Longaker, Michael T., and Rod J. Rohrich, Lauren Greenberg, Heather Furnas, Rpbert Wald, Vivek Bansal, Hisham Seify, Anthony Tran, Jane Weston, Joshua M. Korman, Rodney Chan, David Kaufman, Vipul R. Dev, Joseph A. Mele, Michael Januszyk, Cristy Cowley, Peggy McLaughlin, Bill Beasley, Geoffrey C. Gurtner. 2014. "A randomized controlled trial of the embrace advanced scar therapy device to reduce incisional scar formation." *Plastic and Reconstructive Surgery* 134:536–46. doi: 10.1097/PRS.0000000000000417.

[34] de Souza, Kenia S., and Thiago A. Cantaruti, Geraldo M. Jr Azevedo, Daniel A. de A. Galdino, Claudiney M. Rodrigues, Raquel A. Costa, Nelson M. Vaz, Claudia R. Carvalho. 2015. "Improved cutaneous wound healing after intraperitoneal injection of alpha-melanocyte-stimulating hormone." *Experimental Dermatology* 24:198–203. doi: 10.1111/exd.12609.

[35] Singla, Dinender K., and Reetu D. Singla, Latifa S. Abdelli, Carley Glass. 2015. "Fibroblast growth factor-9 enhances M2 macrophage differentiation and attenuates adverse cardiac remodeling in the infarcted diabetic heart." *PLoS One* 10:e0120739. doi: 10.1371/journal.pone.0120739.

[36] Gay, Denise, and Ohsang Kwon, Zhikun Zhang, Michelle Spata, Maksim V. Plikus, Phillip D. Holler, Mayumi Ito, Zaixin Yang, Elsa Treffeisen, Chang D. Kim, Arben Nace, Xiaohong Zhang, Sheena Baratono, Fen Wang, David M. Ornitz, Sarah E. Millar, George Cotsarelis. 2013. "Fgf9 from dermal [gamma][delta] T cells induces hair follicle neogenesis after wounding." *Nature Medicine* 19:916–23. doi: 10.1038/nm.3181.

[37] Morris, Michael W. Jr, and Myron 3rd Allukian, Benjamin J. Herdrich, Robert C. Caskey, Carlos Zgheib, Junwang Xu, Wanda Dorsett-Martin, Marc E. Mitchell, Kenneth W. Liechty. 2014. "Modulation of the inflammatory response by increasing fetal wound size or interleukin-10 overexpression determines wound phenotype and scar formation." *Wound Repair and Regeneration* 22:406–14. doi: 10.1111/wrr.12180.

[38] Kieran, Ingrid, and Amanda Knock, James Bush, Karen So, Anthony Metcalfe, Rosalind Hobson, Tracey Mason, Sharon O'Kane, Mark Ferguson. 2013. "Interleukin-10 reduces scar formation in both animal and human cutaneous wounds: results of two preclinical and phase II randomized control studies." *Wound Repair and Regeneration* 21:428–36. doi: 10.1111/wrr.12043.

[39] Ding, Jie, and Zengshuan Ma, Hongbin Liu, Peter Kwan, Takashi Iwashina, Heather A. Shankowsky, Donald Wong, Edward E. Tredget. 2014. "The therapeutic potential of a C-X-C chemokine receptor type 4 (CXCR-4) antagonist on hypertrophic scarring in vivo." *Wound Repair and Regeneration* 22:622–630. doi: 10.1111/wrr.12208.

[40] Dulauroy, Sophie, and Selene E. Di Carlo, Francina Langa, Gerard Eberl, Lucie Peduto. 2012. "Lineage tracing and genetic ablation of ADAM12(+) perivascular

cells identify a major source of profibrotic cells during acute tissue injury." *Nature Medicine* 18:1262–70. doi: 10.1038/nm.2848.

[41] Thielitz, Anja, and Robert W. Vetter, Bianca Schultze, Sabine Wrenger, Luca Simeoni, Siegfried Ansorge, Klaus Neubert, Jürgen Faust, Petra Lindenlaub, Harald P. M. Gollnick, Dirk Reinhold. 2008. "Inhibitors of dipeptidyl peptidase IV-like activity mediate antifibrotic effects in normal and keloid-derived skin fibroblasts." *The Journal of Investigative Dermatology* 128:855–66.

[42] Powell, D. W., and R. C. Mifflin, J. D. Valentich, S. E. Crowe, J. I. Saada, A. B. West. 1999. "Myofibroblasts. I. Paracrine cells important in health and disease." *The American Journal of Physiology - Cell Physiology* 277:C1–C19.

[43] Hinz, Boris, and Sem H. Phan, Victor J. Thannickal, Andrea Galli, Marie-Luce Bochaton-Piallat, Giulio Gabbiani. 2007. "The myofibroblast: one function, multiple origins." *The American Journal of Pathology* 170:1807–16.

[44] Desai, Vivek D., and Henry C. Hsia, Jean E. Schwarzbauer. 2014. "Reversible modulation of myofibroblast differentiation in adipose-derived mesenchymal stem cells." *PLoS One* 9:e86865. doi: 10.1371/journal.pone.0086865.

[45] Rinella, Letizia, and Francesca Marano, Laura Berta, Ornella Bosco, Marco Fraccalvieri, Nicoletta Fortunati, Roberto Frairia, Maria G. Catalano. 2016. "Extracorporeal shockwaves modulate myofibroblast differentiation of adipose-derived stem cells." *Wound Repair and Regeneration* 24:275-86. Doi: 10.1111%2Fwrr.12410.

[46] Corcione, Anna, and Federica Benvenuto, Elisa Ferretti, Debora Giunti, Valentina Cappiello, Francesco Cazzanti, Marco Risso, Francesca Gualandi, Giovanni L. Mancardi, Vito Pistoia, Antonio Uccelli. 2006. "Human mesenchymal stem cells modulate B-cell functions." *Blood* 107:367–72. Doi: 10.1182/blood-2005-07-2657.

[47] Di Nicola, Massimo, and Carmelo Carlo-Stella, Michele Magni, Marco Milanesi, Paolo D. Longoni, Paola Matteucci, Salvatore Grisanti, Alessandro M. Gianni. 2002. "Human bone marrow stromal cells suppress T-lymphocyte proliferation induced by cellular or nonspecific mitogenic stimuli." *Blood* 99:3838–43.

[48] Doi, Hanako, and Yuriko Kitajima, Lan Luo, Chan Yan, Seiko Tateishi, Yusuke Ono, Yoshishige Urata, Shinji Goto, Ryoichi Mori, Hideaki Masuzaki, Isao Shimokawa, Akiyoshi Hirano, Tao-Sheng Li. 2016. "Potency of umbilical cord blood- and Wharton's jelly-derived mesenchymal stem cells for scarless wound healing." *Scientific Reports* 6:18844. doi: 10.1038/srep18844.

[49] Sabapathy, Vikram, and Balasubramanian Sundaram, Sreelakshmi VM, Pratheesh Mankuzhy, Sanjay Kumar. 2014. "Human Wharton's Jelly Mesenchymal Stem Cells plasticity augments scar-free skin wound healing with hair growth." *PLoS One* 9:e93726. doi: 10.1371/journal.pone.0093726.

[50] Mizoguchi, Masayuki, and Shigaku Ikeda, Yasushi Suga, Hideoki Ogawa. 2000. "Expression of cytokeratins and cornified cell envelope-associated proteins in

umbilical cord epithelium: A comparative study of the umbilical cord, amniotic epithelia and fetal skin." The *Journal of Investigative Dermatology* 115:133–4. Doi: 10.1046/j.1523-1747.2000.00031-4.x.

[51] Arno, Anna I., and Saeid Amini-Nik, Patrick H. Blit, Mohammed Al-Shehab, Cassandro Belo, Elaine Herer, Col H. Tien, Marc G. Jeschke. 2014. "Human Wharton's jelly mesenchymal stem cells promote skin wound healing through paracrine signaling." *Stem Cell Research & Therapy* 5:28. doi: 10.1186/scrt417.

[52] Jiang, Lei-Wei, and Hongduo Chen, Hongguang Lu. 2016. "Using human epithelial amnion cells in human de-epidermized dermis for skin regeneration." *Journal of Dermatological Science* 81:26–34. doi: 10.1016/j.jdermsci.2015.10.018.

[53] Mahmoudi Rad, Mahnaz, and Niki Mahmoudi Rad, Yasaman Mirdamadi. 2015. "Expression of TGF-beta3 in isolated fibroblasts from foreskin." *Reports of Biochemistry & Molecular Biology* 3:76–81.

[54] Skrzypczyk, Aniela, and Shibashish Giri, Augustinus Bader. 2016. "Generation of induced pluripotent stem cell line from foreskin fibroblasts." *Stem Cell Research* 17:572–5. doi: 10.1016/j.scr.2016.09.014.

[55] Ding, D. C., and W. C. Shyu, S. Z. Lin. 2011. "Mesenchymal stem cells." *Cell Transplantation* 20:5–14. doi: 10.3727/096368910X.

[56] Lee, Dylan E., and Nagi Ayoub, Devendra K. Agrawal. 2016. "Mesenchymal stem cells and cutaneous wound healing: Novel methods to increase cell delivery and therapeutic efficacy." *Stem Cell Research & Therapy* 7:37. doi: 10.1186/s13287-016-0303-6.

[57] Li, Meirong, and Fuxin Luan, Yali Zhao, Haojie Hao, Jiejie Liu, Liang Dong, Xiaobing Fu, Weidong Han. 2015. "Mesenchymal stem cell-conditioned medium accelerates wound healing with fewer scars." *International Wound Journal* 14:64-73. doi: 10.1111/iwj.12551.

[58] Mia, Masum M., and Ruud A. Bank. 2016. "The pro-fibrotic properties of transforming growth factor on human fibroblasts are counteracted by caffeic acid by inhibiting myofibroblast formation and collagen synthesis." *Cell and Tissue Research* 363:775-89. doi: 10.1007/s00441-015-2285-6.

[59] Wang, Weihong, and Mi Zhang, Wei Lu, Xiaojun Zhang, Dandan Ma, Xiangming Rong, Chunyan Yu, Yan Jin. 2010. "Cross-linked collagen-chondroitin sulfate-hyaluronic acid imitating extracellular matrix as scaffold for dermal tissue engineering." *Tissue Engineering. Part C, Methods* 16:269–79. doi: 10.1089/ten.TEC.2009.0161.

[60] Sato, M. 2006. "Upregulation of the Wnt/beta-catenin pathway induced by transforming growth factor-beta in hypertrophic scars and keloids." *Acta Dermato-Venereologica* 86:300–7. Doi: 10.2340/00015555-0101.

[61] Bastakoty, Dikshya, and Sarika Saraswati, Justin Cates, Ethan Lee, Lillian B. Nanney, Pampee P. Young. 2015. "Inhibition of Wnt/beta-catenin pathway

promotes regenerative repair of cutaneous and cartilage injury." *FASEB Journal* 29:4881–92. Doi: 10.1096/fj.15-275941.

[62] Shi, Yan, and Bin Shu, Ronghua Yang, Yingbin Xu, Bangrong Xing, Jian Liu, Lei Chen, Shaohai Qi, Xusheng Liu, Peng Wang, Jinming Tang, Julin Xie. 2015. "Wnt and Notch signaling pathway involved in wound healing by targeting c-Myc and Hes1 separately." *Stem Cell Research & Therapy* 6:120. Doi: 10.1186/s13287-015-0103-4.

[63] Driskell, Ryan R., and Beate M. Lichtenberger, Esther Hoste, Kai Kretzschmar, Ben D. Simons, Marika Charalambous, Sacri R. Ferron, Yann Herault, Guillaume Pavlovic, Anne C. Ferguson-Smith, Fiona M. Watt. 2013. "Distinct fibroblast lineages determine dermal architecture in skin development and repair." *Nature* 504:277–81. Doi: 10.1038/nature12783.

[64] Gurtner, Goeffrey C., and Sabine Werner, Yann Barrandon, Michael T. Longaker. 2008. "Wound repair and regeneration." *Nature* 453:314–21. Doi: 10.1038/nature07039.

[65] Driskell, Ryan R., and Fiona M. Watt. 2015. "Understanding fibroblast heterogeneity in the skin." *Trends in Cell Biology* 25:92–9. doi: 10.1016/j.tcb.2014.10.001.

[66] de la Roche, Marc, and Ashraf E. Ibrahim, Juliusz Mieszczanek, Mariann Bienz. 2014. "LEF1 and B9L shield beta-catenin from inactivation by Axin, desensitizing colorectal cancer cells to tankyrase inhibitors." *Cancer Research* 74:1495–505. doi: 10.1158/0008-5472.CAN-13-2682.

[67] Sen, Chandan K, and Suphadip Ghatak. 2015. "miRNA control of tissue repair and regeneration." The *American Journal of Pathology* 185:2629–40. doi: 10.1016/j.ajpath.2015.04.001.

[68] Cheng, Jie, and Hongbo Yu, Simin Deng, Guofang Shen. 2010. "MicroRNA profiling in mid- and late-gestational fetal skin: implication for scarless wound healing." The *Tohoku Journal of Experimental Medicine* 221:203–9.

[69] Zhao, Feng, and Zhe Wang, Hongxin Lang, Xiaoyu Liu, Dianbao Zhang, Xiliang Wang, Tao Zhang, Rui Wang, Ping Shi, Xining Pang. 2015. "Dynamic Expression of Novel MiRNA Candidates and MiRNA-34 Family Members in Early- to Mid-Gestational Fetal Keratinocytes Contributes to Scarless Wound Healing by Targeting the TGF-beta Pathway." *PLoS One* 10:e0126087. doi: 10.1371/journal.pone.0126087.

[70] Gras, Christiane, and Dominica Ratuszny, Catarina Hadamitzky, Haijiao Zhang, Rainer Blasczyk, Constança Figueiredo. 2015. "miR-145 Contributes to Hypertrophic Scarring of the Skin by Inducing Myofibroblast Activity." *Molecular Medicine* 21:296–304. doi: 10.2119/molmed.2014.00172.

[71] Monaghan, Michael, and Shane Browne, Katja Schenke-Layland, Abhay Pandit. 2014. "A collagen-based scaffold delivering exogenous microrna-29B to modulate extracellular matrix remodeling." *Molecular Therapy* 22:786–96. doi: 10.1038/mt.2013.288.

In: Cutaneous Scars: Biology, Clinics and Management ISBN: 978-1-53615-657-7
Editors: Berna Aksoy, Hasan Mete Aksoy et al. © 2019 Nova Science Publishers, Inc.

Chapter 9

CLINICAL ASPECTS OF SCARS

Zehra Asiran Serdar* and Neslihan Fisek Izci
Department of Dermatology,
Faculty of Medicine, Bahçeşehir University, Istanbul, Turkey

ABSTRACT

Cutaneous wound healing is a complex response to skin injury and disregulation of this process can lead to abnormal scar formation. Scars have distinctive differences from normal tissues in terms of appearance and histopathology. Abnormal scar types show increased contraction, dermal thickening and miyofibroblast staining compared to normal skin and normotrophic scarring. Scars are classified on the basis of differences from normal tissues. In this chapter, we review the spectrum of scar types and their subtypes.

Keywords: acne scars, atrophic scars, clinical types, hypertrophic scars, keloids, normotrophic scars, proliferative scars, striae

1. INTRODUCTION

Scars are a common clinical problem, faced primarily by dermatologists and plastic surgeons. People with abnormal scarring may have physical, cosmetic, psychological and social problems [1]. The exact incidence of scars is not known. They may occur in all skin types worldwide, but *hypertrophic scars* and *keloids* are more common in the black population with a prevalence of 5 - 15% [2, 3].

*Corresponding Author's Email: dr@drzehraserdar.com.

Skin tissue repair results in a broad spectrum of scar types. The *clinical types* range from a normal fine line to a variety of abnormal scars, including widespread scars, *atrophic scars*, scar contractures, *hypertrophic scars* and *keloid* scars [4].

Scars can be classified as proliferative, normotrophic and atrophic. Raised (or *proliferative) scars* include *keloids* and *hypertrophic scars*. *Atrophic scars* include *striae* distensae, scars as a result of acne and burns [5].

2. Proliferative Scars

We describe raised skin scars as *hypertrophic scars* or *keloids*. These are the result of abnormal wound healing of injured or irritated skin in predisposed individuals and represent an exaggerated connective tissue response to trauma, inflammation, surgery or burns [6, 7]. *Hypertrophic scars* and *keloids* are cosmetically distressing and can also cause pruritus, pain or pressure [7, 8].

The first step in scar therapy begins with the simple identification and diagnosis of the problematic abnormal wound healing [1]. Although both *keloids* and *hypertrophic scars* are in the abnormal scarring spectrum, they are not necessarily one and the same [9]. Though *hypertrophic scars* and *keloids* have many common clinical similarities, there are many pathological and biochemical differences that suggest these entities are distinct from each other [10].

They are initially pink-to-purple inflamed lesions that cause pain and pruritus. The overlying epidermis is typically smooth and thin, and in palpation the dermal layer of the lesion is firm. Both types of these lesions may inhibit normal function of adjacent tissues [8, 11]. *Hypertrophic scars* and *keloids* may appear at any site of the body but they are especially frequent on the earlobes, chin, neck, shoulders, upper trunk and lower legs [4, 12].

It is difficult to differentiate *hypertrophic scars* from *keloids*; therefore, it is important to establish criteria to distinguish them. Such criteria is discussed below and summarized in Table 1. [13].

Hypertrophic scars usually develop within 4 weeks after trauma. If epithelialization takes longer than 21 days, the risk of development of *hypertrophic scars* increases independent of age and region [14]. Remaining within the boundaries of the initial injury, they do not extend beyond the general geographic margins of the wound, and have a tendency to regress spontaneously over time after the initial injury [4, 8, 11]. *Hypertrophic scars* commonly occur after burn injury on the trunk and extremites [4]. Initially the lesions are erythematous and raised, evolving over time into pale flatter scars. The incidence rate of hypertrophic scarring has been reported to be as high as 91% following extensive trauma, such as a deep burn injury [8].

Keloids spread beyond the limits of the original injury and invade the surrounding normal skin. They do not regress spontaneously and continue to grow over time. *Keloids* are firm irregularly shaped tumors with a shiny surface, while the overlying epidermis is thinned from pressure and smooth. On the lesion, there may be telangiectasias and focal areas of ulceration. The color is pink-purple to red and may be accompanied by hyperpigmentation. They occur frequently on the sternal region, earlobes, neck, shoulders, upper back and posterior neck [15, 16]. Other common sites include the deltoids, upper limbs, lower limbs and ears [15]. They rarely occur on genitalia, eyelids, palms, soles, or across joints [14]. While *keloids* can occur at any age, they show a peak incidence in patients aged between 15 and 24 years [8].

Table 1. Key features for hypertrophic scars and keloids [11, 14, 17]

	Hypertrophic scars	Keloids
Incidence	Frequent	Rare
Ethnic groups	No predilection	African, American, Asian, Hispanic
Site predilection	Anywhere	Chest, earlobes, shoulders, upper back
Preceeded by injury	Yes	Not always
Onset after injury	Immediate	Delayed
Growth beyond border of original injury	No	Yes
Symptoms	Firm, pruritic, painful	Firm, pruritic, painful
Spontaneous regression	Sometimes; tends to flatten with time	Uncommon
Recurrence	Rare	Common
Treatment response	Good	Poor

3. Normotrophic Scars

Normotrophic scars are the most harmless scars formed as a result of an adequate reaction of the body to injuries. Normal wound healing involves the phases of inflammation, proliferation and remodeling (maturation) phase. Clinically, the outcomes of the remodeling phase are the most important. During remodeling, collagen deposition occurs in an organized fashion, ideally resulting in inconspicuous scar tissue. If the wound completes all stages of healing without deviations, a *normotrophic scar* is formed (Figure 1). Over time, these scars become thin, level with the skin and assume a whitish color. Normally, they do not require any correction except for the aesthetic improvement of the scar appearance [18, 19].

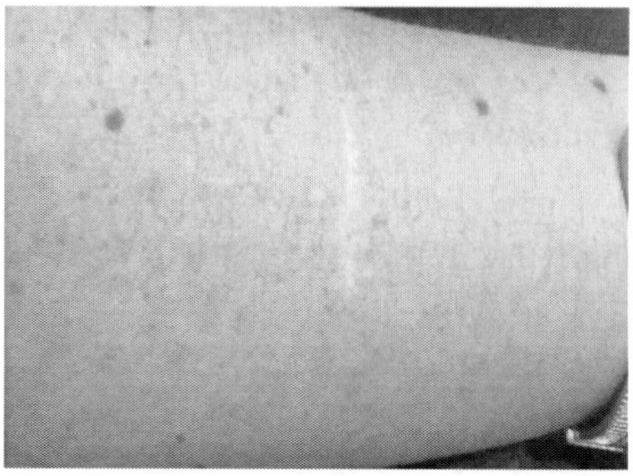

Figure 1. Normotrophic scar located on forearm (Courtesy of Berna Aksoy, MD).

4. Atrophic Scars

4.1. Striae Distensae

(Synonyms: striae atrophicans; stretch marks; linear atrophy)

Striae distensae (SD) are common linear atrophic lesions of the skin which arise due to stretching of the skin. Although they do not cause major medical problems, *striae* represent an aesthetic concern for those affected. Thus, they pose a significant psychological and therapeutic challenge [20].

Striae are usually multiple, symmetric and well-defined linear atrophic scars. There are two forms of SD; *striae* rubrae and *striae* albae. *Striae* rubrae is the acute stage, characterized by erythematous, red-to-violaceous and elevated lines. They are aligned perpendicular to the direction of skin tension and can be mildly pruritic. Vascular changes occur that contribute to the red and erythematous appearance of *striae* rubrae. Over time, the color gradually fades and the lesions become atrophic and hypopigmented (*striae* albae). These *striae* are usually permanent with the skin surface exhibiting a fine wrinkled appearance. Additionally, in *striae* rubrae, collagen fibers become thicker, more densely packed, are arranged in a parellel pattern and show a reduction in elastic fibers. Conversely, *striae* albae have less vascularity and tend to be very pale in colour. *Striae* albae have been described as appearing similar to mature and flattened or stretched dermal scars [21]. The *striae* can measure a few millimeters to a few centimeters in width and several centimeters in length. Most literature has described SD during pregnancy and puberty with reported prevalences varying from 11% to 88% and occurring about twice as frequently in women as in men [11, 20].

SD occur most commonly on the abdomen, breasts, buttocks and thighs [20, 21]. During puberty, rapid increase in size cause *striae*. SD of adolescents have been previously reported to be much more common in girls than in boys. The most common sites in girls are breasts, thighs, hips and buttocks, while in boys they appear on the shoulders, lumbosacral region and thighs [22]. Cho et al. have reported that *striae* of the buttocks, upper thigh and calf run vertically and are correlated with body weight and body mass index (BMI), whereas *striae* of the knee and lower back run horizontally, and those on the knee are correlated with height in boys [22].

Pregnancy, sudden weight gain, adolescent growth spurts and hormonal disturbances are the most frequent causes of SD. The factors that lead to development of *striae* have not been precisely elucidated but many elements, including hormones, genetic predisposition and increased mechanical stress on connective tissue, may play a role. It was found that skin samples with SD show decreased fibroblast metabolism compared to normal skin, with decreased levels of collagen, elastin and fibronectin gene expression. Kasielska et al. reported that history of contraceptive intake and a family history of *striae* are risk factors of SD occurrence, while weight loss can reduce the risk of these lesions [23]. They also occur in a number of pathological conditions such as obesity, Cushing's and Marfan syndromes, and long-term systemic or topical corticosteroid use [22]. The *striae* induced by corticosteroids may be larger and more widely distributed [12]. Sometimes, in those with darker skin, increased melanization will lead to striae cerulae (blue) or striae nigra (black). The colour of SD is linked to the stage of their evolution and to the influence of melanocyte mechanobiology [24].

Striae gravidarum (SG) is a common, disfiguring, gestational skin change, with a reported frequency between 55 and 90%. SG presents as atrophic linear scars that cause distress. SG is often failed to be noticed as a cosmetic concern, which makes the patient burden lesser. SG first appears in the form of pink-to-red bands that become raised, longer, wider and violet-red. After a period (months to years), they tend to fade and become hypopigmented, wrinkled and atrophic, and appear parallel to skin tension lines. SG typically presents itself on the breasts, abdomen, hips and thighs, and can cause itching, burning and discomfort. Up to 90% of SG appears in primigravidas [25].

4.2. Other Atrophic Scars

Infections such as varicella, tertiary syphilis, tuberculids, some deep mycoses (esp. sporotrichosis) and onchocerciasis can result in *atrophic scars* [12].

Varicella (chickenpox) is a common viral disease that causes persistent *atrophic scars*. The post-infectious scars occur in approximately 7% to 18% of cases. Varicella scars are generally atrophic and may be associated with other complications, such as hyperpigmentation and hypopigmentation. Usually resistant to available treatments, varicella scars are typically deep so any treatment may include release of scar tissue by cutting under the surface skin [26, 27].

Cutaneous lupus erythematosus can cause thick, red and scaly rashes on the face, neck and scalp. Over a period of a few months, some of these lesions progress to scarring discoid lesions, while others respond very well to treatment and clear completely. Scars have been seen in the majority of patients. While the face is predominantly affected, scarring also affects the scalp, other hairy areas such as the eyebrows, nonhairy areas, mucosa and nails [28, 29].

Lupus vulgaris and chronic follicular pyodermas leave a combination of atrophy and sclerosis [12].

Exposure to ionizing radiation and injury by cold or heat give rise to poikiloderma that is characterized by atrophy, pigmentation and telangiectasia [12]. In Ehlers – Danlos syndrome, we can confront wide *atrophic scars* that follow injuries [12].

Congenital erosiv and vesicular dermatosis (CEVD) with reticulated supple scarring is a rare congenital condition with unknown aetiology. First described by Cohen and colleagues in 1985, it clinically presents at birth with erythema, vesicles and erosions. The skin heals within the first months of life with soft reticulate scarring which tends to follow the long axes of limbs [30].

Spontaneous atrophic scarring of the cheeks is a very rare disorder that spontaneously develops in young adults. The shallow atrophic lesions with sharp margins may present with linear, rectangular or varioliform shapes. The differential diagnoses are atrophoderma vermiculatum, chickenpox scars and artefact [31].

5. Acne Scarring

Acne scarring is often significant, causing psychological and emotional distress and may result in low self-esteem. Several studies have reported that the prevalance of post-acne scarring is between 11% and 14% in the general population and 49% in patients affected with acne [32]. The nature and extent of this scarring is directly related to the depth, intensity and duration of inflammation [33]. *Acne scars* can be hypertrophic or atrophic depending on being elevated or depressed in relation to the skin surface [34]. In 80 to 90% of cases, there is loss of collagen in the dermis that results in *atrophic scars*. Less commonly, we see hypertrophic and keloidal scars that show excessive deposition of collagen with reduced collagenase activity [34, 35].

Hypertrophic scars are raised, erythematous, firm nodular lesions that remain within the boundaries of the original site of injury (Figure 2). *Keloids* appear as reddish-purple deep papules and nodules, usually extending beyond the borders of the original injury and often continue to grow without regression (Figure 3). Also, *keloids* are frequently resistant to treatment and have a high recurrence rate. They are more common in indivuals with Fitzpatrick skin phototypes IV/V. *Hypertrophic scars* and *keloids* occur predominantly on the anterior chest, shoulders and upper back [34, 36], while the jaw line, posterior neck and other facial areas may also be affected [37].

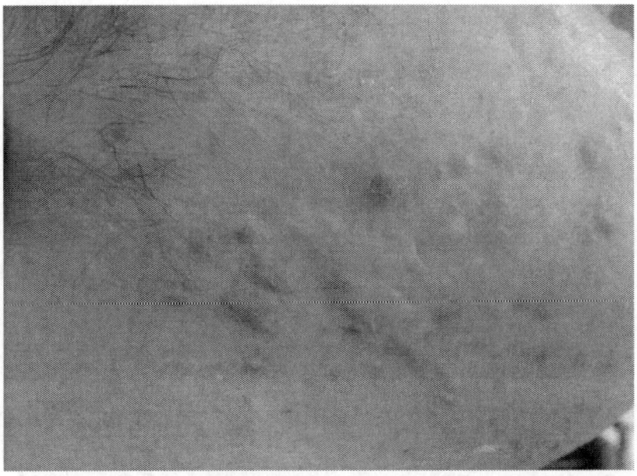

Figure 2. Hypertrophic acne scars along the jawline (Courtesy of Berna Aksoy, MD).

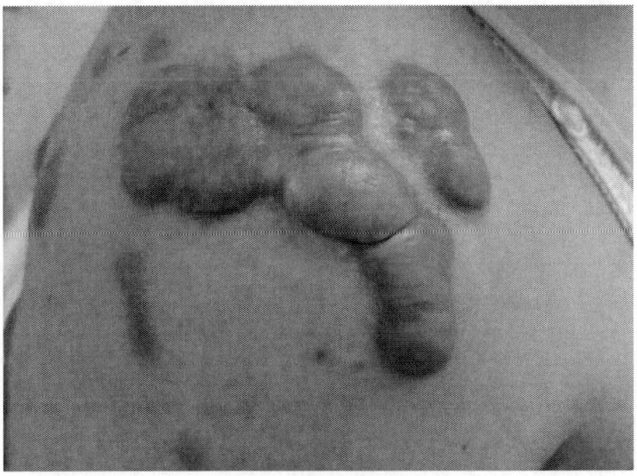

Figure 3. Extensive post-acne keloids located on shoulder (Courtesy of Berna Aksoy, MD).

Atrophic scars occur predominantly on the face (Figure 4) and rarely on the trunk [38]. They are depressed in the skin due to loss of collagen and destructive inflammation in the deep dermis with fibrous contractions. *Atrophic scars* are classified according to depth, width and architecture [37, 38]. Icepıck scars are narrow (less than 2 mm), V-shaped epithelial tracts that are punctiform deep lesions and can be resistant to conventional skin resurfacing options [35, 36, 39]. Boxcar scars are round to oval depressions with sharply demarcated vertical edges, similar to varicella scars. Clinically, they are wider at the surface than icepick scars and do not taper to a point at the base. These scars can be either shallow (0.1 - 0.5 mm) or deep (> 0.5 mm) [39, 40]. Rolling scars are usually wider and may reach up to 5 mm in diameter. Abnormal fibrous anchoring of the dermis to the subcutis leads to superficial shadowing and a rolling or undulating appearance of the overlying skin [40-42].

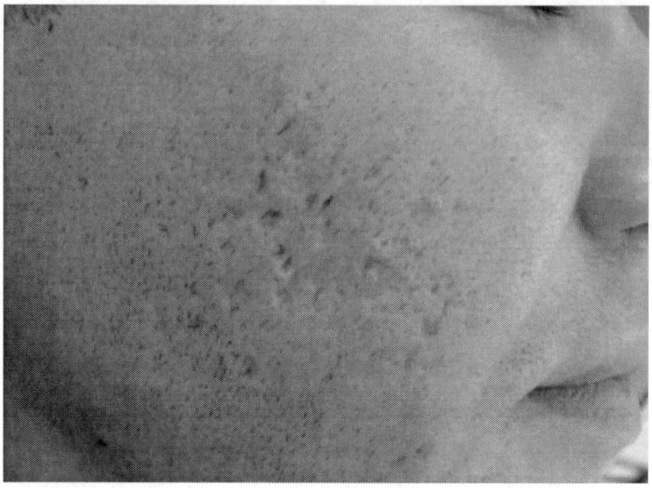

Figure 4. Ice pick and boxcar scars on the cheek (Courtesy of Berna Aksoy, MD).

Key features for acne scars are summarized in Table 2. below:

Table 2. Key features for acne scars (Adapted from [40, 42])

Scar Classification	Clinical Features
Atrophic Scar	Loss of collagen, most common form
Icepick	Deep and narrow (< 2mm) V-shaped epithelial tracts
Boxcar	Shallow (< 0.5 mm) or deep (> 0.5 mm) Round to oval depressions
Rolling	Wide (> 4-5 mm) and shallow Results from dermal tethering to the subcutis
Proliferative Scars	Excess collagen deposition
Hypertrophic	Raised, firm, erythematous papules that do not exceed the margin of the original wound
Keloid	Red to purple papules or nodules that proliferate beyond original injury borders

Conclusion

Scars frequently cause both functional and aesthetic problems. Skin tissue repair results in a broad spectrum of scar types, which can be classified as hypertrophic, normotrophic and atrophic. These scar types have different characteristics from one another, making an exact scar assessment essential for diagnosis and determining the proper therapeutic management strategy.

REFERENCES

[1] Wolfram, Dolores, and Alexander Tzankov, Petra Pülzl, Hıldegunde Piza-Katzer. 2009. "Hypertrophic scars and keloids--a review of their pathophysiology, risk factors, and therapeutic management." *Dermatologic Surgery* 35:171-81. doi: 10.1111/j.1524-4725.2008.34406.x.

[2] van den Broek, Lenie J., and Grace C. Limandjaja, Frank B. Niessen, Susan Gibbs. 2014. "Human hypertrophic and keloid scar models: principles, limitations and future challenges from a tissue engineering perspective." *Experimental Dermatology* 23:382-6. doi: 10.1111/exd.12419.

[3] Mauch, Cornelia, and Karin Scharffetter-Kochanek. 2009. "Connective Tissue Diseases: Hypertrophic Scars and Keloids." In *Braun-Falco's Dermatology*, edited by Burgdorf, Walter H. C., and Gerd Plewig, Helmut H. Wolff, Micheal Landthaler, 688-89. Italy: Springer.

[4] Bayat, Ardeshir, and Duncan A. McGrouther, Mark W. J. Ferguson. 2003. "Skin scarring". *British Medical Journal* 326:88-92.

[5] Chacon, Anna, and Katlein França, Jennifer Ledon, Keyvan Nouri. 2013. "Scars and scarring: Causes, types, and treatment options." In: *Dermatology & Cutaneous Surgery*, 1-24. USA: Nova Science Publishers, Inc.

[6] English, Robert S., and Philip D. Shenefelt. 1999. "Keloids and hypertrophic scars." *Dermatologic Surgery* 25:631-8.

[7] Ogawa, Rei, and Satoshi Akaishi, Shigehiko Kuribayashi, Tsuguhiro Miyashita. 2016. "Keloids and hypertrophic scars can now be cured completeley: Recent Progress in Our Understanding of the Pathogenesis of Keloids and Hypertrophic Scars and the Most Promising Current Therapeutic Strategy". *Journal of Nippon Medical School* 83:46-53. doi: 10.1272/jnms.83.46.

[8] Trace, Anthony P., and Clinton W. Enos, Alon Mantel, Valerie M. Harvey. 2016. "Keloids and Hypertrophic Scars: A Spectrum of Clinical Challenges." *American Journal of Clinical Dermatology* 17:201-23. doi: 10.1007/s40257-016-0175-7.

[9] Limandjaja, G. C., and L. J. van den Broek, T. Waaijman, H. A. van Veen, V. Everts, S. Monstrey, R. J. Scheper, F. B. Niessen, S. Gibbs. 2017. "Increased epidermal thickness and abnormal epidermal differentiation in keloid scars." The *British Journal of Dermatology* 176:116-126. doi: 10.1111/bjd.14844.

[10] Slemp, Alison E., and Richard E. Kirschner. 2006. "Keloids and scars: a review of keloids and scars, their pathogenesis, risk factors, and management.'' *Current Opinion in Pediatrics* 18:396-402. Doi: 10.1097/01.mop.0000236389.41462.ef.

[11] Burton, Claude S., and Vaishali Escaravage. 2008. "Dermal Hypertrophies." In: *Dermatology* edited by Bolognia, Jean L., and Joseph L. Jorizzo, Ronald P. Rapini, Julie V. Schaffer, 1497-501. Spain: Elsevier Limited.

[12] Lovell, Christopher R. 2016. "Acquired Disorders of Dermal Connective Tissue". In *Rook's Textbook of Dermatology* edited by Griffiths, Cristopher, and Jonathan Barker, Tanya Bleiker, Robert Chalmers, Daniel Creamer, 96.6-45. Singapore: Wiley Blackwell.

[13] Rabello, Felibe B., and Cleyton D. Souza, Jayme A. Farina Junior. 2014. "Update on hypertrophic scar treatment." *Clinics* (Sao Paulo) 69:565-73.

[14] Barbul, Adrian, and David T. Efron, Sandra L. Kavalukas. 2015. "Wound Healing." In *Schwartz's Principles of Surgery*, 261-262. USA: The Mc Graw Hill Company.

[15] Chike-Obi, Chuma J., and Patrick D. Cole, Anthony E. Brissett. 2009. "Keloids: pathogenesis, clinical features, and management." *Seminars in Plastic Surgery* 23:178-84. doi: 10.1055/s-0029-1224797.

[16] James, William D., and Timothy G. Berger, Dirk M. Elston. 2006. "Fibrous Tissue Abnormalities" In *Andrew's Disease of the Skin, Clinical Dermatology*, 602-5. Canada: Elsevier Company.

[17] Krieg, Thomas, and Monique Aumailley, Manuel Koch, Mon-Li Chu, Jouni Uitto. 2012. "Collagens, Elastic Fibers, and Other Extracellular Matrix Proteins of the Dermis." In *Fitzpatrick's Dermatology in General Medicine*, edited by Goldsmith, Lowell A., and Stephen I. Katz, Barbara A. Gilchrest, Amy S. Paller, David J. Leffell, Klaus Wolff, 707-10. USA: The Mc Graw Hill Company.

[18] Lenie, Limandjaja, and J. van den Broek, Melanie Breetveld, Taco Waaijman, Stan Monstrey, Edith M. de Boer, Rik J. Scheper, Frank B. Niessen, Susan Gibbs. 2018. "Characterization of in vitro reconstructed human normotrophic, hypertrophic and keloid scar models." *Tissue Engineering*. Part C, Methods 24:242-53. doi: 10.1089/ten.TEC.2017.0464.

[19] Safonov, I. 2012. "Normotrophic scars." In: *Atlas of Scar Treatment and Correction*. Berlin, Heidelberg: Springer.

[20] Hague, Adam, and Ardeshir Bayat. 2017. "Therapeutic targets in the management of striae distensae: A systematic review." *Journal of the American Academy of Dermatology* 77(3): 559-68. doi: 10.1016/j.jaad.2017.02.048.

[21] Ud-Din, S., and D. McGeorge, A. Bayat. 2016. "Topical management of striae distansea (stretch marks): prevention and therapy of striae rubrae and albae." *Journal of the European Academy of Dermatology and Venereology* 30: 211–22. doi: 10.1111/jdv.13223.

[22] Cho, S., and E. S. Park, D. H. Lee, K. Li, J. H. Chung. 2006. "Clinical features and risk factors for striae distensae in Korean adolescents." *Journal of the European Academy of Dermatology and Venereology* 20(9):1108-13. DOI: 10.1111/j.1468-3083.2006.01747.x.

[23] Kasielska-Trojan, Anna, and Bogusław Antoszewski. 2017. "Do body build and composition influence striae distansae occurance and visibility in women?" *Journal of Cosmetic Dermatology* doi: 10.1111/jocd.12455.

[24] Bogdan, Catalina, and Sonia Iurian, Ioan Tomuta, Mirela Moldovan. 2017. "Improvement of skin condition in striae distensae: development, characterization and clinical efficacy of a cosmetic product containing Punica granatum seed oil and Croton lechleri resin extract." *Drug Design, Development and Therapy* 11:521-31. doi: 10.2147/DDDT.S128470.

[25] Farahnik, B., and K. Park, G.Kroumpouzos, J. Murase. 2017. "Striae gravidarum: Risk factors, prevention, and management." *International Journal of Women's Dermatology* 3:77-85. doi: 10.1016/j.ijwd.2016.11.001.

[26] Leung, Alexander K. C., and C. Pion Kao, Reginald S. Sauve. 2001. "Scarring Resulting from Chickenpox." *Pediatric Dermatology* 18:378-80.

[27] Barikbin, Behrooz, and Nelda Saadat, Zahra Akbari, Maryam Yousefi, Parviz Toossi. 2012. "Focal High-Concentration Tricholoroacetic Acid Peeling for treatment of Atrophic Facial Chickenpox Scar." *Dermatologic Surgery* 38: 1662-7. doi: 10.1111/j.1524-4725.2012.02541.x.

[28] Al-Refu, K., and M. Goodfield. 2009. "Scar classification in cutaneous lupus erythematosus." The *British Journal of Dermatology* 161:1052-8. doi: 10.1111/j.1365-2133.2009.09313.x.

[29] Wenzel, Joerg, and Manfred Uerlich, E. Wörrenkämper, Thomas Tueting. 2005. "Scarring skin lesions of discoid lupus erythematosus are characterized by high numbers of skin-homing cytotoxic lymphocytes associated with strong expression of the type I interferon-induced protein MxA." The *British Journal of Dermatology* 153:1011-5. Doi: 10.1111/j.1365-2133.2005.06784.x.

[30] Y. Y. Vun, M. M. Malik, G. M. Murphy, B. O'Donnell. 2005. "Congenital erosive and vesicular dermatosis." *Clinical and Experimental Dermatology* 30:146-8. Doi: 10.1111/j.1365-2230.2004.01670.x.

[31] Kuflik, Julianne H., and Robert A. Schwartz, Kenneth A. Becker, W. Clark Lambert. 2005. "Atrophia maculosa varioliformis cutis." *International Journal of Dermatology* 44:864-6. Doi: 10.1111/j.1365-4632.2004.02220.x

[32] Chathra, Namitha, and Venkataram Mysore. 2018. "Resurfacing of facial acne scars with a new variable-pulsed Er:YAG laser in Fitzpatrick skin types IV and V." *Journal of Cutaneous and Aesthetic Surgery* 11:20-5. doi: 10.4103/JCAS.JCAS_4_18.

[33] Hirsch, Ranella J., and Amy B. Lewis. 2001. "Treatment of Acne Scarring". *Seminars in Cutaneous Medicine and Surgery* 20:190-8.

[34] Hay, Rania Abdel, and Khalid Shalaby, Hesham Zaher, Vanessa Hafez, Ching-Chi Chi, Sandra Dimitri, Ashraf F Nabhan, Alison M Layton. 2016. "Interventions for acne scars." *Cochrane Database of Systematic Reviews* 4:CD011946. doi: 10.1002/14651858.CD011946.pub2.

[35] Connolly, Deirdre, and Ha Linh Vu, Kavita Mariwalla, Nazanin Saedi. 2017. "Acne Scarring- Pathogenesis, Evaluation, and Treatment Options". The *Journal of Clinical and Aesthetic Dermatology* 10:12–23.

[36] Sobanko, Joseph F., and Tina S. Alster. 2012. "Management of Acne Scarring, Part I. A Comparative Review of Laser Surgical Approaches." *American Journal of Clinical Dermatology* 13:319-30. doi: 10.2165/11598910-000000000-00000.

[37] Goodman, Greg J. 2003. "Post acne scarring: a review." *Journal of Cosmetic & Laser Therapy* 5:77-95.

[38] Basta-Juzbasic, Aleksandra. 2010. "Current Therapeutic Approach to Acne Scars." *Acta Dermatovenerologica Croatica* 18:171-5.

[39] Levy, Lauren L., and Joshua A. Zeichner. 2012. "Management of Acne Scarring, Part II." *American Journal of Clinical Dermatology* 13:331-40. doi: 10.2165/11631410-000000000-00000.

[40] Jacob, Carolyn I., and Jeffrey S. Dover, Micheal S. Kaminer. 2001. "Acne scarring: a classification system and review of treatment options." The *Journal of American Academy of Dermatology* 45:109-17. Doi: 10.1067/mjd.2001.113451

[41] Riviera, Albert E. 2008. "Acne scarring: A review and current treatment modalities." The *Journal of American Academy of Dermatology*; 59: 659-76. doi: 10.1016/j.jaad.2008.05.029.

[42] Bhargava, Shashank, and Paulo R. Cunha, Jennifer Lee, George Kroumpouzos. 2018. "Acne Scarring Management: Systematic Review and Evaluation of the Evidence." *American Journal of Clinical Dermatology* 19: 459-77. doi: 10.1007/s40257-018-0358-5.

In: Cutaneous Scars: Biology, Clinics and Management ISBN: 978-1-53615-657-7
Editors: Berna Aksoy, Hasan Mete Aksoy et al. © 2019 Nova Science Publishers, Inc.

Chapter 10

CLINICAL ASPECTS OF ATROPHIC SCARS: SURGICAL, POST-ACNE AND STRIAE

Aysun Sikar Akturk[*]
Department of Dermatology,
Faculty of Medicine, Kocaeli University, Kocaeli, Turkey

ABSTRACT

Cutaneous scars are common after surgical manipulation of the skin. Scars may affect patients' psychological, social and physical lives. Scars are classified into widespread scars, atrophic scars, scar contractures, hypertrophic scars and keloid scars. Atrophic scars are dermal depressions that generally occur as a result of collagen destruction following skin diseases such as acne, infections like varicella, or after burns or surgery. In this section, clinical aspects of atrophic scars such as surgical scars, post-acne scars and striae will be reviewed.

Keywords: acne scar, atrophic scar, striae, surgical scar, widespread scar

1. INTRODUCTION

Tissue loss including dermis and lower skin layers that occur following events such as burns, trauma, injury and surgery heal with the formation of scars [1-5]. The healing process of tissue loss consists of three different phases; 1. hemostasis and inflammation, 2. proliferation and 3. remodeling. These phases are the consequences of many cellular

[*]Corresponding Author's Email: aysun9442@hotmail.com.

and biochemical processes and various signaling pathways following tissue injury. Collagen produced by fibroblasts is one of the most important components in wound healing [1, 4-6]. Complete wound healing usually takes up to 12 to 18 months [7]. However, in some cases it may take years for a wound to heal completely [8]. Delay in one of these phases of wound healing results in delay in wound healing and abnormal scar formation [1, 4].

Scars may be associated with a number of physical comorbidities including hypertrichosis, dyshidrosis, tenderness, pain, pruritus, dysesthesias and functional impairments such as contractures. In addition, people with abnormal skin scarring may face physical, aesthetic, psychological and social consequences and these may be associated with substantial emotional and financial costs [2, 5, 9-11].

Before doing a scar revision various factors such as nutritional status, medical history of patients, smoking, tension of wound edges, infection and hematoma should be considered [7, 8, 11]. Usually scars fade and become much less noticeable, but sometimes they may get even larger. All new scar tissues usually look red, are raised above the skin and fairly hard to the touch. The scars' color gets lighter and they become softer in time. The characteristics of an ideal scar which makes it cosmetically favourable are as follows: 1. it should have similar color and contour as the surrounding skin; and 2. it should be on the same level as the skin [7, 9]. However, scars can not yet be made to disappear completely [9].

Scars are classified as *widespread scars*, *atrophic scars*, scar contractures, hypertrophic scars, and keloid scars [9, 12]. Scars that are difficult to categorize are known as intermediate scars. Widespread and *atrophic scars* are associated with a failure of production of scar tissue. While *widespread scars* are usually seen after surgery, *atrophic scars* are seen not only after surgery but also after burns, acne, infections and trauma [2, 9]. *Atrophic scars* are dermal depressions that occur as a result of collagen destruction during the inflammatory response to skin insults such as acne and varicella [13].

In this section, clinical aspects of *atrophic scars* (surgical, post-acne) and striae will be reviewed.

2. Surgical Scars (Incisional Scars)

Each year in the world 100 million people acquire scars, majority as a result of (55 million) elective operations and (25 million) operations after trauma [2, 9]. Scar formation from surgical procedures is an unavoidable risk, despite measures taken by both the surgeon and patient during the perioperative period [14]. During the perioperative and postoperative periods surgeons' and patients' roles in scar prevention and reduction are of great importance [6, 14]. Understanding these modifiable factors of incisional scar response should include knowledge and experience of incision design, atraumatic handling of soft tissue, hemostasis, aseptic techniques and tension reducing approaches in both the short and long term postoperative setting [6, 11]. Personal factors affecting postoperative scar formation are age, ethnicity, previous medical history, blood flow, skin tension and area of incision [3, 6, 8, 11, 15].

Different scar types may be seen due to surgical procedures. After surgery, *widespread* (stretched) *scars* occurs more frequently than other scar types. *Widespread scars* occur in the midline after surgical incision and develop when fine lines of surgical scars become gradually stretched and widened. This usually happens during the three-week period following surgery. They are typically flat, pale, soft and symptomless scars (Figure 1). They are often seen after knee or shoulder surgery [9].

Hypertrichosis within scars have been reported in postoperative patients with knee replacement surgery and in patients with surgical scars who require the use of orthopedic casts and splints [2].

3. Atrophic Acne Scars

Acne vulgaris is a chronic inflammatory skin disease of the pilosebaceous unit. Scarring can occur as a result of damage during the healing of active acne [16, 17].

Figure 1. Widespread (stretched) surgical scar on the arm.

Acne scars, a permanent complication of acne vulgaris, are a problem of major concern and may affect acne patients' quality of life. The scarring process may occur at any stage of acne and correlates with the severity of the acne [18].

In the remodelling phase of the wound healing process, imbalance between construction and demolition causes *acne scars*. There are two basic types of scars; atrophic and hypertrophic. While collagen tissue growth results in hypertrophic scarring, tissue damage and/or loss results in *atrophic scars* [19]. *Atrophic scars* constitute 80-90% of *acne scars*. *Atrophic acne scars* are subclassified as "ice pick", "boxcar" and "rolling" scars according to the depth and size of destruction. Ice pick scars represents 60% - 70%, boxcar scars 20% - 30% and rolling scars 15% - 25% of total scars. Sometimes these different types of *atrophic scars* may be observed in the same patient and it might be very difficult to differentiate between them [16, 17]:

a. Ice pick scars: They are "V" shaped, narrow (< 2 mm) and have sharp edges and a very narrow base. They are deep scars that extend into the dermis or subcutaneous tissue. The surface reminds us of appearance of the damage caused by an ice crusher; so it is wide on the top, and narrow at the base (Figure 2).
b. Boxcar scars: These scars are wider than icepick, "U" shaped and have a round, polygonal or linear wide surface with a large flat bottom part. There is epidermal atrophy at the scar floor (Figure 3).
c. Rolling scars: They are slightly inclined, "M" shaped, angular, wavy and are not sharply bordered. They are tense and 4-5 mm or wider in size. Fibrous anchoring extends to the subcutis from the dermis and this results in superficial shadowing and undulating. The epidermis is not atrophic at the floor (Figure 4) [17, 19].

4. Striae

Striae (stretch marks, striae distensae, striae atrophicans, striae gravidarum) which are a form of scarring on the skin are a cosmetic problem, mostly among women. They are commonly seen during and after pregnancy. It is known that genetic, hormonal and physical factors are significant in the formation of *striae*. The incidence of *striae* is reported to be between 11% and 88% in the literature [20, 21]. *Striae* gravidarum is a type of *striae* that occurs during pregnancy. It usually occurs after the 24th week of gestation [20, 21].

In addition to pregnancy, other reasons for *striae* include obesity, puberty, Cushing syndrome and use of systemic or topical corticosteroids. *Striae* are frequently located on the abdomen, breasts, thighs and in the gluteal region [20]. Itching and burning may occur during formation of *striae* [21].

There are two clinical and histopathological forms; *striae* rubrae and *striae* albae.

Striae rubrae are clinically seen as flat, erythematous and violaceous bands. *Striae* albae are a permanent form of *striae* which are white, wrinkled and atrophic (Figure 5) [20].

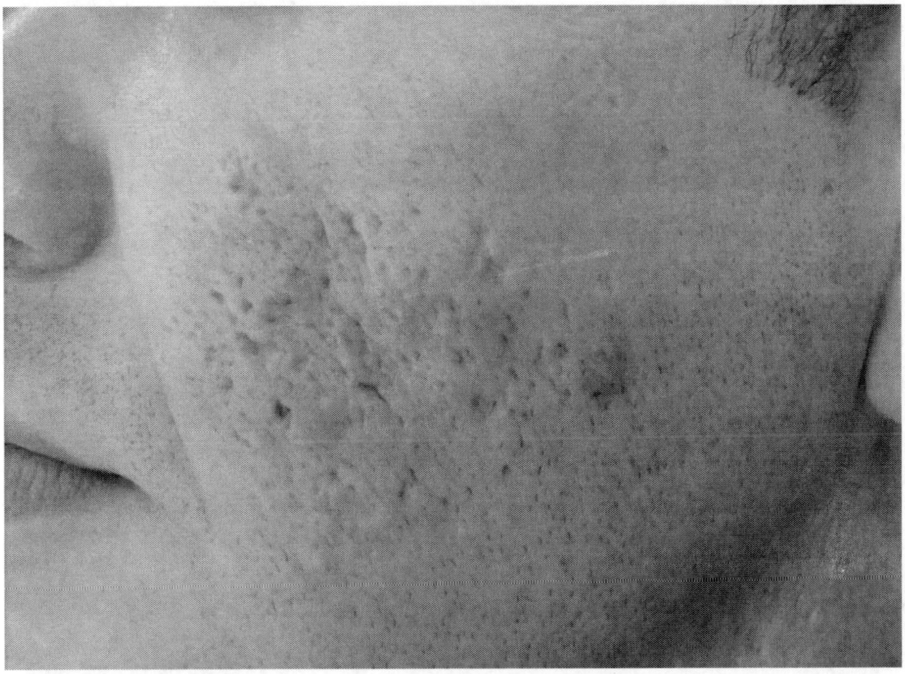

Figure 2. Icepick scars on the cheek (Courtesy of Berna Aksoy, MD).

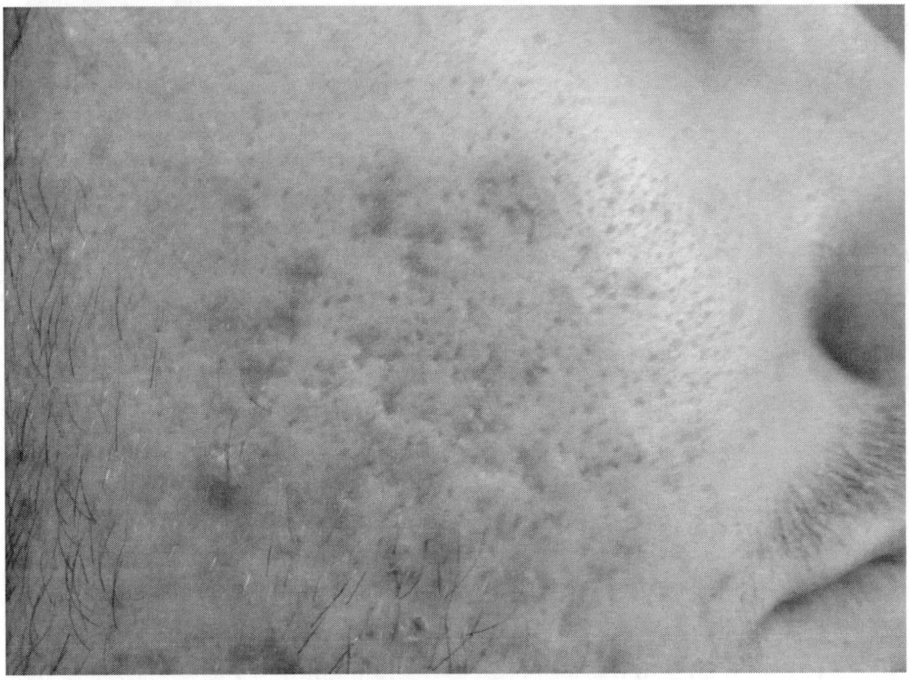

Figure 3. Boxcar and icepick scars on the cheek (Courtesy of Berna Aksoy, MD).

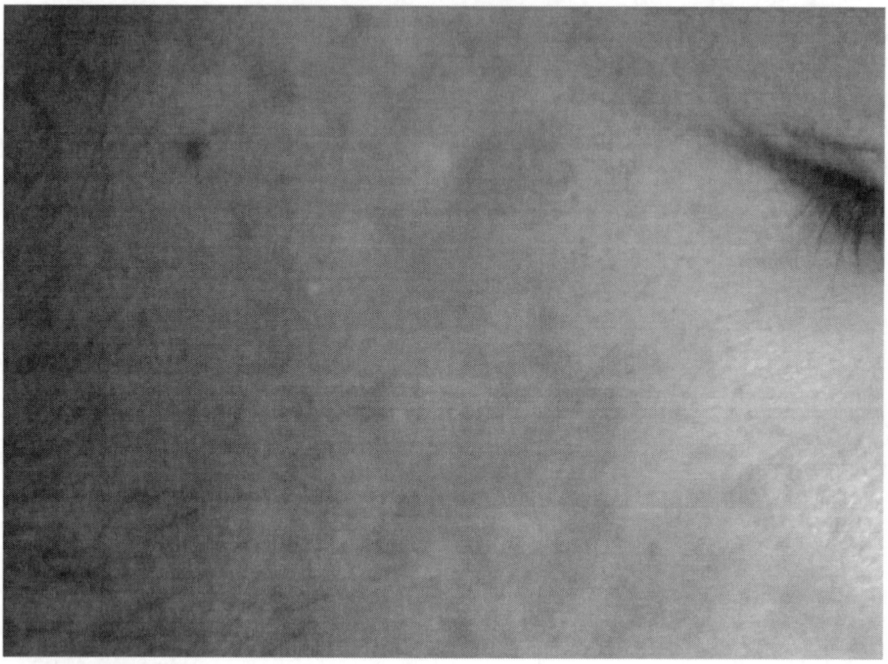

Figure 4. Rolling scars on the cheek (Courtesy of Erol Koc, MD).

Figure 5. Striae albae (striae distensae) because of puberty located on the skin of the torso of a 17-year-old boy.

CONCLUSION

Cutaneous scars are common after surgical manipulation of the skin. Scars may effect patients' psychological, social and physical lives. Atrophic scars are dermal depressions that generally occur as a result of collagen destruction during inflammatory skin diseases such as acne or varicella, or after burns or surgery.

REFERENCES

[1] Greaves, Nicholas S. and Kevin J. Ashcroft, Mohamed Baguneid, Ardeshir Bayat. 2013. 'Current understanding of molecular and cellular mechanisms in fibroplasia and angiogenesis during acute wound healing'. *Journal of Dermatological Science,* 72:206 - 17. doi: 10.1016/j.jdermsci.2013.07.008.

[2] Krakowski, Andrew C. and Christine R. Totri, Matthias B. Donelan, Peter R. Shumaker. 2016. 'Scar Management in the Pediatric and Adolescent Populations'. *Pediatrics,* 137:e20142065. doi: 10.1542/peds.2014-2065.

[3] Gauglitz, G. G. and J. Pötschke, M. T. Clementoni. 2018. 'Therapy of scars with lasers'. *Hautarzt,* 69:17 - 26. doi: 10.1007/s00105-017-4072-7.

[4] Kasuya, Akira and Yoshiki Tokura. 2014. 'Attempts to accelerate wound healing'. *Journal of Dermatological Science,* 76:169 - 72. doi: 10.1016/ j.jdermsci. 2014.11.001.

[5] Kerwin, Leonard Y. and Abdel K. El Tal, Mark A. Stiff, Tarek M. Fakhouri. 2014. 'Scar prevention and remodeling: a review of the medical, surgical, topical and light treatment approaches'. *International Journal of Dermatology,* 53:922 - 36. doi: 10.1111/ijd.12436.

[6] Son, Daegu and Aram Harijan. 2014. 'Overview of surgical scar prevention and management'. *Journal of Korean Medical Science,* 29:751 - 7. doi: 10.3346/ jkms.2014.29.6.751.

[7] Garg, Shilpa and Naveen Dahiya, Somesh Gupta. 2014. 'Surgical scar revision: an overview'. *Journal of Cutaneous and Aesthetic Surgery,* 7: 3 - 13. doi: 10.4103/ 0974-2077.129959.

[8] Burke, M. 1998. 'Scars. Can they be minimised'? *Australian Family Physician,* 27:275 - 8.

[9] Bayat, A. and D. A. McGrouther, M. W. J. Ferguson. 2003. 'Skin scarring'. *BMJ,* 326(7380):88 - 92. Doi: 10.1136/bmj.326.7380.88.

[10] Zhang, Junqian and Christopher J. Miller, Victoria O'Malley, Eric B. Bowman, Jeremy R. Etzkorn, Thuzar M. Shin, Joseph F. Sobanko. 2018. 'Patient and Physician Assessment of Surgical Scars: A Systematic Review'. *JAMA Facial Plastic Surgery,* 20:314 - 23 doi: 10.1001/jamafacial.2017.2314.

[11] Kelekçi, Kıymet H. and Şemsettin Karaca, Emine Demirel, Raziye Desticioğlu, Ayşe M. Biçer, Onur Er, Serpil Aydoğmuş. 2015. 'Risk factors for scar formation after surgical incision'. *Turkderm,* 49:213 - 7. Doi: 10.4274/turkderm.39225.

[12] Perry, Donna M. and Duncan A. McGrouther, Ardeshir Bayat. 2010. 'Current tools for noninvasive objective assessment of skin scars'. *Plastic and Reconstructive Surgery,* 126:912 - 23. doi: 10.1097/PRS.0b013e3181e6046b.

[13] Khatri, Khalil A. and Danielle L. Mahoney, Melissa J. McCartney. 2011. 'Laser scar revision: a review.' *Journal of Cosmetic and Laser Therapy,* 13:54 - 62. doi: 10.3109/14764172.2011.564625.

[14] Eilers, Robert E. and Edward V. Ross, Joel L. Kohen, Arisa E. Ortiz. 2016. 'A combination approach to surgical scars'. *Dermatologic Surgery,* 42:150 - 6. doi: 10.1097/DSS.0000000000000750.

[15] Konda, S. and K. Potter, V. Z. Ren, A. L. Wang, A. Srinivasan, S. Chilukuri. 2017. 'Techniques for optimizing surgical scars, Part 1: wound healing and depressed/atrophic scars'. *Skinmed,* 15:271 - 6.

[16] Fabbrocini, Gabriella and M. C. Annunziata, V. D. Arco, V. De Vita, G. Lodi, M. C. Mauriello, F. Pstore, G. Monfrecola. 2010. 'Acne scars: pathogenesis, classification and treatment'. *Dermatology Research and Practice,* 2010:893080. doi: 10.1155/2010/893080.

[17] Connolly, Deirdre and Ha L. Vu, Kavita Mariwalla, Nazanin Saedi. 2017. 'Acne scarring: pathogenesis, evaluation, and treatment options', The *Journal of Clinical and Aesthetic Dermatology,* 10:12 - 23.

[18] Al Taweel, Abdul-Aziz I. and Abdul-Aziz A.-S. Al Refae, Ahmed M. Hamed, Asmaa M. Kamal. 2018. 'Comparative study of the efficacy of Platelet-rich plasma combined with carboxytherapy vs. its use with fractional carbon dioxide laser in atrophic acne scars'. *Journal of Cosmetic Dermatology,* doi: 10.1111/jocd.12561.

[19] Jacob, Carolyn I. and Jeffrey S. Dover, Michael S. Kaminer. 2001. 'Acne scarring: a classification system and review of treatment options'. *Journal of the American Academy of Dermatology,* 45:109 - 17. Doi: 10.1067/mjd.2001.113451.

[20] Al-Himdani, S. and S. Ud-Din, S. Gilmore, A. Bayat. 2014. 'Striae distensae: a comprehensive review and evidence-based evaluation of prophylaxis and treatment'. The *British Journal of Dermatology,* 170:527 - 47. doi: 10.1111/bjd.12681.

[21] Farahnik, B. and K. Park, G. Kroumpouzos, J. Murase. 2017. 'Striae gravidarum: Risk factors, prevention, and management'. *International Journal of Women's Dermatology,* 3:77 - 85. doi: 10.1016/j.ijwd.2016.11.001.

In: Cutaneous Scars: Biology, Clinics and Management ISBN: 978-1-53615-657-7
Editors: Berna Aksoy, Hasan Mete Aksoy et al. © 2019 Nova Science Publishers, Inc.

Chapter 11

CLINICAL ASPECTS OF PROLIFERATIVE SCARS: HYPERTROPHIC SCAR AND KELOIDS

Elif Yildirim[*]
Department of Dermatology, Faculty of Medicine,
SANKO University, Gaziantep, Turkey

ABSTRACT

Keloids and hypertrophic scars are both raised scars and can be hard to distinguish from each other clinically. It is important to distinguish between hypertrophic scars and keloids clinically, since different treatment modalities are required depending on the diagnosis. In this chapter clinical aspects of proliferative scars are summarized.

Keywords: hypertrophic scars, keloids, proliferative scars

1. INTRODUCTION

It is important to distinguish between *hypertrophic scars* and *keloids* clinically, since different treatment modalities are required depending on the diagnosis. But *keloids* and *hypertrophic scars* are both raised *proliferative scars* and can be hard to distinguish from each other clinically (Table 1) [1].

[*]Corresponding Author's Email: elifalper27@gmail.com.

Table 1. Key features of hypertrophic scars and keloids

	Hypertrophic Scars	Keloid
Preceded by injury	Yes	Not always
Onset	Immediate (4-8 weeks after injury)	Delayed
Confined to wound margin	Yes	No
Spontaneous resolution	Sometimes, gradual	Rare
Treatment response	Good	Poor (recurrence after surgery)
Predilection sites	Shoulders, neck, presternum, knees and ankles	Anterior chest, shoulders, earlobes, upper arms and cheeks

2. Hypertrophic Scars

Hypertrophic scars are often firm, red, raised (typically <4mm), inflamed, itchy, and even painful. They usually occur within 4 to 8 weeks of injury that is earlier in comparison to keloids [2]. Unlike *keloids*, *hypertrophic scars* remain confined within the boundaries of the injury, their sizes are directly proportional to that of injury and they are more responsive to surgical excision [2].

The location of the wound on the body is of great significance in the formation of *hypertrophic scars*. Scars that cross joints or skin creases at right angles such as shoulders, neck, presternum, knees and ankles [3-5] are especially prone to form hypertrophic scarring, possibly because of the constant mechanical tension forces that occur [6].

Widespread *hypertrophic scars* typically occur after burn injury on the trunk and extremities. They are elevated above skin surface, widespread, and sometimes pruritic. Scars are confined to the boundaries of the burn injury (Figure 1). Linear *hypertrophic scars* have a rope-like appearance and are associated with surgery or trauma (Figure 2) [7].

Hypertrophic scars are estimated to occur in 40% to 70% of patients following surgery and up to 91% of patients following burn injuries, depending on the wound depth [8].

Hypertrophic scars have an initial rapid growth phase for up to 6 months, and then they tend to gradually regress. Although it may take years, they end up with flat scars with no further symptoms [3, 9].

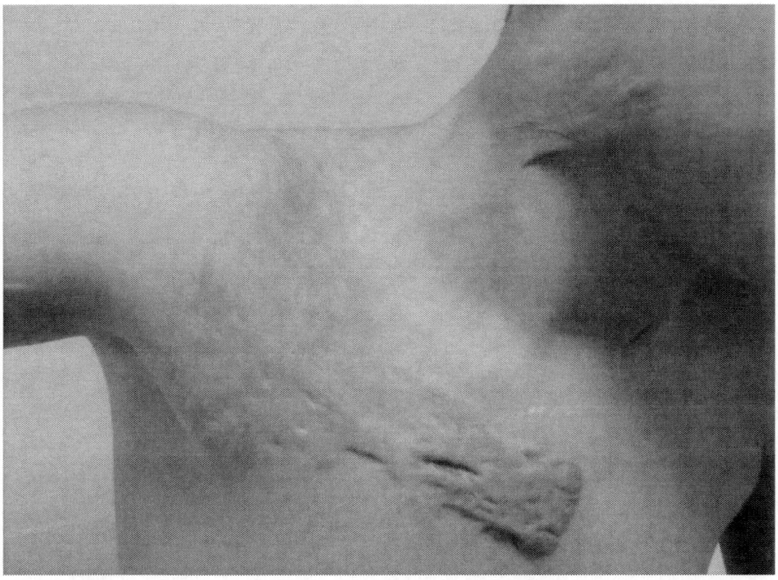

Figure 1. Hypertrophic scars following burn injury (Courtesy of Berna Aksoy, MD).

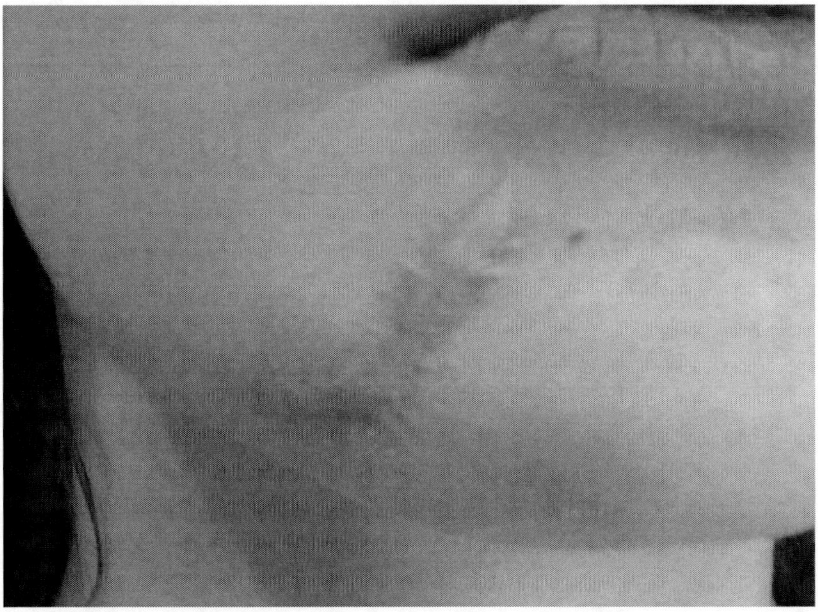

Figure 2. Hypertrophic scar following surgical repair of a deep traumatic laceration (Courtesy of Berna Aksoy, MD).

3. Keloids

Keloids appear as dense fibrous outgrowths which are firm, mildly tender or pruritic, bosselated and well demarcated tumours. Their sizes are variable from 2 to 3mm papules to large pendulous tumours. The epithelium is thinned, may exhibit telangiectasia and there may be focal areas of ulceration [8, 10]. The color is also variable from mildly erythematous in new lesions to dull red or paler in older lesions. They may also be accompanied by hyperpigmentation [11]. The borders of the tumor are well demarcated but irregular in outline and may have claw-like projections. Lesions are usually devoid of hair follicles and other functioning adnexal glands. On examination, these elevated, firm, protuberant nodules or plaques are not confined to the boundaries of the inciting injury and extend beyond the boundaries of injury, causing disfigurement [10, 12].

The reported incidence of *keloid* scars in retrospective series ranges between 4.5 and 16% [13, 14]. While *keloids* can occur at any age, they show a peak incidence in patients aged between 15 and 24 years [15, 16].

Although *keloids* may occur everywhere on body, certain body regions show increased susceptibility to *keloids*. The deltoid, presternal (sternotomy) [17], upper back regions (acne), shoulders (vaccinations) (Figure 3.1.) [18], earlobes (piercing) (Figure 3.2.) [19] and cheeks (acne) [20] seem to be the most commonly affected sites [21]. *Keloid* formation of the eyelids, genitalia, palms, or soles is unusual [21].

Shape of lesions varies from evenly contored symmetric protrusions with regular margins to irregular claw-like projections. *Keloids* on the ears, neck, and abdomen often grow as pedunculated large lobules, whereas those on the central chest, upper back, and extremities are usually raised with a flat surface, the base being wider than the top resembling a butterfly shape (Figure 3.3.) [22].

The most commonly reported symptom, pruritus, frequently occurs at the edges of lesions, while the second most common symptom, pain, primarily occurs in the central aspect of the lesions [23].

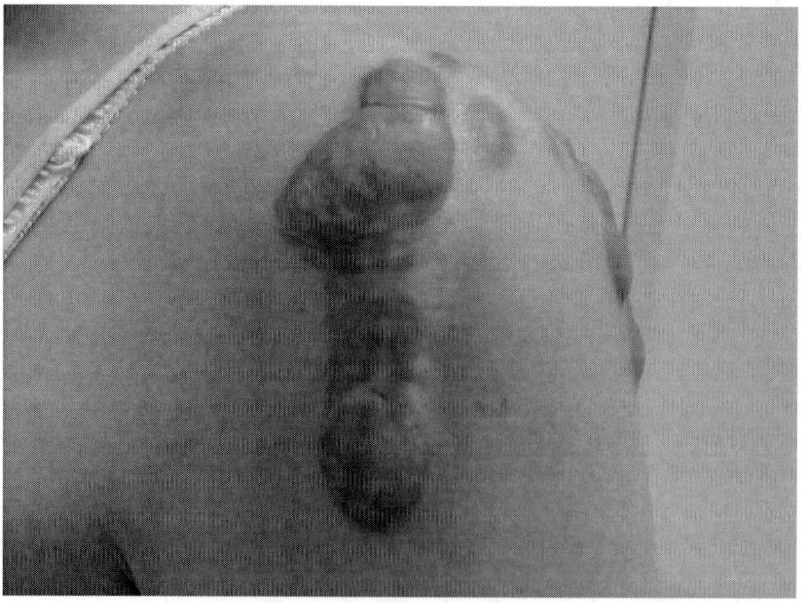

Figure 3.1. Extensive keloids on the shoulder following acne (Courtesy of Berna Aksoy, MD).

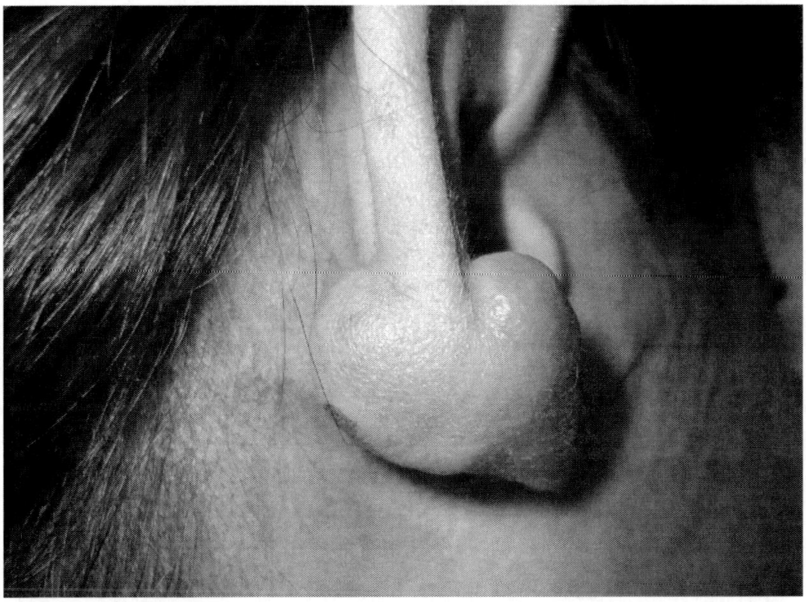

Figure 3.2. Earlobe keloids (Courtesy of Berna Aksoy, MD).

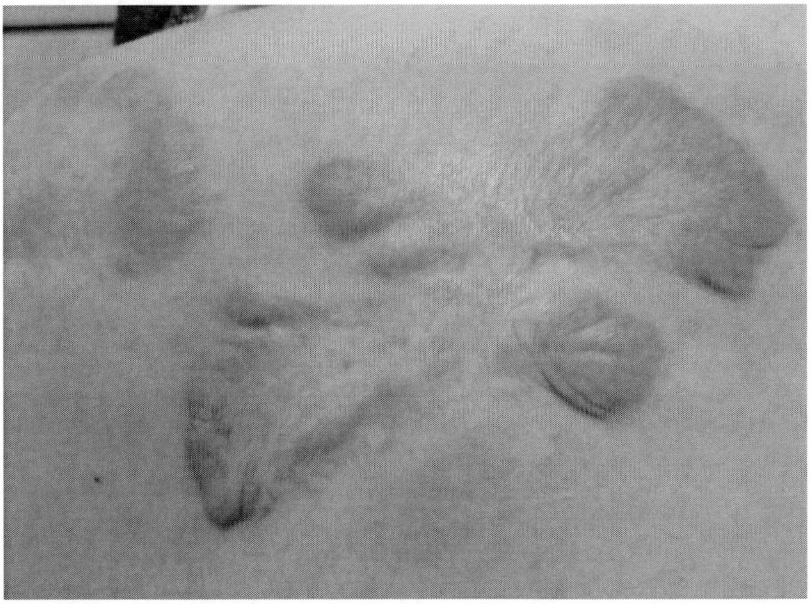

Figure 3.3. Keloids located on the upper back (Courtesy of Berna Aksoy, MD).

Hyperemia, dysesthesia, continued growth, restriction of movement or other functional impairments, and cosmetic disfigurement are also among important sequelae [15]. Many patients are affected both physically and psychologically due to cosmetic problems, functional impairments and subjective symptoms including pruritus and pain. Patients usually report a severe negative impact on quality of life [24].

Keloids, in contrast to *hypertrophic scars*, may develop up to several years after minor injuries and even arise spontaneously on the mid chest in the absence of any known injury. *Keloids* also persist, usually for long periods of time, and do not regress spontaneously [12].

Conclusion

Keloids and hypertrophic scars are both raised proliferative scars and can be hard to distinguish from each other clinically. Hypertrophic scars develop shortly after inciting injury, are confined to the boundaries of previous injury and show spontaneous regression with time. On the contrary keloids develop long after inciting injury, extend beyond the boundaries of previous injury, can develop spontaneously, do not regress and even progress with time.

References

[1] Van den Broek, Lenie J. and Grace C. Limandjaja, Frank B. Niessen, Susan Gibbs. 2014. "Human hypertrophic and keloid scar models: principles, limitations and future challenges from a tissue engineering perspective". *Experimental Dermatology,* 23:382 - 6. doi: 10.1111/exd.12419.

[2] Wheeland, R. G. 1996. "Keloids and hypertrophic scars". In *Cutaneous Medicine and Surgery,* edited by Arndt, K. A. and J. K. Robinson, P. E. Leboit, B. U. Wintroub, 900 - 5. Philadelphia: Saunders Elsevier.

[3] Hawkins, H. K. 2007. "Pathophysiology of the burn scar". In *Total Burn Care,* edited by Herndon, D. N., 608 - 19. Philadelphia: Saunders Elsevier.

[4] From, L. and D. Assad. 1993. "Neoplasms, pseudoneoplasms, and hyperplasia of supporting tissue origin". In *Dermatology in General Medicine,* edited by Jeffers, J. D. and M. R. Englis, 1198 - 9. New York: McGraw-Hill.

[5] Muir, I. F. 1990. "On the nature of keloid and hypertrophic scars". *British Journal of Plastic Surgery,* 43:61 - 9.

[6] Rudolph, R. 1987. "Wide spread scars, hypertrophic scars and keloids". *Clinics in Plastic Surgery,* 14:253 - 60.

[7] Ghazawi, Feras M. and Ramin Zargham, Mirko S. Gilardino, Denis Sasseville, Fatemeh Jafarian. 2018. "Insights into the Pathophysiology of Hypertrophic Scars and Keloids: How Do They Differ?" *Advances in Skin and Wound Care,* 31:582 - 95. doi: 10.1097/01.ASW.0000527576.27489.0f.

[8] Gauglitz, Gerd G. and Hans C. Korting, Tatiana Pavicic, Thomas Ruzicka, Marc G. Jeschke. 2011. "Hypertrophic scarring and keloids: pathomechanisms and current

and emerging treatment strategies". *Molecular Medicine,* 17:113 - 25. doi: 10.2119/ molmed.2009.00153.

[9] Alster, T. S. and T. B. West. 1997. "Treatment of scars: a review". *Annals of Plastic Surgery,* 39:418 - 32.

[10] Rabello, Felipe B. and Cleyton D. Souza, Jayme A. F. Ju´nior. 2014. "Update on hypertrophic scar treatment". *Clinics* (Sao Paulo), 69:565 - 73.

[11] Al-Attar, Ali and Sarah Mess, John M. Thomassen, C. Lisa Kauffman, Steven P. Davison. 2006. "Keloid pathogenesis and treatment". *Plastic and Reconstructive Surgery,* 117:286 - 300.

[12] Murray, John C. 1994. "Keloids and hypertrophic scars". *Clinics in Dermatology,* 12:27 - 37.

[13] Wolfram, Dolores and Alexandar Tzankov, Petra Pülzl, Hildegunde Piza-Katzer. 2009. "Hypertrophic scars and keloids—a review of their pathophysiology, risk factors, and therapeutic management". *Dermatologic Surgery,* 35:171 - 81.

[14] Alhady, S. M. and K. Sivanantharajah. 1969. "Keloids in various races. A review of 175 cases". *Plastic and Reconstructive Surgery,* 44:564 - 6.

[15] Yedomon, G. H. and H. Adegbidi, F. Atadokpede, F. Akpadjan, E. J. Mouto, F. do Ango-Padonou. 2012. "Keloids on dark skin: a consecutive series of 456 cases". *Medecine et Sante Tropicales,* 22:287 - 91. doi: 10.1684/mst.2012.0052.

[16] Trace, Anthony P. and Clinton W. Enos, Alon Mantel, Valerie M. Harvey. 2016. "Keloids and Hypertrophic Scars: A Spectrum of Clinical Challenges". *American Journal of Clinical Dermatology,* 17:201 - 23.

[17] Manuskiatti, Woraphong and Richard E. Fitzpatrick. 2002. "Treatment response of keloidal and hypertrophic sternotomy scars: comparison among intralesional corticosteroid, 5-fluorouracil, and 585-nm flash lamp pumped pulsed-dye laser treatments". *Archives of Dermatology,* 138:1149 - 55.

[18] Coop, C. A. and S. M. Schaefer, R. W. England. 2007. "Extensive keloid formation and progression after each vaccination". *Human Vaccines,* 3:127 - 9.

[19] Lane, Joshua E. and Jennifer L. Waller, Loretta S. Davis L. S. 2005. "Relationship between age of ear piercing and keloid formation". *Pediatrics,* 115:1312 - 4.

[20] Niessen, Frank B. and Paul H. M. Spauwen, Joost Schalkwijk, Moshe Kon. 1999. "On the nature of hypertrophic scars and keloids: a review". *Plastic and Reconstructive Surgery,* 104:1435 - 58.

[21] English, Robert S. and Philip D. Shenefelt. 1999. "Keloids and hypertrophic scars". *Dermatologic Surgery,* 25:631 - 8.

[22] Kelly, A. P. 1988. "Keloids". *Dermatologic Clinics,* 6:413 - 24.

[23] Lee, Siong-See and Gil Yosipovitch, Yiong-Huak Chan, Chee-Leok Goh. 2004. "Pruritus, pain, and small nerve fiber function in keloids: a controlled study". *Journal of American Academy of Dermatology,* 51:1002 - 6.

[24] Bock, Oliver and Gerhard Schmid-Ott, Peter Malewski, Ulrich Mrowietz. 2006. "Quality of life of patients with keloid and hypertrophic scarring". *Archives of Dermatological Research,* 297:433 - 8.

In: Cutaneous Scars: Biology, Clinics and Management ISBN: 978-1-53615-657-7
Editors: Berna Aksoy, Hasan Mete Aksoy et al. © 2019 Nova Science Publishers, Inc.

Chapter 12

SCAR SCALES

Ilkay Ozer[1] and Meltem Onder[2,*]
[1]Department of Dermatology and Venerology, Meram Faculty of Medicine, Necmettin Erbakan University, Konya, Turkey
[2]Department of Dermatology, Faculty of Medicine, Gazi University, Ankara, Turkey

ABSTRACT

Scars can cause functional, aesthetic and psychological problems, and also can affect quality of life significantly. Scaling of a scar is extremely important in order to assess treatment efficacy and/or morbidity associated with scarring. The randomization of qualitative and quantitative measurement tools is crucially important in scaling of scars. Ideal assessment of scarring should include subjective and objective assessment tools together, the scale of choice should be easily applicable by the practitioners, it should yield consistent results in a short time. Different scar scales are summarized in this chapter.

Keywords: scale, scar scaling

1. INTRODUCTION

Scars can cause functional, aesthetic and psychological problems, and affect quality of life depending on their localization and nature [1, 2]. Scars can develop following any type of trauma, burn, surgical procedures or inflammatory skin diseases, and they are an important comorbidity since they may result in financial burden and impairment of an

[*]Corresponding Author's Email: meltemonder@yahoo.com.

individual's quality of life [3]. Although *scar scaling* is extremely important in order to assess treatment efficacy and/or morbidity associated with scarring, there is still no consensus regarding which *scale* to use [4].

2. The Purpose and Importance of Scar Scaling

The randomization of qualitative and quantitative characteristics of measurements in *scar scaling* is crucially important. There are tools such as ultrasonography and these tools can assess parameters such as topographic structure, flexibility, color, thickness, perfusion and stiffness, and and there are tools such as Optical Coherence Tomography, Pneumatometer, durometer, spectrophotometer which can perform three-dimensional measurements of skin surface topography. But the use of these tools is ineffective both in terms of cost and time, and they are not capable of assessing all aspects of scarring [4-7].

For an ideal assessment of scarring; the subjective and objective assessment should be performed together, the scar *scale* of choice should be easily applicable by the practitioners, it should not yield contradictory results and should provide results in a short time [8, 9].

The first assessment of scarring was performed by Garcia-Velasco et al. in order to evaluate hypertrophic burn scar treatment. Color (white, pink or purple, red), consistency (soft, moderately hard, hard) and thickness (flat, slightly raised, prominent) were evaluated individually, and scored between 1 and 3, but these were not merged into a single *scale* [4, 10].

In 1988, Smith et al. used color photographs of scars in order to determine the surface (smooth, partly irregular, mostly irregular), thickness (slight, moderate, severe), color (no difference, slightly darker, much darker) and general cosmetic shape (none, very slight, slight, moderate, severe, and very severe) of scars. However, it was noted that there was a high level of difference between assessment values among the observers in this scar assessment [4, 11]. The first *scale* defined in the literature for assessing scars was introduced in 1990, and there have been attempts to develop many new methods of *scar scaling* since then [12].

Different scar *scales* are summarized in Table 1 and in the following sections.

3. Vancouver Scar Scale and Modified Vancouver Scar Scale (VSS)

Initially used by Sullivan in 1990 for scoring burn scars, this method is currently one of the most commonly used scoring methods [13, 14]. Vascularization, pigmentation, scar height, and flexibility are assessed in this *scar scaling* method, and the total score ranges from 0 to 13 (Table 1) [4, 13].

Table 1. Scar scales

Scar scale	Parameters	
Vancouver Scar Scale (1990)	Vascularity	Normal 0
		Pink 1
		Red 2
		Purple 3
	Pigmentation	Normal 0
		Hypopigmentation 1
		Hyperpigmentation 2
	Height	Flat 0
		< 2 mm 1
		2-5 mm 2
		> 5 mm 3
	Pliability	Normal 0
		Supple 1
		Yielding 2
		Firm 3
		Ropes 4
		Contracture 5
Seattle Scale (1997)	Surface	Smooth: - 1
		Normal: 0
		Rough: (1 to 4)
	Thickness	Thinner: 1
		Normal: 0
		Thicker: (1 to 4)
	Border	Depressed: - 1
		Normal: 0
		Raised: (1 to 4)
	Color	Hypopigmented: - 1
		Normal: 0
		Hyperpigmented: (1 to 4)
Manchester Scar Scale (1998)	Visual Analog Scale	
	0 Poor <————————————————————> Excellent 10	
	Color	Perfect 1
		Slight mismatch 2
		Obvious mismatch 3
		Gross mismatch 4
	Matte vs shiny	Matte 1
		Shiny 2
	Contour	Flush with surrounding skin 1
		Slightly proud/Indented 2
		Hypertrophic 3
		Keloid 4
	Distortion	None 1
		Mild 2
		Moderate 3
		Severe 4
	Texture	Normal 1
		Just palpable 2
		Firm 3
		Hard 4

Table 1. (Continued)

Scar scale	Parameters
Hamilton Scale (1998)	Rate the thickness or height of scar: None: 0 Slight: 1 Moderate: 2 Severe: 3 Surface irregularity: Smooth:0 ¼ of scar area irregular: 1 ½ of scar area irregular: 2 ¾ of scar area irregular: 3 majority of the scar irregular: 4 Vascularity: Normal: 0 Light to medium pink: 1 Deep pink to light red: 2 Medium to deep red: 3 Purplish: 4 Color: Normal: 0 Slightly darker: 1 Darker: 2 Much darker: 3
Patient and Observer Scar Assessment Scale (2004)	Observer component: Normal skin 1<---------------------------------------> 10 Worst scar imaginable Vascularization: Pale Pink Red Purple Mix Pigmentation: Hypo Mix Hyper Thickness: Thicker Thinner Relief: More relief Less relief Mix Pliability: Supple Stiff Mix Surface area: Expansion Contraction Mix Overall opinion 1<--->10 Patient component: No, no complaints: 1<---------------------------------->10 Yes, worst imaginable Is the scar painful? Is the scar itching? No, as normal skin 1<---------------------------------->10 Yes, very different Is the color of the scar different? Is the scar more stiff? Is the thickness of the scar different? Is the scar irregular?
Long distance assesment (2004)	Color: Pale Pink Red Thickness yes-no Contractures yes-no Range of motion restricted or not; General level of activity restricted or not; Breakdowns of graft sites yes-no

Scar scale	Parameters
Matching Assessment of Scars and Photographs (2005)	Surface -1<------------------>4 Border height -1<----------------->4 Thickness -1<----------------->4 Color -1<----------------->4 Pigmentation -1<------->1 Overall opinion abour scar 0<---------------->4
Stony Brook Scar Evaluation Scale (2007)	Width > 2 mm - < 2mm (0 – 1 points) Height Elevated - depressed (0 – 1 points) Color Darker - same or lighter (0 – 1 points) Hatch marks or suture marks Present - absent (0 – 1 points) Overall appearance Poor - good (0 – 1 points) Total score from 0 to 5 points

Although VSS has been initially developed for burn scars, over time its use has spread to other scar types such as hypertrophic, and atrophic linear scars [7, 15-17]. This method of scoring has significant limitations such as inadequate level of assessment of large and irregular scars, lack of patient assessment of subjective symptoms such as pain and itching, and lower hypopigmentation scores compared to hyperpigmentation scores during the assessment of pigmentation [18, 19]. Therefore, it should be noted that it was not designed to indicate the severity of the burn scar, but to indicate the presence or absence of the pathological condition [9]. In order to clear up these limitations, Baryza et al. reported that the inter-observer reliability could be improved by modifying the pigmentation assessment [4, 20]. Forbes-Duchart et al. pointed out the difference in pigmentation among individuals with different skin color, and have suggested that there should be a different assessment according to skin color [21]. Another important modification is the regulation of pigmentation (differentiation as normal and severe hypo/hyper-pigmentation) and height assessment, and the addition of a visual analogue scale (VAS) [12, 22, 23].

4. Seattle Scale

Seattle *scale* developed by Yeong et al. in 1997 is a photographic scar assessment [24]. In this scoring *scale*, scar is compared to the adjacent intact skin, and scar surface, thickness, border, height, and color differences are assessed [4, 24]. In this *scale*, a scoring system ranging from -1 to 4 is used (0 is the normal value), and the biggest disadvantage of this method is that hypopigmentation and atrophic scar appearance may get negative points, thus decreasing the total score (Table 1) [9].

5. Manchester Scar Scale

Developed by Beausang et al. in 1998 by using the assessment of contour, radiance (matte or shiny), color, texture and distortion, this scale uses VAS and photographs [19, 25]. The authors noted that due to vascular changes it was difficult to distinguish color change from pigmentation, and they combined these two parameters into "color" assessment (perfect, slight mismatch, obvious mismatch, major mismatch) (Table 1) [9]. This *scale* is based on clinical and photographic characteristics, and histopathological confirmation of the scar assessment has been attempted [12, 25].

Clinical evaluation was compared with histopathologic examination (orientation, density and maturity of collagen fibers and epidermal changes), and a high level of correlation was observed [25]. It has also been reported that MSS can provide an effective assessment in evaluating linear scars [9, 12]. In this *scale*, other scar characteristics such as angiogenesis or melanin concentration cannot be assessed, and the effect of patient-reported symptoms, such as pain and itching, on quality of life is not assessed. These factors prevent this *scale* from becoming the gold standard [9].

6. Hamilton Scale

Developed by Crowe et al. in 1998, this less known *scar scaling* method is based on rating of photographs (Table 1) [26]. It is based on the assessment of various parameters such as surface irregularity, thickness, color and vascularity merely by using the examination of photographs [9, 26]. In contrast to the Seattle scar scale, Hamilton scar *scale* does not employ a negative scoring system, and new observers have high reliability as expected from experienced observers [26]. Although this *scale* has a high level of inter-observer reliability, a photo-based assessment is performed rather than a real-time assessment, and the subjective symptoms of the patient are not evaluated, which are considered as its limitations [12, 26].

7. Patient and Observer Scar Assessment Scale (POSAS)

Defined by Draaijers et al. in 2004 for burn scars, this *scale* is one of the commonly used scar *scales* [13, 27]. Since it takes into consideration both patient and observer assessment, it has been reported to be a more valuable method of scar measurement compared to the scales that include only observer or patient assessment (Table 1) [27-29]. In a study, scar assessment scores were compared between the patients and the clinicians, and it was observed that patients' scores were lower compared to those of the observers.

This once again emphasized the importance of both observer and patient assessment in *scar scaling* [30]. In addition to the assessment of vascularization, pigmentation, elasticity, thickness, relief, and surface area by the observer (rated between 1 and 10), the patient also assesses color, flexibility, thickness, relief, itching and pain and rates these parameters again in between 1 and 10 [31]. In 2005, the surface area assessment which had not been originally included was added to the *scale*, and it was reported that this *scar scaling* method, developed initially for burn scars, could also be used in linear scars and keloid scars owing to this addition [32, 33].

This POSAS system is an improved scar scoring method that assesses pain and itching, however, it does not take the effect of these symptoms on the quality of life into consideration [5]. It has been reported that the modified POSAS *scale*, which was developed to overcome this shortcoming, may contribute greatly to the assessment of scars as a result of the addition of the assessment of effects of scars on daily quality of life, such as pain and itching [28].

8. Long Distance Assessment

This scar *scale*, which was used by Smith et al. for the burn care routine of children hospitalized in long-distance hospitals in 2004, introduced the use of video conferencing system in the assessment of scars [34]. Six variables are assessed in this scoring system: color, scar thickness, contractures (assessed by patients following verbal instructions), limitation of movement (rated by patient and patient relatives), general activity, scar breakdown (scar depression) (Table 1). It was reported that the results were comparable to the results of face to face contact with patients [4, 34].

9. Matching Assessment of Scars and Photographs (MAPS)

Developed in 2005, this *scale* is the modified version of the Seattle scale [35]. It is based on the use of VAS, which assesses pain and itching, with the addition of assessing five parameters including edge height, thickness, color and pigmentation, surface and localization (Table 1) [9, 35]. It has been reported that the assessment of photographs may provide better information about the effectiveness of scar management due to the use of recorded data [35]. It has been noted that an extensive pre-training is not needed in order to use this *scale* [9].

10. Stony Brook Scar Evaluation Scale

Defined by Singer et al. in 2007, this *scale* includes an addition to the visual analog scoring, and is based on the assessment of width, height or depression, color, presence of suture marks and general appearance, each of which is scored from 0 to 1 giving the overall score from 0 (worst) to 5 (best) (Table 1) [36]. It has been reported that this score may not be adequate in assessing scars at a late stage since it was originally designed to assess scars at an early stage, and this scar *scale* can be used in the postoperative evaluation of keloid scars [36, 37]. This scoring system was designed to facilitate the assessment of wound healing and histopathologic examination of scars. Its limitation is that it does not include patient assessment of subjective symptoms [4].

11. Visual Analog Scale and Dermatology Life Quality Index

Visual analogue *scale* and dermatology life quality index were not originally developed with the purpose of *scar scaling*, and yet they have found their place among other scar *scales* to assess the effects of scar symptoms such as itching and pain on quality of life [12, 38].

VAS was developed to score subjective pain experience. In this *scale*, patients rank their pain intensity by putting a mark on a 10 cm long line (painless state 0, worst imaginable pain experience 10) in order to assess their pain experience [39]. As a *scar scaling*, digital photographs are assessed in four dimensions (pigmentation, vascularity, acceptability and observer comfort), and individual scores are summed up to get a single overall score ranging from "excellent" to "poor" [5]. It has demonstrated high observer reliability and consistency [5, 40]. It has been suggested that VAS can be used effectively both in monitoring and the evaluation of treatment as a *scar scaling* method [40, 41].

Dermatology Life Quality Index (DLQI), developed in 1994, is a scoring system used to assess the quality of life of individuals with dermatologic conditions [42]. Studies have reported that scars may cause behavioral and psychological morbidities such as physical discomfort and social dysfunction, thus affecting quality of life negatively [43]. It has been reported that the DLQI *scale*, which assesses parameters such as pain, itching and feeling of embarrassment, can also be a useful method in scar assessment [44, 45]. Similar to VAS, DLQI is not a system developed for scar assessment, and using these two *scales* together with other scar *scales* is recommended since these *scales* are effective methods for determining morbidity in scar scoring [12].

CONCLUSION

Several scar scoring methods have been developed since the introduction of Vancouver scar scale in 1990. Each has its benefits as well as its limitations, and there is still no scoring system which can be defined as the gold standard in the strictest sense. Currently, there is no scoring scale that examines both objective and subjective aspects of scars as well as their impact on the quality of life. There is a need for scales that can assess these parameters together.

REFERENCES

[1] Falder, Sian, and Allyson Browne, Dale Edgar, Emma Staples, Joy Fong, Suzanne Rea, Fiona Wood. 2009. "Core outcomes for adult burn survivors: a clinical overview." *Burns* 35:618-41. doi: 10.1016/j.burns.2008.09.002.

[2] Van Loey, Nancy E. E., and Maarten J. M. Van Son. 2003. "Psychopathology and psychological problems in patients with burn scars: epidemiology and management." *American Journal of Clinical Dermatology* 4:245-272. Doi: 10.2165/00128071-200304040-00004

[3] Sen, Chandan K., and Gayle M. Gordillo, Sashwati Roy, Robert Kirsner, Lynn Lambert, Thomas K. Hunt, Finn Gottrup, Geoffrey C. Gurtner, Michael T. Longaker. 2009. "Human skin wounds: a major and snowballing threat to public health and the economy." *Wound Repair and Regeneration* 17:763-771. doi: 10.1111/j.1524-475X.2009.00543.x.

[4] Brusselaers, Nele, and Ali Pirayesh, Henk Hoeksema, Jozef Verbelen, Stijn Blot, Stan Monstrey. 2010. "Burn scar assessment: a systematic review of different scar scales." The *Journal of Surgical Research* 164:e115-123. doi: 10.1016/j.jss.2010.05.056.

[5] Fearmonti, Regina, and Jennifer Bond, Detlev Erdmann, Howard Levinson. 2010. "A review of scar scales and scar measuring devices." *Eplasty* 10:e43.

[6] Kaartinen, Ilkka S., and Petri O. Valisuo, Vladimir Bochko, Jarmo T. Alander, Hannu O. Kuokkanen. 2011. "How to assess scar hypertrophy--a comparison of subjective scales and Spectrocutometry: a new objective method." *Wound Repair and Regeneration* 19:316-23. doi: 10.1111/j.1524-475X.2011.00679.x.

[7] Poetschke, Julian, and Hannah Schwaiger, Gerd G. Gauglitz. 2017. "Current and Emerging Options for Documenting Scars and Evaluating Therapeutic Progress." *Dermatologic Surgery* 43:S25-S36. doi: 10.1097/DSS.0000000000000698.

[8] Powers, P. S., and S. Sarkar, D. B. Goldgof, C. W. Cruse, L. V. Tsap. 1999. "Scar assessment: current problems and future solutions." The *Journal of Burn Care & Rehabilitation* 20:54-60.

[9] van der Wal, M. B., and P. D. Verhaegen, E. Middelkoop, P. P. van Zuijlen. 2012. "A clinimetric overview of scar assessment scales." *Journal of Burn Care & Research* 33:e79-87. doi: 10.1097/BCR.0b013e318239f5dd.

[10] Garcia-Velasco, M, and R. Ley, D. Mutch, N. Surkes, H. B. Williams. 1978. "Compression treatment of hypertrophic scars in burned children." *Canadian Journal of Surgery* 21:450-2.

[11] Smith, G. M., and D. M. Tompkins, M. E. Bigelow, A. Y. Antoon. 1988. "Burn-induced cosmetic disfigurement: can it be measured reliably?" The *Journal of Burn Care & Rehabilitation* 9:371-5.

[12] Nguyen, Tuyet A., and Stephanie I. Feldstein, Peter R. Shumaker, Andrew C. Krakowski. 2015. "A review of scar assessment scales." *Seminars in Cutaneous Medicine and Surgery* 34:28-36. doi: 10.12788/j.sder.2015.0125.

[13] Bae, Seong H., and Yong C. Bae. 2014. "Analysis of frequency of use of different scar assessment scales based on the scar condition and treatment method". *Archives of Plastic Surgery* 41:111-5. doi: 10.5999/aps.2014.41.2.111.

[14] Sullivan, T., and J. Smith, J. Kermode, E. McIver, D. J. Courtemanche. 1990. "Rating the burn scar." The *Journal of Burn Care & Rehabilitation* 11:256-60.

[15] Choi, Yuri, and Ji H. Lee, Yeon H. Kim, Yong S. Lee, Hang-Seok Chang, Cheong S. Park, Mi R. Roh. 2014. "Impact of postthyroidectomy scar on the quality of life of thyroid cancer patients." *Annals of Dermatology* 26:693-9. doi: 10.5021/ad.2014.26.6.693.

[16] Kim, Hyun K., and Mi K. Park, Beom J. Kim, Myeung N. Kim, Chan W. Kim, Sung E. Kim. 2012. "The treatment of keloids with pneumatic technology: a pilot study." *International Journal of Dermatology* 51:1502-7. doi: 10.1111/j.1365-4632.2012.05607.x.

[17] Kwon, S. Y., and S. D. Park, K. Park. 2014. "Comparative effect of topical silicone gel and topical tretinoin cream for the prevention of hypertrophic scar and keloid formation and the improvement of scars." *Journal of the European Academy of Dermatology and Venereology* 28:1025-33. doi: 10.1111/jdv.12242.

[18] Durani, Piyush, and D. A. McGrouther, M. W. J. Ferguson. 2009. "Current scales for assessing human scarring: a review." *Journal of Plastic, Reconstructive & Aesthetic Surgery* 62:713-20. doi: 10.1016/j.bjps.2009.01.080.

[19] Roques, C., and L. Teot. 2007. "A critical analysis of measurements used to assess and manage scars." The *International Journal of Lower Extremity Wounds* 6:249-53. DOI: 10.1177/1534734607308249.

[20] Baryza, M.J., and G. A. Baryza. 1995. "The Vancouver Scar Scale: an administration tool and its interrater reliability." The *Journal of Burn Care & Rehabilitation* 16:535-8.

[21] Forbes-Duchart, Lisa, and Sheryle Marshall, Anne Strock, Juliette E. Cooper. 2007. "Determination of inter-rater reliability in pediatric burn scar assessment using a modified version of the Vancouver Scar Scale." *Journal of Burn Care & Research* 28:460-7. Doi: 10.1097/BCR.0b013E318053D3BB

[22] Nedelec, B., and H. A. Shankowsky, E. E. Tredget. 2000. "Rating the resolving hypertrophic scar: comparison of the Vancouver Scar Scale and scar volume." The *Journal of Burn Care & Rehabilitation* 21:205-12.

[23] Nedelec, Bernadette, and Jose A. Correa, Grazyna Rachelska, Alexis Armour, Leo LaSalle. 2008. "Quantitative measurement of hypertrophic scar: intrarater reliability, sensitivity, and specificity." *Journal of Burn Care & Research* 29:489-500. doi: 10.1097/BCR.0b013e3181710869.

[24] Yeong, E. K., and R. Mann, L. H. Engrav, M. Goldberg, V. Cain, B. Costa, M. Moore, D. Nakamura, J. Lee. 1997." Improved burn scar assessment with use of a new scar-rating scale." The *Journal of Burn Care & Rehabilitation* 18:353-5.

[25] Beausang, E., and H. Floyd, K. W. Dunn, C. I. Orton, M. W. J. Ferguson. 1998. "A new quantitative scale for clinical scar assessment." *Plastic and Reconstructive Surgery* 102:1954-61.

[26] Crowe, J. M., and K. Simpson, W. Johnson, J. Allen. 1998. "Reliability of photographic analysis in determining change in scar appearance." The *Journal of Burn Care & Rehabilitation* 19:183-6.

[27] Draaijers, Lieneke J., and Fenike R. Tempelman, Yvonne A. Botman, Wim E. Tuinebreijer, Esther Middelkoop, Robert W. Kreis, Paul P. M. van Zuijlen. 2004. "The patient and observer scar assessment scale: a reliable and feasible tool for scar evaluation." *Plastic and Reconstructive Surgery* 113:1960-5.

[28] Fearmonti, Regina M., and Jennifer E. Bond, Detlev Erdmann, L. Scott Levin, Salvatore V. Pizzo, Howard Levinson. 2011. "The modified Patient and Observer Scar Assessment Scale: a novel approach to defining pathologic and nonpathologic scarring." *Plastic and Reconstructive Surgery* 127:242-247. doi: 10.1097/PRS.0b013e3181f959e8.

[29] Tyack, Zephanie, and Megan Simons, Anneliese Spinks, Jason Wasiak. 2012. "A systematic review of the quality of burn scar rating scales for clinical and research use." *Burns* 38:6-18. doi: 10.1016/j.burns.2011.09.021.

[30] Collins, Lindsey K., and Thomas J. Knackstedt, Pamela Ganger, Emily Scherer, Faramarz H. Samie. 2017. "Applying a Visual Assessment Tool to Facial Linear Scars." *Facial Plastic Surgery* 33:97-101. doi: 10.1055/s-0036-1597684.

[31] van der Wal, Martijn B., and Wim E. Tuinebreijer, Monica C. Bloemen, Pauline D. Verhaegen, Esther Middelkoop, Paul P. M. van Zuijlen. 2012. "Rasch analysis of

the Patient and Observer Scar Assessment Scale (POSAS) in burn scars." *Quality of Life Research* 21:13-23. doi: 10.1007/s11136-011-9924-5.

[32] van der Wal, Martijn B., and Wim E. Tuinebreijer, Asa Lundgren-Nilsson, Esther Middelkoop, Paul P. M. van Zuijlen. 2014. "Differential item functioning in the Observer Scale of the POSAS for different scar types." *Quality of Life Research* 23:2037-45. doi: 10.1007/s11136-014-0637-4.

[33] van de Kar, Annekatrien L., and Leonard U. Corion, Mark J. Smeulders, Lieneke J. Draaijers, Chantal M. A. M. van der Horst, Paul P. M. van Zuijlen. 2005. "Reliable and feasible evaluation of linear scars by the Patient and Observer Scar Assessment Scale." *Plastic and Reconstructive Surgery* 116:514-22.

[34] Smith, A. C., and R. Kimble, J. Mill, D. Bailey, P. O'Rourke, R. Wootton. 2004. "Diagnostic accuracy of and patient satisfaction with telemedicine for the follow-up of paediatric burns patients." *Journal of Telemedicine and Telecare* 10:193-8. Doi: 10.1258/1357633041424449

[35] Masters, Margot, and Margaret McMahon, Birgit Svens. 2005. "Reliability testing of a new scar assessment tool, Matching Assessment of Scars and Photographs (MAPS)." The *Journal of Burn Care & Rehabilitation* 26:273-84.

[36] Singer, Adam J., and Blavantray Arora, Alexander Dagum, Sharon Valentine, Judd E. Hollander. 2007. "Development and validation of a novel scar evaluation scale." *Plastic and Reconstructive Surgery* 120:1892-7. Doi: 10.1097/01.prs. 0000287275.15511.10

[37] Furtado, F., and B. Hochman, L. M. Ferreira. 2012. "Evaluating keloid recurrence after surgical excision with prospective longitudinal scar assessment scales." *Journal of Plastic, Reconstructive and Aesthetic Surgery* 65:e175-81. doi: 10.1016/j.bjps.2012.02.005.

[38] Quinn, James V., and George A. Wells. 1998. "An assessment of clinical wound evaluation scales." *Academic Emergency Medicine* 5:583-6.

[39] Scott, Jane, and E. C. Huskisson. 1976. "Graphic representation of pain." *Pain* 2:175-84.

[40] Duncan, Jonathan A., and Jeremy S. Bond, Tracey Mason, Anna Ludlow, Peter Cridland, Sharon O'Kane, Mark W. J. Ferguson. 2006. "Visual analogue scale scoring and ranking: a suitable and sensitive method for assessing scar quality?" *Plastic and Reconstructive Surgery* 118:909-18. Doi: 10.1097/01.prs. 0000232378.88776.b0

[41] Martin, Daniel, and Nisha Umraw, Manuel Gomez, Robert Cartotto. 2003. "Changes in subjective vs objective burn scar assessment over time: does the patient agree with what we think?" The *Journal of Burn Care & Rehabilitation* 24:239-44. DOI: 10.1097/01.BCR.0000075842.55039.03

[42] Finlay, A. Y., and G. K. Khan. 1994. "Dermatology Life Quality Index (DLQI)--a simple practical measure for routine clinical use." *Clinical and Experimental Dermatology* 19:210-6.

[43] Brown, B. C., and S. P. McKenna, K. Siddhi, D. A. McGrouther, A. Bayat. 2008. "The hidden cost of skin scars: quality of life after skin scarring." *Journal of Plastic, Reconstructive & Aesthetic Surgery* 61:1049-58. doi: 10.1016/j.bjps.2008.03.020.

[44] Balci, Didem D., and Tacettin Inandi, Cigdem A. Dogramaci, Ebru Celik. 2009. "DLQI scores in patients with keloids and hypertrophic scars: a prospective case control study." *Journal der Deutschen Dermatologischen Gesellschaft* 7:688-92. doi: 10.1111/j.1610-0387.2009.07034.x.

[45] Mazharinia, Nazila, and Shahin Aghaei, Zahra Shayan. 2007. "Dermatology Life Quality Index (DLQI) scores in burn victims after revival." *Journal of Burn Care & Research* 28:312-7. Doi: 10.1097/BCR.0B013E318031A151.

In: Cutaneous Scars: Biology, Clinics and Management ISBN: 978-1-53615-657-7
Editors: Berna Aksoy, Hasan Mete Aksoy et al. © 2019 Nova Science Publishers, Inc.

Chapter 13

ACNE SCAR SCALES

Neslihan Fisek Izci*
Department of Dermatology, Faculty of Medicine,
Bahçeşehir University, Istanbul, Turkey

ABSTRACT

Acne is a common disorder with a high prevalence among adolescents, and it frequently results in scars. Evaluating a scar's type and severity is a very important step in choosing the best treatment option. Several scales have been developed to classify acne scars and evaluate their types and severities. In this chapter, we review the most frequently used grading systems for postacne scarring.

Keywords: Acne scars, atrophic scars, grading, postacne scarring, scale

1. INTRODUCTION

Acne has a high prevalence (90–95%) among adolescents, and up to 12–14% of adults suffer from persistent acne lesions [1]. Scarring is a major and common long-term complication of acne. The prevalence of *postacne scarring* is estimated to be 1–11% in the general population [2]. All types of acne, from papulopustular to nodulocystic, can cause persistent scarring. Scarring can occur at any stage of the disease, and it is believed that early treatment of inflammatory and nodulocystic acne is the best way to prevent scars [3, 4]. *Acne scars* have been linked to physical and psychological distress,

*Corresponding Author's Email: neslifisek@gmail.com.

especially in adolescents suffering from poor self-esteem, depression, anxiety, embarrassment, anger, low academic performance, body image alterations and unemployment [2, 4].

2. The Purpose and Importance of Acne Scar Scaling

The nature and extent of *postacne scarring* is directly related to the initial inflammation's depth, intensity and duration [5]. *Acne scars* can be hypertrophic or atrophic, depending on their elevation or depression in relation to the skin's surface [6]. In 80 to 90% of cases, there is a loss of collagen in the dermis that results in *atrophic scars*. Less commonly, we see hypertrophic and keloidal scars, which show both excessive deposition of collagen and reduced collagenase activity [7, 8].

Based on the variety of scar subtypes, many therapy options are available [9]. There are several frequently used methods for evaluating and *grading* active acne lesions that allow for the benefits of treatment to be assessed. Evaluating the scar's type and severity is an important step in selecting the most appropriate therapeutic option [4]. In addition, evaluation allows comparisons to be made before and after treatment. Most dermatologists believe that systematic nomenclature is important for describing *acne scars;* however, in one study, only 39% of dermatologists were satisfied with the currently available classification systems [9]. Jacob et al. categorized *atrophic scars* into three subtypes: *ice pick, boxcar* and *rolling*. Sometimes, all of these subtypes can be observed in the same patient, and it can be difficult to differentiate between them. Therefore, some authors have proposed *acne scar grading* systems of varying complexities [4, 9]. Several of these systems will be described in detail below.

3. Goodman and Baron's Qualitative Global Scarring Grading System

This qualitative global scarring *grading* system is simple and universally accepted. In this system, four different grades are used to identify *postacne scarring* (Table 1). These grades may be further subdivided into focal areas of involvement. This system aims to establish a simple index of severity that can be compared over time between clinicians, and it can be used daily due to its quickness. It subdivides *acne scars* into Grades 1–4 based on the scars' severity (macular, mild, moderate or severe, respectively).

- *Grade 1* is macular acne scar seen as erythematous, hyperpigmented or hypopigmented lesions that are often localized to the epidermis or superficial dermis. Hyperpigmentation often occurs due to the post-inflammatory effect of acne and may settle with time, although it may require months or even years to be resolved. Hypopigmented areas, on the other hand, often represent end points of scar healing in acne and may not improve with time.

Table 1. Goodman and Baron's Qualitative Global Scarring Grading System

Grade	Level of disease	Characteristics	Examples of scars
1	Macular disease	Erythematous, hyper- or hypopigmented flat marks visible to the patient or observer and irrespective of distance.	Erythematous, hyper- or hypopigmented flat marks
2	Mild disease	Mild atrophy or hypertrophy that may not be obvious at social distances of 50 cm or greater and may be covered adequately by makeup, the normal shadow of shaved beard hair in males or normal body hair when the location is extrafacial.	Mild rolling or small, soft papular
3	Moderate disease	Moderate atrophic or hypertrophic scarring that is obvious at social distances of 50 cm or greater and is not covered easily by makeup, the normal shadow of shaved beard hair in males, or body hair when the location is extrafacial; however, it is still able to be flattened by manual stretching of the skin.	More significant rolling, shallow boxcar or mild-to-moderate hypertrophic or papular scars
4	Severe disease	Severe atrophic or hypertrophic scarring that is obvious at social distances of 50 cm or greater, is not covered easily by makeup or the normal shadow of shaved beard hair in males or body hair (extrafacial locations), and is not able to be flattened by manual stretching of the skin.	Punched out atrophic (deep boxcar), ice pick, bridges and tunnels, gross atrophy, dystrophic scars, significant hypertrophic scars or keloids

- *Grade 2* describes mildly atrophic or hypertrophic scars that may not be overly visible from a conversational distance of 50 cm or more. Makeup can often cover these marks. Mild rolling, atrophic-type scars and mild papular scars can be classified into this category.
- *Grade 3* comprises moderate acne scarring with significant contour abnormality. These scars can be flattened through stretching but cannot be easily covered with makeup. Examples include rolling scars, shallow boxcar scars and mild-to-moderate hypertrophic and papular scars.
- *Grade 4* represents the most severe and noticeable form of acne scarring. These lesions cannot be flattened through stretching, and they cannot be hidden by makeup. This type of scarring includes all deep atrophic and non-distensible scars (ice pick and deep boxcar scars), bridges and tunnels, dystrophic scars and severe cases of hypertrophic and keloid scars.

This *grading* system further categorizes scarring according to its distribution, with focal involvement of a single cosmetic area categorized as 'A' and two to three areas of discrete involvement categorized as 'B'.

The Qualitative Scarring *Grading* System proposed by Goodman and Baron appears simple and universally acceptable in cases with mild acne scarring with respect to the different scarring patterns and the easy-to-comprehend *grading* system. However, in severe cases, different patterns are often present simultaneously; thus, it may be difficult to differentiate and appropriately grade these scars using this scale [10, 11].

4. Goodman and Baron's Quantitative Global Scarring Grading System

In 2006, Goodman and Baron developed a scale for the global severity of acne scarring known as the Quantitative Global Scarring *Grading* System for *postacne scarring*. This assessment tool is based on both the type and number of scars, taking them into account based on a points system instead of a category system. The system's numerical scoring scale is subdivided based on scar severity as follows: macular and mild atrophic scars receive 1 point, moderately atrophic scars receive 2 points, severely atrophic scars receive 3 points and hyperplastic scars receive 4 points. The severity score is then multiplied by a factor depending on the lesion count (1 point if the lesion count < 10, 2 points if the lesion count is 11–20 and 3 points if the lesion count > 20).

The final score ranges from 0 to 84. A summary of the quantitative *grading* scale is shown in Table 2. The complexity of this *grading* system may pose a limitation regarding its use.

Table 2. Goodman and Baron's Quantitative Global Scarring Grading System

Grade (type)		No. of lesions		
		1–10	11–20	>20
A	Milder scarring (1 point each) Macular erythematous or pigmented Mildly atrophic dish-like	1 pts	2 pts	3 pts
B	Moderate scarring (2 points each) Moderately atrophic dish-like Punched out with shallow bases and small scars (< 5 mm) Shallow but broad atrophic areas	2 pts	4 pts	6 pts
C	Severe scarring (3 points each) Punched out with deep but normal bases, small scars (< 5 mm) Punched out with deep and abnormal bases, small scars (< 5 mm) Linear or troughed dermal scarring Deep and broad atrophic areas	3 pts	6 pts	9 pts
D	Hyperplastic papular scars	2 pts	4 pts	6 pts
E	Hyperplastic keloidal or hypertrophic scars	Area < 5 cm^2 6 pts	Area 5–20 cm^2 12 pts	Area > 20 cm^2 18 pts

One study evaluated the inter-rater reliability of the Goodman et al. Quantitative Global Acne Scarring *Grading* System and found a difference in inter-rater agreeability based on training level [12]. This system lacks reproducibility in clinical applications; therefore, a more objective *grading* system is necessary [11].

5. Echelle d'Evaluation Clinique des Cicatrices d'Acne (ECCA) Scale

A second quantitative *scale* is the Echelle d'Evaluation Clinique des Cicatrices d'Acne (ECCA) *scale* developed by Dreno et al. This *grading* system is based on the total number and individual types of scars (Table 3). Dreno et al. sought to create a standardized *scale* to use in clinical practice with the aim of standardizing discussions on scar treatment.

In this *grading* system, the scar is subdivided into types based on its morphology, and the grade is calculated by multiplying the semiquantitative scar score with an appropriate weighting factor. Principally, this *scale* identified six types of scars and assigned each of them a score that indicates its disfiguring impact: the weighting factor. The total score is the sum of the scar type and the extent of the lesion. Scores range from 0 to 540.

Despite the high inter-investigator reliability reported by Dreno et al.'s study, this *scale* has imperfections. The clinical relevance of the total score range and the scale's restriction of use to the face are some of the scale's limitations. Also, the *scale* is complex, requiring a 30-minute training session [11, 13].

6. The Global Scale for Acne Scar Severity (SCAR-S)

Tan et al. developed a six-category global severity *scale* (SCAR-S) for *grading postacne scarring* on the face, chest and back. Most other scales focus only on facial scarring, require individual scars to be counted or were developed to direct repair strategies; therefore, Tan et al. set out to develop a practical *scale* that was more inclusive. They evaluated SCAR-S with regard to acne severity and patient-reported scar severity. This *scale* does not require lesion counting, parallels the categories of a global acne severity *scale* and can be used in the context of evaluating overall acne severity. Furthermore, the SCAR-S includes both atrophic and hypertrophic scars as well as the face, chest and back.

Acne scar severity is evaluated using a 6-point and 6-category global system based on a global evaluation *scale* modified for *postacne scarring* (Table 4). The six categories range from 'clear' to 'extremely severe', and their scores range from 0 to 5. The scale is independently applied to the face, chest and back, and the scores are then combined to obtain a composite score.

Patients' self-assessments of *acne scarring* were significantly correlated with clinician evaluations for both facial SCAR-S and overall SCAR-S scores ($p < 0.001$), with r values of 0.31 and 0.30, respectively [11, 14].

Table 3. Echelle d'Evaluation Clinique des Cicatrices d'Acne (ECCA) Scale

Description	Weighting factor (a)	Semi-quantitative score (b)	Grading (a x b)
Ice pick/V-shaped atrophic scars, diameter of less than 2 mm, and punctiform	15	0 = no scars 1 = a few scars (<5) 2 = a limited number of scars (5–20) 3 = many scars (>20)	/______/
Boxcar/U-shaped atrophic scars, diameter of 2–4 mm, with sheer edges	20	0 = no scars 1 = a few scars (<5) 2 = a limited number of scars (5–20) 3 = many scars (>20)	/______/
Rolling/M-shaped atrophic scars, diameter of more than 4 mm, superficial and with irregular surfaces	25	0 = no scars 1 = a few scars (<5) 2 = a limited number of scars (5–20) 3 = many scars (>20)	/______/
Superficial elastolysis	30	0 = absent 1 = mild 2 = moderate 3 = intense	/______/
Subgrading 1			/______/
Hypertrophic inflammatory scars of less than two years of age	40	0 = no scars 1 = a few scars (<5) 2 = a limited number of scars (5-20) 3 = many scars (>20)	/______/
Keloid or hypertrophic scars of more than two years of age	50	0 = no scars 1 = a few scars (<5) 2 = a limited number of scars (5-20) 3 = many scars (>20)	/______/
Subgrading 2			/______/
Global score (subgradings 1 + 2) (0–540)			/______/

Table 4. The Global Scale for Acne Scar Severity (SCAR-S)

Category	Score	Description
Clear	0	No visible acne scars
Almost clear	1	Scars barely visible from 2.5 m away
Mild	2	Easily recognizable; less than half of the affected area (e.g., the face, back or chest) is involved
Moderate	3	More than half of the affected area (e.g., the face, back or chest) is involved
Severe	4	The entire area is involved
Very severe	5	The entire area has prominent atrophic or hypertrophic scars

CONCLUSION

A consensus regarding acne scar evaluation is currently lacking. Although several acne grading scales have been developed, they have many limitations. Thus, it is necessary to develop a well-validated, gold standard scale for use in both clinical practice and research trials. An objective measure of scar severity should be a component of global acne severity evaluations.

REFERENCES

[1] Fabbrocini, Gabriella and M. C. Annunziata, V. D'Arco, V. D. Vita, G. Lodi, M. C. Mauriello, F. Pastore, G. Monfrecola. 2010. "Acne Scars: Pathogenesis, Classification and Treatment''. *Dermatology Research and Practice,* 2010: 893080. doi: 10.1155/2010/893080.

[2] Fife, Douglas. 2016. "Evaluation of Acne Scars: How to Assess Them and What to Tell the Patient". *Dermatologic Clinics,* 34:207 - 13. doi: 10.1016/ j.det.2015.11.009.

[3] Cachafeiro, Thais H. and Gabriela F. Escobar, Gabriela Maldonado, Tania F. Cestari. 2014. "Translation into Brazilian Portuguese and validation of the

"Quantitative Global Scarring Grading System for Post-acne Scarring". *Anais Brasileiros de Dermatologica,* 89:851 - 3.

[4] Fabbrocini, Gabriella and Valerio De Vita, Antonella Cozzolino, Claudio Marasca, Caterina Mazzella, Ambra Monfrecola. 2012. "The Management of Atrophic Acne Scars: Overview and New Tools. "*Journal of Clinical and Experimental Dermatology Research,* S5:001. doi:10.4172/2155-9554.S5-001.

[5] Hirsch, R. J. and A. B. Lewis. 2001. "Treatment of Acne Scarring". *Seminars in Cutaneous Medicine and Surgery,* 20:190 - 8. Doi: 10.1053/sder.2001.27557.

[6] Chathra Namitha and Venkataram Mysore. 2018. "Resurfacing of facial acne scars with a new variable-pulsed Er:YAG laser in Fitzpatrick skin types IV and V". *Journal of Cutaneous and Aesthetic Surgery,* 11:20 - 5. doi: 10.4103/JCAS.JCAS_4_18.

[7] Abdel Hay, Rania and Khalid Shalaby, Hesham Zaher, Vanessa Hafez, Ching-Chi Chi, Sandra Dimitri, Ashraf F. Nabhan, Alison M. Layton. 2016. "Interventions for acne scars". *Cochrane Database of Systematic Reviews,* 4:CD011946. doi: 10.1002/14651858.

[8] Connolly, Deirdre and Ha L. Vu, Kavita Mariwalla, Nazanin Saedi. 2017. "Acne Scarring - Pathogenesis, Evaluation and Treatment Options". *Journal of Clinical and Aesthetic Dermatology,* 10:12 - 23.

[9] Petukhova, Tatyana A. and Negar Foolad, Neha Prakash, Vivian Y. Shi, Victoria R. Sharon, Lyndsay O'Brecht, Ifrah A. Ali, Stephanie Feldstein, Justin Halls, Qinlu Wang, Chin-Shang Li, Raja K. Sivamani. 2016. "Objective volumetric grading of postacne scarring". *Journal of the American Academy of Dermatology,* 75:229 - 31. doi: 10.1016/j.jaad.2016.03.002.

[10] Goodman, Greg J. and Jennifer A. Baron. 2006. "Postacne scarring: a qualitative global scarring grading system". *Dermatologic Surgery,* 32:1458 - 66. Doi: 10.1111/j.1524-4725.2006.32354.x.

[11] Clark, Ashley K. and Suzana Saric, Raja K. Sivamani. 2018. "Acne scars: How do we grade them?" *American Journal of Clinical Dermatology,* 19:139 - 44. doi: 10.1007/s40257-017-0321-x.

[12] Goodman, Greg J. and Jennifer A. Baron. 2006. "Postacne scarring--a quantitative global scarring grading system". *Journal of Cosmetic Dermatology,* 5:48 - 52. Doi: 10.1111/j.1473-2165.2006.00222.x.

[13] Dreno, B. and A. Khammari, N. Orain, C. Noray, C. Mérial-Kieny, S. Méry, T. Nocera. 2007. "ECCA grading scale: an original validated acne scar grading scale for clinical practice in dermatology". *Dermatology,* 214:46-51. Doi: 10.1159/000096912.

[14] Tan, Jerry K. L. and Jing Tang, Karen Fung, Aditya K. Gupta, D. Richard Thomas, Sheetal Sapra, Charles Lynde, Yves Poulin, Wayne Gulliver, Rolf J. Sebaldt. 2010. "Development and validation of a Scale for Acne Scar Severity (SCAR-S) of the face and trunk". *Journal of Cutaneous Medicine and Surgery,* 14:156 - 60. Doi: 10.2310/7750.2010.09037.

In: Cutaneous Scars: Biology, Clinics and Management
Editors: Berna Aksoy, Hasan Mete Aksoy et al.
ISBN: 978-1-53615-657-7
© 2019 Nova Science Publishers, Inc.

Chapter 14

DERMATOSES DEVELOPING ON SCAR TISSUE

Mualla Polat*[*] *and Tekden Karapinar
Department of Dermatology,
Faculty of Medicine, Bolu Abant Izzet Baysal University, Bolu,Turkey

ABSTRACT

While numerous diseases have been reported to emerge from scar tissues formed on the skin (most often resulting from burns, but also due to trauma, laceration, chronic venous ulcer, fistula, chickenpox and vaccination), the exact mechanism of this transformation is still unknown. The majority of these diseases are skin neoplasms, which often develop on burn scars. In this chapter, malignancies and other dermatoses that develop on scar tissue will be discussed.

Keywords: BCC, herpes zoster, malignancies, melanoma, morphea, neoplasms, pyoderma gangrenosum, sarcoidosis, sarcoma, SCC

1. INTRODUCTION

Many dermatoses can develop on the scar, especially on burn scars. The exact mechanism of development of them is still unknown. The majority of these disorders are skin cancers, which often develop on burn scars. In this chapter, various *neoplasms* and other dermatoses that can develop on scar tissue will be discussed.

[*]Corresponding Author's Email: polatmualla@gmail.com.

2. NEOPLASMS

Skin *malignancies* are the most common *malignancies* worldwide, with approximately 2-3 million keratinocytic skin cancer cases and 132,000 melanoma cases occurring each year. The most important environmental cause for skin cancer is exposure to ultraviolet (UV) radiation. In addition, scar tissue resulting from vaccination, burns, and other injuries can also cause skin cancer. For non-white ethnicities, scar tissue is thought to be a more common cause of skin cancer than UV exposure [1, 2].

Malignancies caused by burn scars were first described in the 1st century A.C. by Celsus. Later, Marjolin defined chronic ulcers developing on scar tissue [3], and Da Costa coined the term "Marjolin's ulcer" to describe the malignant transformation of skin wounds, and in particular, scar tissue [4]. Malignant transformations have been reported in various chronic scars, including chronic venous stasis ulcers, osteomyelitis, vaccination areas, pilonidal sinuses, urinary fistula, chronic hydradenitis suppurativa, frost bite, and skin graft donor regions [5]. Ewing underscored some features of tumors that develop on scars [3], including presence of scar tissue, presence of tumor at scar borders, lack of tumor presence at the site prior to scar, tumor histology consistent with skin tissue and cell types observed in scar tissue, and adequate interval between burn scar and tumor development.

The pathogenesis of skin *neoplasms* developing on chronic scar is thought to be different than that of other skin *neoplasms*, although this is not clearly known. In addition, factors influencing malignant transformation, recurrence, and metastatic spread have not yet been clearly elucidated.

It is thought that malignant degeneration results from recurring ulceration and healing of the scar tissue [3]. Other processes that play a role in malignant transformation include carcinogenic toxin formation in the scar tissue, having scar tissue that disturbs immunological mechanisms controlling new tumor formation, and having weak lymphatic regeneration in the scar, which results in reduction of antibody movement towards the damaged area. None of these aforementioned processes is believed to induce carcinogenesis on its own, but they are believed to accelerate the process [6].

The most common malignancy observed on burn scars is epidermoid carcinoma, followed by basal cell carcinoma and malignant melanoma. Sarcomas very rarely develop on burn scars [7]. Skin cancers developing on burn scars are reported to have higher rates of recurrence (16%) and mortality (21%) as well as poorer prognosis [4].

2.1. Squamous Cell Carcinoma (Epidermoid Carcinoma)

Squamous cell carcinoma (*SCC*) is defined as a malignant skin tumor originating from keratinocytes present in the epidermis [8]. The etiopathogenesis of SCC may include solar injury, arsenic exposure, thermal injury, chronic radiation, viral factors, and immune suppression.

Although the incidence of skin cancers in the general population varies between countries, the most common skin cancer is basal cell carcinoma (BCC) (70%), followed by *SCC* (15%) and melanoma. However, *SCC* is the most common (75%) skin cancer that develops on scar tissue [2], in particular, on burn scars. It has been reported that the interval between injury and onset of malignancy is on average 31 years, and the most commonly affected areas are the lower extremities (43.7%), upper extremities (22.4%), trunk (11.5%), and head (22.4%) [4].

Various explanations as to why *SCC* develops on scar tissue have been hypothesized. First, it has been proposed that burn tissues are immunologically unique [3]. There is evidence indicating that HLA-DR4 may be related to cancer development, while some researchers reported that patients with scar carcinoma have abnormalities in the p53 gene. Recent advances at the molecular level have led to research showing that scar *SCC* cases have Fas gene mutations in the apoptosis function region, which can contribute to neoplastic transformation [3]. It has been noted that carcinomas emerging primarily from burn scars develop as a result of decreased resistance to infections, while ulcers form due to weakened vascularity. In addition, one theory suggests that liberated tissue toxins can act as carcinogens, and therefore, the scar tissue may be more susceptible to the harmful effects of UV radiation [9]. Crawley et al. noted that some patients have lymphocytic infiltrate around the tumor; they hypothesized that this infiltrate may form an immunological connection with the tumor, restricting its spread, and therefore leading to better survival [10].

The age of onset between *SCC* emerging from normal tissue and scar tissue is quite different, as the age of onset from normal tissue is 65-70 years, while it is 50 years from scar tissue. *SCC* emerging from both normal and scar tissue is more common among males than females. *SCC* occurs on the head at a rate of 80-90%, while *SCC* emerging from scar tissue is more common in the extremities (rate of 60-70%). The average interval between a premalignant lesion to the onset of *SCC* is 10 years, whereas this time is approximately 30 years in cases of scar *SCC*. Skin *SCC* accounts for 16% of all skin malignancies, while scar *SCC* accounts for 75% of malignancies developing on scar tissue. Skin *SCC* rates of recurrence, metastasis, and mortality are 1.3-18%, 0.5-16%, and 1%, respectively, while the same rates for scar *SCC* are 10-37%, 35%, and 21%, respectively [4]. Interestingly, Koh et al. reported a case of pseudoangiomatous *SCC*, which is a very rare and aggressive variant of *SCC* that develops on a burn scar [11].

The development of *SCC* on scars other than burn scars has been reported. For example, Friedman et al. reported a case of a 62 year old female who developed *SCC* 59 years after getting a Leishmania scar on her right cheek [9].

In cases where the lesion is small and mobile, large surgical resection (at least 2 cm surgical border) is the most effective treatment of *SCC* that developed on a scar.

Amputation is an alternative option in cases where malignant cells have invaded very deep, making excision impossible [5]. There is very little published information regarding radiation treatment of Marjolin ulcers. However, radiation therapy has been used in cases when excision is not appropriate or when the patient declines surgical treatment [5].

2.2. Basal Cell Carcinoma

Basal cell carcinomas (*BCC*) originate from the basal cell layer of the epidermis. They are the most common skin malignancies, accounting for 75-80% of all skin cancers. Of all *BCC*s, 70-80% develop on the head and neck region [12]. *BCC* typically occurs in the fifth or sixth decades of life. It is characterized by destructive local growth, and metastasis is rare. There are five types of *BCC*, which depend on its clinical and histomorphological features, as follows: superficial, nodular, morpheaform, fibroepitheliomatous, and infundibulocystic [13]. While actinic injury is the main risk factor for *BCC* [14], trauma/burns also play a role in its development. *BCC*s are believed to develop from superficial burns, whereas SCCs tend to emerge from deeper and thicker burns [15].

*BCC*s account for 12% of all neoplasms that develop on scars. On the other hand, only 0.5% of *BCC*s develop on scar tissues [16]. *BCC*s that emerge from burn scars are often localized to the head and neck region. Less frequently, *BCC* can develop on the extremities and the chest [17].

There is not a clear connection between scar and malignancy; the mechanism of neoplasm development is not clearly understood. However, some researchers have hypothesized that reduced blood flow to the adnexa and epidermis as well as atrophy may play a role. In addition, it should be noted that scars are more susceptible to the destructive effects of actinic radiation, and the majority of these tumors have been associated with chronic solar dermatosis [17]. Keratosis (Figure 1) or fissure development may be seen in scars prior to the development of carcinoma. However, indurated, ulcerated, and elevated plaque formation should be considered as an indication of carcinoma [14].

The average age of onset for *BCC* developing on normal skin is 60 years, and is 55 years for *BCC* developing on scar tissue. The development of *BCC* on both normal and scar tissues is more frequent among males, and *BCC* is often localized to the head. *BCC* from normal tissue and scar tissue have similar general characteristics [4]. One study reported that 18% of 60 tumors developing on the legs, arms, scalp, and trunk showed signs of scars, while this rate was only 0.77% for other areas. Treves and Pack detected burn scar in only 7 of the 1,374 *BCC* cases they examined. Also in that study, scar tissue was detected in 6 of 42 patients who were followed up with a diagnosis of *BCC* [14].

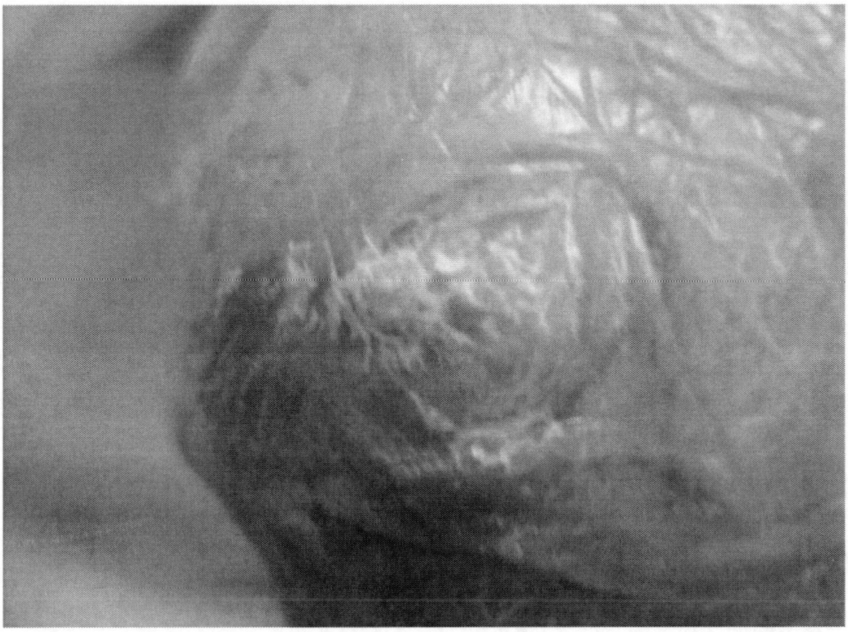

Figure 1. Scar keratosis developed on burn scar tissue on the elbow of a male patient (Courtesy of Berna Aksoy, MD).

There are a limited number of reports regarding the development of *BCC* on burns, vaccination scars, Leishmaniasis, cutaneous lupus, lupus vulgaris, epidermolysis bullosa, and surgical ulcer (such as Marjolin's ulcer). The cause of malignant transformation is still being studied. However, the elasticity and vascular structure of the scar lesion can cause the epithelium to become more sensitive to trauma and malignancy. Scar formation may disturb the epithelial-stromal relationship (e.g., local immune factors, cytokines, growth factors, and other messengers) and increase the production of stromal elements, such as metalloproteinases. In addition, the scar tissue often loses several immunological protective mechanisms, which may provide the right environment for malignant transformation and invasion [16].

In addition to burn scars, *BCC* has also been reported to develop on vaccination scars. Polat et al. and Nielsen [16, 18] reported that *BCC* cases can develop from Bacillus Calmette–Guerin (BCG) vaccine scars; Pace and Degaetano [1] indicated that they can develop from influenzae vaccine scars; and Goncalves, Riley and Zelickson [19-21] reported that *BCC* may develop from smallpox vaccine scars. Further, Smith et al. reported that *BCC* developed from a BCG vaccine scar in one patient and from a hepatitis A-typhus vaccine scar in another patient [22], while Curry et al. reported a case with *BCC* and dermatofibroma developing from a smallpox vaccine scar [23].

Surgical excision is recommended for lesions that fail to heal with conservative treatment. Mohs surgery is required when borders are obscure, such as in morpheaform BCCs [15].

2.3. Malignant Melanoma

*Melanoma*s originate from melanocytes, which are dendritic cells localized to the skin's basal layer. The incidence of *melanoma*s is increasing worldwide. *Melanoma*s account for 3% of all skin cancers and 65% of all skin cancer-related deaths. Risk factors for *melanoma*s include red hair color, light skin color, history of three or more sun burns before 20 years of age, recurring sun exposure, family history of *melanoma*, history of actinic keratosis, previous history of *melanoma*, and solarium use [24].

The pathogenesis of *melanoma* development on scars is still unclear. Some studies suggest that a carcinogenic toxin is produced at the site of the scar. Alternatively, some authors state that scars create an environment that is more susceptible to neoplastic growth [25]. Histologically, an intense fibrous reaction is observed in scar areas. This fibrous reaction disturbs the normal course of blood and lymphatic vessels, leading to reduced blood flow and subsequently reduced nutrition and oxygenation. This may potentially lead to regional immunodeficiency and a decrease in the vital capacity of immune cells, therefore providing the grounds for malignant transformation of melanocytes and neoplastic growth [25].

The first case of malignant *melanoma* (MM) developing on a burn scar was reported by Giblin et al. in 1965 [26, 27]. This was followed by a report from Gellin and Epstein in 1975, which revealed the development of MM in a fireman 9 years after he experienced burns. SCC and MM developing from burn scars were found to be similar in terms of lesion site, gender, and age distribution, while the rate of metastasis was reported to differ (30% in SCC and 75% in MM). The reason for the lower metastasis rate in SCC is thought to be due to the fact that the tumor is restricted within the scar tissue because of lymphatic fibrosis. Since MM developing on scar tissue has a high rate of metastasis, MM has more significance than SCC [27].

The mean age for *melanoma* diagnosis is 55.8 years. One important factor for *melanoma* emerging from burn scars is the interval between the date of injury and the *melanoma* diagnosis. This time can vary from 0 to 71 years, with an average of 43.8 years. Therefore, patients with burn scars should be followed-up for a long time in order to determine the possible development of malignancy [25]. Riberi et al. emphasized the importance of burn treatment, and noted that the early excision of necrotic scars and grafting can reduce the risk of neoplastic proliferation. Patients should be followed-up more carefully, especially when burn wounds are not properly surgically cleaned or are left to heal secondarily [25].

The recommended treatment for *melanoma* is lymph node dissection accompanied by large excision, which is performed via grafting [28]. Ryan et. al. reported that they successfully treated five patients with advanced stage cutaneous *melanoma* using the combination of 5-fluorouracil and surgery [29]. Hwang et al. treated a patient with lentigo maligna *melanoma* on the right arm with large excision and a split-thickness skin graft [30]. Further, Orlet et. al. treated an 87 year old patient with Clark stage 4 MM with large excision and skin grafting [31].

2.4. Sarcomas

*Sarcoma*s are solid tumors originating from bone or soft tissue. Only a small portion of primary mesenchymal tumors originate from the dermal layer. *Sarcoma*s have a more aggressive course and a higher risk of metastasis compared to SCC or BCC [32]. Chronic burn scars are well-known for their potential for malignant transformation. SCC, BCC, and MM are observed on burn scars with decreasing frequency, but it is very rare for sarcomas to develop on scar tissue [33].

The exact pathogenesis of malignant transformation is not known. Fleming and Rezek [34] suggested that the deep tissues are subjected to less trauma and have less tissue regeneration than the epidermis, which could play a role [33]. It is known that there is a long latent period between injury and development of malignancy. In their review, Can et al. reported the average interval between burn injury and tumor diagnosis in burn-related sarcomas was 35.7 years (range: 3-71 years) [33].

In 1941, Fleming and Rezek [34] reported a case that developed fibrosarcoma 49 years after burn scar development, which is the first reported case of a *sarcoma* developing on a scar. However, Gargan et al. [35] re-examined the photomicrographs from Fleming's article, and stated that according to the current pathological classification, that patient may have had malignant fibrous histiocytoma. Arons et al. [36] reported the second case of fibrosarcoma developing on a scar, which was localized to the scalp, while Greager et. al. reported the third fibrosarcoma case developing on a burn scar [37]. Since then, several other cases of fibrosarcoma developing on burn scar have been reported. Ozyagan et al. reported a 39 year-old female case with fibrosarcoma developing on scar tissue at the scalp [7]. Yamamura et al. reported a rare malignant fibrous histiocytoma that developed on a burn scar on the left arm of a 29 year-old male patient [38]. Gargan et al. [35] and Cocke and Tomlinson [39] also reported malignant fibrous histiocytoma cases, while Horton et. al [40] and Nishimoto et. al. [41] reported cases with liposarcoma developing on scar tissue. Other rare tumors emerging from scar tissue include carcinosarcoma [40], osteogenic sarcoma [42], malignant schwannoma [43], mesenchymal malignancy [44], and leiomyosarcoma [33].

Fibrosarcoma is more frequently observed on scar tissue, and this is thought to be due to the fact that scar tissue contains an abundant number of fibroblasts [7]. Of the four burn fibrosarcomas reported in the literature, three were localized to the head and neck region; therefore, it is concluded that the head and neck region is the most common localization for fibrosarcoma originating from burn scar [7].

Scar-related epithelial cancers are known to have a more aggressive behavior compared to those developing on normal tissue. However, it is not clear whether scar-related *sarcomas* are more aggressive than similar tumors originating from healthy skin. Large excision is the recommended treatment for scar-related epithelial cancer and sarcomas [7].

2.5. Others

2.5.1. Plasmacytoma

It is well-known that malignant tumors can develop on scar tissue. In addition, plasmacytomas may develop on trauma and scar areas as well. There are few reported cases of multiple myeloma being associated with development of plasmacytoma in trauma areas. The exact mechanism for plasmacytoma development on trauma sites is not known [45]. Cotter and Enright reported the case of a 76 year-old male patient who had monoclonal gammopathy for 14 years, and developed plasmacytomas on incision scars used to treat the right humerus bone traumatic fractures and on the sternotomy incision scar [46]. Li et al. described the development of a plasmacytoma on the left infraclavicular area 1 year after the implantation of a pacemaker in a 89 year-old male patient [45].

2.5.2. Traumatic Neuroma

Traumatic neuromas are benign lesions that most often develop after a surgical operation. These are not true neoplasms. Traumatic neuromas represent the nerve's healing response to induced damage, and often occur as a palpable nodule. They develop secondary to irregular nerve and connective tissue proliferation, which happens when the body tries to regenerate injured tissue following complete or partial nerve laceration due to an accident or surgical trauma [47].

Traumatic neuromas rarely develop on scar tissue. Most of the reported cases developed on mastectomy scars. In their 2012 literature review, Li et al. reported 10 cases with co-existing breast cancer and traumatic neuroma [47]. Baltalarlı et al. reported the case of a 54 year-old female with traumatic neuroma developing on a mastectomy scar [48].

2.5.3. Atypical Fibroxanthoma

Atypical fibroxanthoma is a rare neoplasm that typically presents as a painless, hard, skin-colored/brown, often ulcerated, and usually immobile nodule. This condition is often a result of fibrocytic or myofibrocytic differentiation that develops rapidly (within months) in the sun-exposed areas of elderly individuals. UV exposure, radiation, and immunosuppression are the most likely risk factors. Despite its malignant histopathological appearance, atypical fibroxanthoma often has a benign course and rarely metastasizes [49]. Its etiopathogenesis is not clearly known, and its diagnosis is made by the exclusion of other malignant tumors. It is believed to be a superficial variant of malignant fibrous histiocytoma. It has also been proposed to be a different variant of squamous cell carcinoma [50]. Local excision is curative for most patients [49].

Francesco et al. reported the case of a 69 year old male with discoid lupus erythematosus (DLE) for 20 years who developed atypical fibroxanthoma on the DLE scar localized to the left temporal area [49]. The authors hypothesized that local immunosuppression due to the scar as well as UV exposure were the underlying environmental factors for tumor development [49].

Ito et al. reported two cases of atypical fibroxanthoma. One of these was on the sun-exposed left cheek area of a 95 year-old woman, and the other was on a burn scar localized on the upper back area of a 93 year-old men [50]. The authors noted that the latter developed on a burn scar that was not exposed to the sun, and they did not detect any immunohistochemical differences between the two cases [50].

3. Other Dermatoses

3.1. Sarcoidosis

Sarcoidosis is a multi-system disease characterized by non-caseating granulomas. Its etiology is not clearly known [51]. This disease is more common between the ages of 20-29 years in both sexes, and in women older than 50 years of age [52]. *Sarcoidosis* can affect the lungs, lymph nodes, liver, spleen, phalangeal bones, parotid glands, eyes and skin. Cutaneous symptoms are common and may be the initial signs of the systemic inflammatory process [53]. Skin involvement is seen in 25% of *sarcoidosis* cases. Cutaneous *sarcoidosis* may present with numerous polymorphous signs and can mimic various diseases [51]. In 20-35% of *sarcoidosis* cases, cutaneous involvement manifests as disease-specific and non-specific lesions. Disease-specific lesions include macules, papules, plaques, nodules, lupus pernio, scar, alopecia, ulcerations, and hypopigmentations accompanied by histopathological non-caseating granulomas. Scar *sarcoidosis* occurs in areas with increased scar tissue thickness, that is a result of infiltration by sarcoidal granulomas, and is characterized by a more erythematous and violaceous discoloration of the scar (Figure 2). The prevalence of scar *sarcoidosis* varies between 5.4% and 13.8%. It is a rarer form of *sarcoidosis* compared to the other cutaneous types [52].

The pathogenesis of scar *sarcoidosis* is not known. However, it has been proposed that the activated T-cell mediated immune response targeting foreign bodies persisting in the tissue after trauma in genetically susceptible individuals plays a role [53-55]. Dal

Sacco et al. suggested that scar *sarcoidosis* may be a special form of patergy, similar to the patergy reaction in Behçet's disease [56].

Scar *sarcoidosis* can develop on surgical scars, fresh tattoos, on herpes zoster or burn scars, vaccine scars, intravenous or intramuscular injection sites, and at sites where injection is made for desensitization. It can manifest as an infiltration of older wounds, or as small red-brown colored nodules developing around these areas [52, 57]. The diagnosis of scar *sarcoidosis* is often missed because it is typically confused with hypertrophic scar. Further, *sarcoidosis* responds to intralesional steroid treatment. Therefore, this rare form of *sarcoidosis* should be considered when an unexpected change or growth occurs in an otherwise inactive scar, and should always be evaluated via histopathological examination [58].

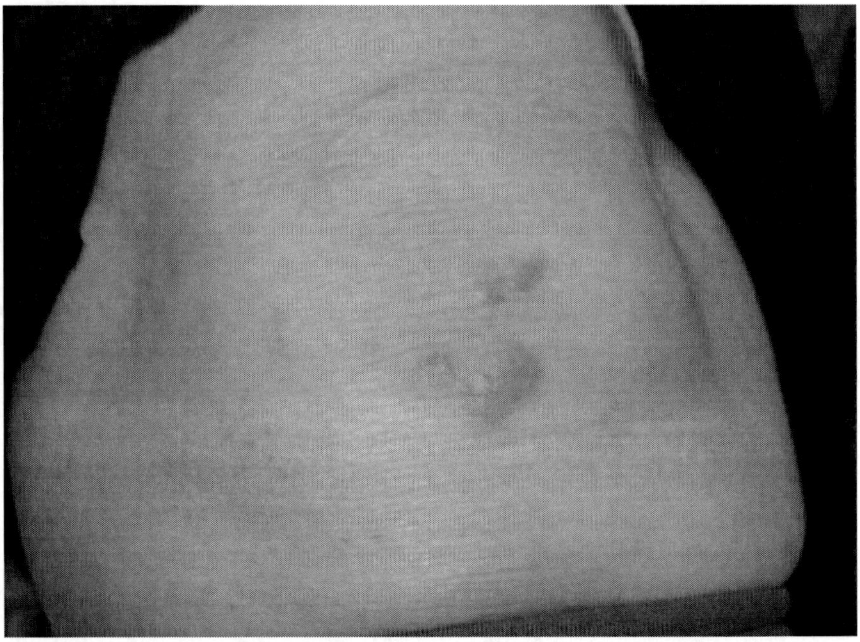

Figure 2. Sarcoidosis of scars, which are due to a traffic accident 35 years ago, on the knee of a 58 year old female (Courtesy of Berna Aksoy, MD).

Some believe that scar *sarcoidosis* is correlated with systemic disease activity. In fact, cases with scar *sarcoidosis* had more frequent pulmonary parenchymal involvement than those with accompanying erythema nodosum lesion. Because of this, systemic involvement signs should be carefully questioned and investigated in cases with a diagnosis of scar *sarcoidosis* [52, 57].

The differential diagnosis of scar *sarcoidosis* includes foreign body-type granulomatous reaction, hypertrophic scar tissue, and keloid. However, studies have shown the presence of polarized material in 5% of cases with *sarcoidosis*, and therefore, it should be noted that this polarized material does not exclude the diagnosis of *sarcoidosis* [52, 59].

In some cases, scar *sarcoidosis* may be the first and only skin finding of systemic *sarcoidosis*. Since obtaining biopsy from skin is easier than obtaining biopsy from internal organs, this underscores the importance of cutaneous signs [52].

Scar *sarcoidosis* may heal spontaneously. However, topical steroids, tacrolimus, or hydroxychloroquine are known effective therapeutic agents [60]. The treatment of systemic *sarcoidosis* depends on the severity of the disease; prednisone is the most commonly used treatment [51].

3.2. Morphea

Morphea is characterized by local collagen accumulation in the skin, has an unknown etiology, and resembles scleroderma. It has been proposed that *morphea* begins with unidentified antigens that interact with host's immune system. Reported triggers include trauma, radiotherapy, BCG vaccine, pregnancy, Borrelia burgdorferi infections, silicone prosthesis implantation, viral factors, toxic factor and neurogenic factors [61].

Although trauma has been reported to be a trigger for *morphea*, the exact mechanism remains unknown. Trauma-related vascular injury and fibroblast activation may explain the pathogenesis of *morphea* development due to trauma. However, the exact cause of immunological activation and the development of *morphea* in patients with trauma induced scar remains unknown. Schaffer emphasized that radiation-related neoantigens are important in the development of radiation-induced *morphea* [62].

Morphea developing on a scar has been rarely reported in the literature. Terao et al. reported the case of a 56 year-old female developing *morphea* on a surgical scar 1 year after laparoscopic cholecystectomy. The authors noted that the surgical procedure caused dermal cell modification, which may have led to immune activation, or it may have been due to a foreign antigen [61].

3.3. Pyoderma Gangrenosum

Pyoderma gangrenosum (PG) is a neutrophilic dermatosis characterized by painful and progressive ulcerations. Its etiology is not fully understood. PG may occur after a systemic disease (e.g., rheumatoid arthritis or inflammatory bowel disease) or trauma. Surgical debridement may worsen the condition, leading to large ulcerations and scars

[63]. The Patergy phenomenon may explain the development of PG following minor injuries or surgical operations in cases who do/do not have systemic autoimmune disease [64].

PG developed on a scar has been rarely reported in the literature. Castillo et al. reported a 47 year-old male developing PG on an arteriovenous fistula scar on the right arm associated with hemodialysis [64]. Segaran et al. reported a 31 year-old healthy female who developed PG on the operation scar 7 years after breast reduction surgery [63].

3.4. Herpes Zoster

Herpes zoster is a common dermatologic disease caused by the reactivation of the varicella zoster virus. It usually affects one side and is characterized by painful vesicles on the sensory dermatomes [65]. Weakened cellular immune system and advanced age are among the known risk factors. Clinical reports and case series have indicated that mechanical trauma is a possible risk factor. *Herpes zoster* rashes have been reported following cryosurgery, liver biopsy, axillary nerve blockade, spinal surgery, intubation and massage over the dermatomes that underwent trauma [65]. Trauma and surgical operations are known to reactivate the *herpes zoster* virus, although the mechanism remains unclear [66].

The development of *herpes zoster* on a scar is rare. Reported cases in the literature include a 35 year-old female patient who developed a *herpes zoster* lesion at the level of the left 7th rib following osteoblastic osteosarcoma surgery [66], a 74 year-old male patient who developed a lesion at the right lower lung lobe cutaneous area following surgery performed for lung metastasis of rectum cancer [67], and a 29 year-old male patient who developed *herpes zoster* at the left periorbital area following trauma [65].

Conclusion

Many dermatoses can develop on the scar, especially on burn scars. Malignancies (SCC, BCC, malignant melanoma, sarcomas, and other neoplasms) develop more frequently on scars, but many other dermatoses can also occur such as sarcoidosis, morphea, pyoderma gangrenosum and herpes zoster. Burn scar tissue has a greater risk of malignancy development and should be followed up for a long time. Excision and grafting of deep burns, and close follow-up of non-healing ulcerated burn scars are essential for the prevention and early detection of burn scar neoplasms.

REFERENCES

[1] Pace, Alistair, and James Degaetano. 2004. 'Basal cell carcinoma developing in an influenza vaccine scar.' The *Australasian Journal of Dermatology* 45:75-6.

[2] Wallingford, Sarah C., and Catherine M. Olsen, Elsemieke Plasmeijer, Adele C. Green. 2011. 'Skin cancer arising in scars: a systematic review.' *Dermatologic Surgery* 37:1239-44. doi: 10.1111/j.1524-4725.2011.02060.x.

[3] Kowal-Vern, Areta, and Bryan K. Criswell. 2005. 'Burn scar neoplasms: a literature review and statistical analysis.' *Burns* 31:403-13. DOI: 10.1016/j.burns. 2005.02.015.

[4] Huang, Chun-Yuan, and Chung-Ho Feng, Yen-Chang Hsiao, Shiow S. Chuang, Jui-Yung Yang. 2010. 'Burn scar carcinoma.' The *Journal of Dermatological Treatment* 21:350-6. doi: 10.3109/09546630903386580.

[5] Ozek, Cuneyt, and Ruhi Cankayali, Ufuk Bilkay, Ulvi Guner, Hakan Gundogan, Ecmel Songur, Yalcin Akin, Arman Cagdas. 2001. 'Marjolin's ulcers arising in burn scars.' The *Journal of Burn Care & Rehabilitation* 22:384-9.

[6] Gül, Ülker, and Arzu Kılıç, Nilüfer Halilzade. 2004. 'The Rate, Demographic and Clinical Features of the Squamous Cell Carcinoma Developing on Burn Scar.' *Turkiye Klinikleri Journal of Dermatology* 14:119-22.

[7] Ozyazgan, Irfan, and Olgun Kontaş. 1999. 'Burn scar sarcoma.' *Burns* 25:455-8.

[8] Cavaliere, Raymond, and Danielle M. Mercado, Malary Mani. 2018. 'Squamous Cell Carcinoma From Marjolin's Ulcer of the Foot in a Diabetic Patient: Case Study.' The *Journal of Foot and Ankle Surgery* 57:838-43. doi: 10.1053/j.jfas. 2017.11.016.

[9] Friedman, Robin, and Sonali Hanson, Leonard H. Goldberg. 2003. 'Squamous cell carcinoma arising in a Leishmania scar.' *Dermatologic Surgery* 29:1148-9.

[10] Crawley, W. A., and A. L. Dellon, J. J. Ryan. 1978. 'Does Host Response Determine the Prognosis in Scar Carcinoma?' *Plastic and Reconstructive Surgery* 62:407-14.

[11] Koh, Sung H., and Suk J. Oh, Huan Chun, Seon G. Kim. 2014. 'Pseudoangio-sarcomatous squamous cell carcinoma developing on a burn scar: a case report and review of the literature.' *Burns* 40:e47-e52. doi: 10.1016/j.burns.2014.02.019.

[12] Goder, M., and R. Kornhaber, D. Bordoni, E. Winkler, J. Haik, A. Tessone. 2016. 'Cutaneous basal cell carcinoma arising within a keloid scar: a case report.' *Onco Targets and Therapy* 9:4793. doi: 10.2147/OTT.S113724.

[13] Jones, M., and M. Bresch, D. Alvarez, A. Böer. 2009. 'Keloidal basal cell carcinoma: not a distinctive clinicopathological entity.' The *British Journal of Dermatology* 160:127-31. doi: 10.1111/j.1365-2133.2008.08828.x.

[14] Connolly, J. 1960. 'Basal cell carcinoma occurring in burn scars.' *Canadian Medical Association Journal* 83(27):1433.

[15] Kannan, Ruben Y., and Gulriaz K. Rauf. 2010. 'Acute burn scar basal cell carcinoma.' *Annals of Plastic Surgery* 64:321-2. doi: 10.1097/SAP.0b013e3181a72f29.

[16] Polat, Mualla, and Ali H. Parlak, Oguz Hasdemir, Çetin Boran. 2009. 'Basal cell carcinoma in a bacillus Calmette–Guérin scar.' *International Journal of Dermatology* 48(5):542-3. doi: 10.1111/j.1365-4632.2009.03930.x.

[17] Koga Y., and Y. Sawada. 1997. 'Basal cell carcinoma developing on a burn scar.' *Burns* 23(1):75-7.

[18] Nielsen, T. 1979. 'Basal cell epithelioma in a BCG vaccination scar.' *Archives of Dermatology* 115(6):678.

[19] Goncalves, J. A. 1966. 'Malignant change in smallpox vaccination scars.' *Archives of Dermatology* 93:229-30.

[20] Riley, K. A. 1970. 'Basal Cell Epithelioma in Smallpox Vaccination Scar: Report of a Case.' *Archives of Dermatology* 101:416-7.

[21] Zelickson, A. S. 1968. 'Basal cell epithelioma at site and following smallpox vaccination: report of a case.' *Archives of Dermatology* 98:35-6.

[22] Smith, V., and C. Soon, B. Dharma, E. Eltigani, A. Bedlow, R. Carr. 2008. 'Basal cell carcinomas arising in travel vaccination scars.' *Clinical and Experimental Dermatology* 33:515-6. doi: 10.1111/j.1365-2230.2008.02750.x.

[23] Curry, Jonathan L., and Steven J. Goulder, Brian J. Nickoloff. 2008. 'Occurrence of a basal cell carcinoma and dermatofibroma in a smallpox vaccination scar.' *Dermatologic Surgery* 34:132-4. Doi: 10.1111/j.1524-4725.2007.34021.x.

[24] Dzwierzynski, William W. 2013. 'Managing malignant melanoma.' *Plastic and Reconstructive Surgery* 132:446e-60e. doi: 10.1097/PRS.0b013e31829ad411.

[25] Ribero, Simone, and Marcella Grassi, Virginia Caliendo, Danilo Lauro, Giuseppe Macripò. 2012. 'Melanoma arising on a scar 10 years after a burn: management and review of the literature.' *Annals of Plastic Surgery* 69:27-9. doi: 10.1097/SAP.0b013e318250f084.

[26] Kikuchi, Hidezumi, and Takaaki Nishida, Motoki Kurokawa, Mitsuru Setoyama, Atsushi Kisanuki. 2003. 'Three cases of malignant melanoma arising on burn scars.' The *Journal of Dermatology* 30:617-24.

[27] Goldberg, Neil S., and June K. Robinson, Carol Peterson. 1985. 'Gigantic malignant melanoma in a thermal burn scar.' *Journal of the American Academy of Dermatology* 12:949-52.

[28] Sheff, Jordan S., and Thomas A. Pane. 2009. 'Spindle cell melanoma arising from decades-old burn scar.' *Plastic and Reconstructive Surgery* 124:274e-5e. doi: 10.1097/PRS.0b013e3181b98e1a.

[29] Ryan, Robert F., and Martin S. Litwin, Edward T. Krementz. 1981. 'A new concept in the management of Marjolin's ulcers.' *Annals of Surgery* 193:598.

[30] Hwang, Kun, and Jin Y. Han, Se I. Lee. 2004. 'Multiple malignant melanomas at different burn scar areas: a case report.' *Dermatologic Surgery* 30:562-5. Doi: 10.1111/j.1524-4725.2004.30179.x.

[31] Orlet, Hermann K., and Joseph Still, Edward Law, Charles Gertler. 2001. 'Malignant melanoma in a burn scar.' *Annals of Plastic Surgery* 46:59-61.

[32] Patt, Joshua C., and Nikkole Haines. 2016. 'Soft tissue sarcomas in skin: presentations and management.' *Seminars in Oncology* 43:413-8. doi:10.1053/j.seminoncol.2016.02.026.

[33] Can, Zeki, and Sarper Yilmaz, Ali R. Erçöçen, Ilker Apaydin, Isinsu Kuzu. 1998. 'Sarcoma developing in a burn scar: case report and review of the literature.' *Burns* 24:68-71.

[34] Fleming, R. M., and P. R. Rezek. 1941. 'Sarcoma developing in an old burn scar.' *American Journal of Surgery* 54:457-65.

[35] Gargan, T. J., and L. Mitchell, W. Plaus. 1988. 'Burn scar sarcoma.' *Annals of Plastic Surgery* 20:477-80.

[36] Arons, M. S., and J. Lynch, S. Lewis, T. Blocker Jr. 1965. 'Scar tissue carcinoma Part I. A clinical study with special reference to burn scar carcinoma.' *Annals of Surgery* 161:170.

[37] Greager, J. A., and K. Reichard, J. P. Campana, T. K. D. Gupta. 1994. 'Fibrosarcoma of the head and neck.' *American Journal of Surgery* 167:437-9.

[38] Yamamura, T., and K. Aozasa, T. Honda, A. Takada, M. Maeda, S. Sano. 1984. 'Malignant fibrous histiocytoma developing in a burn scar.' The *British Journal of Dermatology* 110:725-30.

[39] Cocke, W., and J. Tomlinson. 1993. 'Malignant fibrous histiocytoma developing in burn scar of the ear.' *Burns* 19:241-3.

[40] Horton, C. E., and H. H. Crawford, H. G. Love, R. A. Loeffler. 1958. 'The malignant potential of burn scar.' *Plastic and Reconstructive Surgery and Transplantation Bulletin* 22:348-53.

[41] Nishimoto, S., and T. Matsushita, K. Matsumoto, S. Adachi. 1996. 'A rare case of burn scar malignancy.' *Burns* 22:497-9.

[42] Drut, Ricardo, and Leonardo Barletta. 1975. 'Osteogenic sarcoma arising in an old burn scar.' *Journal of Cutaneous Pathology* 2:302-6.

[43] Scott, J., and R. Morris, A. McPhaden, S. Knight, M. Webster. 1996. 'Malignant schwannoma in a burn scar.' *Burns* 22:494-6.

[44] Çeliköz, B., and M. Demiriz, N. Selmanpakoglu. 1997. 'A shorter lag period of mesenchymal malignancy on Marjolin's ulcer.' *Burns* 23:72-4.

[45] Li, Anthony, and Alexander Chen, Mark Gallagher, Pawel Kaczmarek, Brendan Tinwell, James Sneddon, Sandeep Cliff. 2013. 'Primary cutaneous plasmacytoma occurring after pacemaker implantation and recurring in scar tissue.' *Dermatology Online Journal* 19:3.

[46] Cotter, Melanie, and Helen Enright. 2003. 'Plasmacytoma occurring in scar tissue.' *British Journal of Haematology* 121:680.

[47] Li, Quan, and Er-li Gao, Yin-long Yang, Hong-ye Hu, Xiao-qu Hu. 2012. 'Traumatic neuroma in a patient with breast cancer after mastectomy: a case report and review of the literature.' *World Journal of Surgical Oncology* 10:35.

[48] Baltalarli, B., and N. Demirkan, B. Yağci. 2004. 'Traumatic neuroma: unusual benign lesion occurring in the mastectomy scar.' *Clinical Oncology (Royal College of Radiologists)* 16:503-4.

[49] De Francesco, V., and E. Errichetti, E. Pegolo, G. Stinco. 2014. 'Atypical fibroxanthoma arising in a scar of discoid lupus erythematosus.' *Journal of Cutaneous Medicine and Surgery* 18:353-5. Doi: 10.2310/7750.2013.13144.

[50] Ito, Ayako, and Nanako Yamada, Yuichi Yoshida, Shinichi Morino, Osamu Yamamoto. 2011. 'Myofibroblastic differentiation in atypical fibroxanthomas occurring on sun-exposed skin and in a burn scar: an ultrastructural and immunohistochemical study.' *Journal of Cutaneous Pathology* 38:670-6. doi: 10.1111/j.1600-0560.2011.01708.x.

[51] Aktimur, Recep, and Sude H. Aktimur, Elif Çolak, Ömer Alıcı, Mehmet D. Demirağ. 2014. 'Old-scar mass and changing surgical perspective: Sarcoidosis.' *Turkish Journal of Surgery* 31:47-8. doi: 10.5152/UCD.2014.2693.

[52] Gerçeker Türk, Bengu, and Tugce Özkapu, Meltem Türkmen, Alican Kazandı, Can Ceylan. 2013. 'Scar sarcoidosis.' *Turkderm* 47:66-8. Doi: 10.4274/turkderm.68736.

[53] Kocak, Cengiz, and Ergin Yücel, Nazlı D. Namdar, Hasan Tak. 2015. 'A case of scar sarcoidosis developing in an old scar area on the forehead.' *Acta Dermatovenerologica Alpina, Pannonica, et Adriatica* 24:61-3.

[54] Zampino, Maria R., and Monica Corazza, Alessandro Borghi, Andrea Marzola, Annarosa Virgili. 2009. 'HLA typing in an IFN-α-induced scar sarcoidosis: possible pathogenetic and clinical implications.' *Acta Dermato-Venereologica* 89:661-2. doi: 10.2340/00015555-0724.

[55] Fetil, Emel, and Turna İlknur, Oguz Kilinç, Banu Lebe, Ergun Kuşku, Ali T. Güneş. 2006. 'Scar Sarcoidosis After Years From Traumatic Injury.' *Turkiye Klinikleri Journal of Dermatology* 16:186-9.

[56] Dal Sacco, D., and E. Cozzani, Aurora Parodi, A. Rebora. 2005. 'Scar sarcoidosis after hyaluronic acid injection.' *International Journal of Dermatology* 44:411-2. Doi: 10.1111/j.1365-4632.2005.01930.x.

[57] Yanardağ, Halil, and Ömer N. Pamuk, Tuncer Karayel. 2003. Cutaneous involvement in sarcoidosis: analysis of the features in 170 patients. *Respiratory Medicine* 97:978-82.

[58] Lodha, Saurabh, and Miguel Sanchez, Stephen Prystowsky. 2009. 'Sarcoidosis of the skin: a review for the pulmonologist.' *Chest* 136:583-96. doi: 10.1378/chest.08-1527.

[59] McKee, P., and E. Calonje, S. Granter. 2005. *Pathology of the skin*. China: Elsevier Mosby.

[60] Aksoy, Berna, and H. Mete Aksoy, Onat Akin, İsmail Yüksekol. 2011. 'Topikal Takrolimus Tedavisine Çok Iyi Yanit Veren Skar Sarkoidozu/Scar Sarcoidosis with an Excellent Response to Treatment with Topical Tacrolimus.' *Turkderm* 45:219-21. Doi: 10.4274/turkderm.81567.

[61] Terao, Mika, and Hiroyuki Murota, Misa Song, Ichiro Katayama. 2006. 'Case of morphea occurring on a scar after laparoscopy.' The *Journal of Dermatology* 33:722-3. Doi: 10.1111/j.1346-8138.2006.00168.x.

[62] Schaffer, J. V., and C. Carroll, I. Dvoretsky, M. J. Huether, M Girardi. 2000. 'Postirradiation morphea of the breast presentation of two cases and review of the literature.' *Dermatology* 200:67-71. Doi: 10.1159/000018322

[63] Segaran, A., and M. Mohammad, J. Sterling, C. Malata. 2013. 'Pyoderma gangrenosum arising in a breast reduction scar: seven years post-procedure.' *Journal of Plastic, Reconstructive & Aesthetic Surgery* 66:e370-e2. doi: 10.1016/j.bjps.2013.05.016.

[64] Castillo, R., and G. Cañadas-De La Fuente, H. Husein-ElAhmed, J. Cantero-Hinojosa. 2011. 'Pyoderma gangrenosum developing over an arteriovenous fistula scar.' *Internal Medicine Journal* 41:436-7. doi: 10.1111/j.1445-5994.2011.02479.x.

[65] Choi, Hwan J., and Jun H. Kim, Young M. Lee. 2012. 'Herpes zoster developing within recent subciliary incision scar.' The *Journal of Craniofacial Surgery* 23:930-1. doi: 10.1097/SCS.0b013e31824ddf72.

[66] Yamamoto, Toshiyuki. 2016. 'Herpes zoster occurring on scars: two cases.' *European Journal of Dermatology* 26:396-7. Doi: 10.1684/ejd.2016.2783.

[67] Lorant, A. 1968. 'Effect of surgical scar on herpes zoster.' *New England Journal of Medicine* 278:397.

In: Cutaneous Scars: Biology, Clinics and Management ISBN: 978-1-53615-657-7
Editors: Berna Aksoy, Hasan Mete Aksoy et al. © 2019 Nova Science Publishers, Inc.

Chapter 15

COMPLICATIONS OF CUTANEOUS SCARRING: CLINICAL ASPECTS

Evren Odyakmaz Demirsoy[1,*] and Emrah K. Yasar[2]
[1]Deparment of Dermatology,
[2]Dcpartment of Plastic and Reconstructive Surgery,
Faculty of Medicine, Kocaeli University, Kocaeli, Turkey

ABSTRACT

Some scars can cause various physical, aesthetic, and psychological complications depending on their location, size or type. Pruritus and pain are the most common unpleasant symptoms associated with scars. Some scars are unstable or develop contracture or malignant transformation at the worst. These scar complications are discussed in this chapter.

Keywords: scar carcinoma, complication, contracture, malignancy, Marjolin's ulcer, scar neoplasm, unstable scars

1. INTRODUCTION

Scars develop almost after every dermal injury. Fortunately, most of these scars are stable, harmless, and clinically insignificant if aesthetic anxiety is ignored. However, some scars can cause various physical, aesthetic and psychological *complication*s depending on their location, size or type. Pruritus and pain are the most common

*Corresponding Author's Email: evrenodyakmaz@yahoo.com.

unpleasant symptoms associated with scars and diminish the quality of life. Conversely, some scars are unstable and keep losing the healed skin over them again and again; this could lead to secondary infections and malignancy. Malignant transformation is the worst outcome associated with a scar [1, 2]. These unpleasant outcomes are discussed in this chapter.

2. Psychological Complications

Every type of scar, even the clinically insignificant ones, causes some level of anxiety associated with aesthetic concerns in patients. However, excessive scars (hypertrophic scars and keloids) particularly affect patients psychologically. Studies have revealed that scars can cause anxiety, depression, post-traumatic stress reactions, loss of self- esteem, and stigmatization, thus leading to a diminished quality of life [3-6].

3. Unstable Scars

The term "*unstable scars*" is used to define scars which are associated with frequent loss of covering skin over the scar.

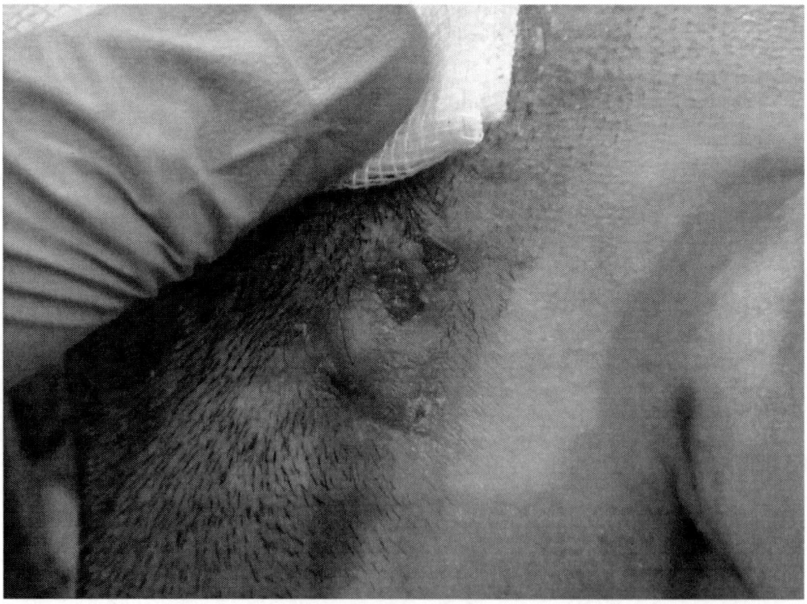

Figure 1. Unstable scar located on the retroauricular region of the scalp (Courtesy of Berna Aksoy, MD).

They usually occur in trauma-prone areas such as the surface of joints, skin creases or bony prominences as a consequence of poor quality of dermal component of the scar tissue (Figure 1). These unstable scar areas have a tendency to develop malignant behavior [7, 8]. Thus, the possibility of neoplastic transformation should always be considered and histopathological examination should always be performed if ulcers on scars do not heal.

4. CONTRACTURES

Contracture is a general term that defines the lack of movement of tissues which are otherwise expected to be mobile [9]. Wound contraction is a physiologic component of wound healing and involves interactions between fibroblasts, myofibroblasts, and collagen. This healing process reduces the size of the wound and is a beneficial mechanism when the tissue loss is minimal or in a non-critical area [8]. However, if the tissue loss is excessive or if the scar is deep or located over a joint surface, then this process may result in physical deformity and functional limitations. Location, extent, and depth of injury affect the extent and severity of contracture formation [10]. Scar contractures are particularly seen following serious burns. Burn scar contractures can lead to poor functional and cosmetic outcomes as well as possible psychological consequences. Contractures are the most common cause of functional deficits in burn patients (Figure 2) [10, 11].

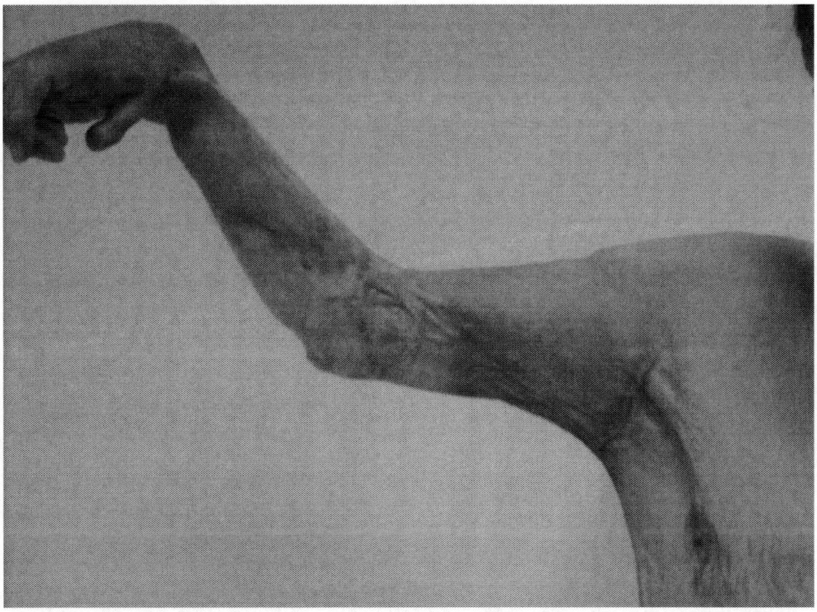

Figure 2. Hand, elbow and shoulder contractures that were treated with surgical operations in a burn victim (Courtesy of Berna Aksoy, MD).

Prolonged skin *contracture* may lead to shortening of musculotendinous units and neurovascular structures. Unstable ulcers are usually seen on these scars [8].

Special measures, such as silicon sheets, pressure garments, and range-of-motion exercises should be taken with the aim of maintaining the flexibility of the joint, particularly when scars are located in *contracture* prone areas. Surgical intervention to release the tension at the joints may be recommended for patients nonresponsive to all the above measures [10].

5. Malignancies Arising in Scars

The potential of development of *malignancies* in burn scars has been known for a long time, with the earliest observations by Celsus dating back to the first century. These scars were named "*Marjolin's ulcers*" after a French academic surgeon, Jean-Nicolas Marjolin, who documented chronic ulcers arising from scar tissue for the first time. Although this term was initially used for squamous cell carcinoma (SCC) that occurred on burn scars, it is now used for all neoplasms developing from scar tissues, chronic ulcers, and skin disorders with chronic inflammation [12].

Because of the lack of population-based studies, the magnitude of risk of skin cancer development on scars is not known. Skin cancer arising on scars with the exception of burn scars has not been epidemiologically investigated. Burn *scar carcinomas* comprise the majority of all recorded *scar neoplasms* and it is estimated that 2% of SCCs and 0.03% of basal cell carcinomas (BCC) arise from burn scars [12].

5.1. Etiology

Marjolin's ulcers mostly arise from burn scars. However, they are also associated with non-healing ulcers and scars caused by chronic inflammatory processes. These chronic inflammatory conditions include osteomyelitis, venous ulcers, vaccinations, snake bites, lupus, pilonidal abscesses, pressure sores, spinal cord injury, dermatitis artefacta, and chronic wounds of epidermolysis bullosa [12-17].

5.2. Pathogenesis

Although the pathogenesis of *scar carcinomas* is not fully understood, various etiological factors have been implicated. It is possible that the pathogenesis is linked with multiple factors which are environmental, immunological, and genetic in nature [12].

Abnormal biological activity of keratinocytes due to prolonged healing is a major risk factor of *scar carcinomas*. Scar site is associated with avascular tissue and obliterated lymphatics. So the normal tissue surveillance for cellular mutation at these sites is decreased and makes these scars immunologically vulnerable. Consequently, tumors at these sites can grow to overwhelming sizes before breaking through the burn scar barrier and confronting an unsuspecting immune system [18,19].

After the malignant cells reach the regional lymph nodes, rapid growth occurs, probably due to the first contact of tumor cells with the immune system at this location rather than the primary lesion site. As a possible consequence of this mechanism, *scar carcinomas* are more aggressive and prone to metastasis [18, 19]. Mutations in genes responsible for cell division and apoptosis have been reported in patients with *Marjolin's ulcer* [20, 21].

It is proposed that deeper tissues are subject to milder trauma and undergo less tissue regeneration compared with epidermis and superficial dermis, mesenchymal malignancies are rare for this reason. BCC is more likely to occur if the burn is superficial and skin adnexa are spared.

Many of the burn *scar neoplasms* occur in individuals with deeper burns, which destroy hair follicles and sebaceous glands; so, these patients no longer have basal cells available in the burned area [22].

Healing by secondary intention, non-healing wounds, and fragile scars that are easily traumatized and ulcerated are the risk factors for the development of scar neoplasms [22].

5.3. Histological Type

The most common type of malignancy arising in scars is SCC, followed by BCC [22]. Malignant melanoma, sarcomas (osteogenic sarcoma, liposarcoma, fibrosarcoma, dermatofibrosarcoma, leiomyosarcoma, malignant fibrous histiocytoma, and malignant schwannoma), adenocarcinoma, and carcinoma in situ are the other reported *scar neoplasms* [18, 22-26].

A meta-analysis reviewed 1078 cases of burn *scar neoplasm* with 71% of the cases being SCC, 12% BCC, 6% melanoma, 5% sarcoma, and 4% other neoplasms [22].

5.4. Clinical Presentation

Although *Marjolin's ulcers* are rare, they frequently behave as an aggressive skin cancer type, and hence, early diagnosis, which directly affects patients' life expectancy, is very crucial. Certain changes such as nodule formation, induration or ulceration at the scar site may herald malignant transformation [19].

Marjolin's ulcers usually present as non-healing ulcers on a long-term scar. Two types of ulcers may be seen in malignant transformation: flat ulcer with elevated margins and surrounding indurations (Figure 3) or, less commonly, exophytic ulcers resembling granulation tissue [19].

Therefore, malignant transformation should be suspected when ulcers exist for more than 3 months or have elevated margins, excessive granulation tissue, an easily bleeding surface, drainage of foul-smelling pus, or an increase in size. If there is a clinical suspicion of *malignancy*, biopsy should be performed from multiple sites to avoid overlooking neoplastic transformation [19].

Although all parts of the body can be affected; lower extremities are the most frequently affected site, followed by the head region. The face, neck, and scalp are the most frequently affected sites for BCC [22].

The latency period, defined as the time between initial injury and confirmation of *malignancy*, tends to be long, being usually about 36 years. However, the reported values for this duration range from four weeks to 75 years [12]. The latency period is inversely proportional to the patients' age at the time of initial injury. Younger patients tend to develop *malignancy* after a much longer period of time [14].

Marjolin's ulcers are more common in men than in women, and the typical age at the time of diagnosis is the fifth decade of life [22].

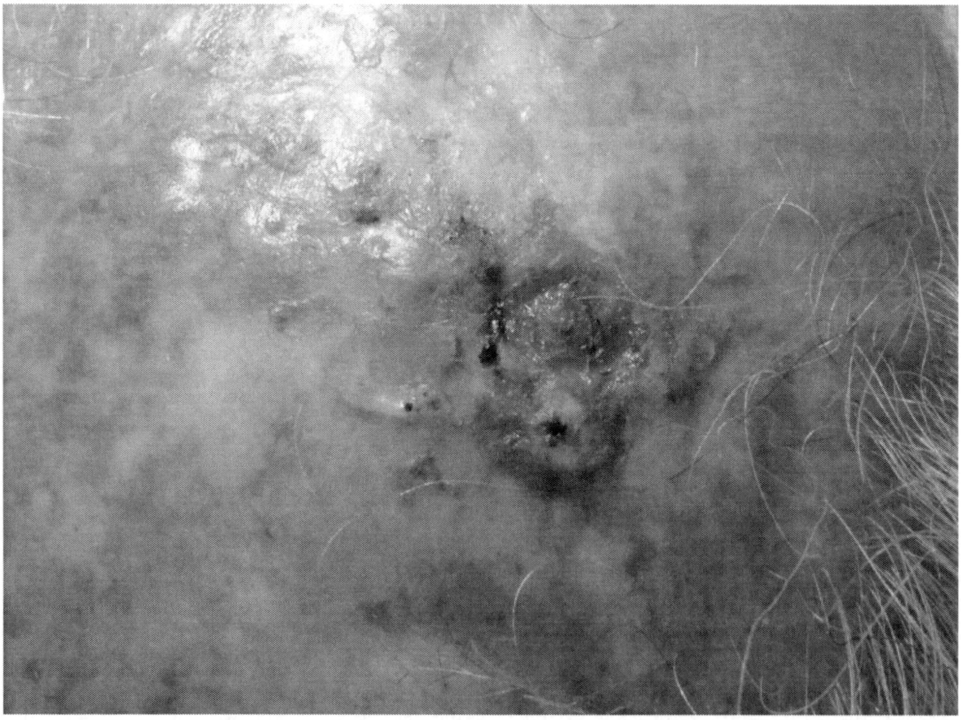

Figure 3. Marjolin's ulcer located on a long standing burn scar of the scalp (Courtesy of Berna Aksoy, MD).

5.5. Treatment and Prognosis

Providing stable healing via skin grafting or flap would be the best preventive treatment option for the burn *scar neoplasm* because slowly healing and ulcerated burns are more prone to malignant transformation [18, 22].

Marjolin's ulcers tend to be more aggressive than other forms of skin cancer, and hence, their treatment should be performed in a multi-disciplinary fashion considering patients' clinical presentations. Metastasis is the most important prognostic factor.

Wide local excision and wound coverage with skin grafting or flaps are the optimal treatment choices. If there is a clinically palpable lymph node, lymph node resection is recommended, except for cases of melanoma, wherein sentinel lymph node biopsy should be performed regardless of the presence of palpable lymph nodes. In some cases, extremity amputation may be necessary. Additional treatment methods like local radiation therapy or chemotherapy are recommended in patients with unfavorable prognostic factors or metastases [14, 19].

CONCLUSION

Most of the scars are stable, harmless, and clinically insignificant. Some scars can cause various physical, aesthetic and psychological complications, or be unstable, or develop contracture and at worst malignant transformation may occur. These scar complications are important and challenging, and should be managed by a multidisciplinary approach.

REFERENCES

[1] Monstrey, S. and E. Middelkoop, J. J. Vranckx, F. Bassetto, U. E. Ziegler, S. Meaume, L. Teot. 2014. "Updated scar management practical guidelines: non-invasive and invasive measures". *Journal of Plastic, Reconstructive and Aesthetic Surgery,* 67:1017 - 25. doi: 10.1016/j.bjps.2014.04.011.

[2] Bayat, A. and D. A. McGrouther and M. W. Ferguson. 2003. "Skin scarring". *BMJ,* 326(7380):88 - 92.

[3] Robert, R. and W. Meyer, S. Bishop, L. Rosenberg, L. Murphy, P. Blakeney. 1999. "Disfiguring burn scars and adolescent self-esteem". *Burns,* 25:581 - 5.

[4] Bock, O. and G. Schmid-Ott, P. Malewski, U. Mrowietz. 2006. "Quality of life of patients with keloid and hypertrophic scarring". *Archives of Dermatological Research,* 297:433 - 8. doi: 10.1007/s00403-006-0651-7.

[5] Taal, L. and A. W. Faber. 1998. "Posttraumatic stress and maladjustment among adult burn survivors 1 to 2 years postburn. Part II: the interview data". *Burns,* 24:399 - 405.

[6] Reinholz, M. and J. Poetschke, H. Schwaiger, A. Epple, T. Ruzicka, G. G. Gauglitz. 2015. "The dermatology life quality index as a means to assess life quality in patients with different scar types". *Journal of the European Academy of Dermatology and Venereology,* 29:2112 - 9. doi: 10.1111/jdv.13135.

[7] Meaume, S. 2002. "Chronic wound scars". *Wound Repair and Regeneration,* 10: 103 - 6.

[8] Goel, A. and P. Shrivastava. 2010. "Post-burn scars and scar contractures". *Indian Journal of Plastic Surgery,* 43:S63-S71. doi: 10.4103/0970-0358.70724.

[9] Fergusson, D. and B. Hutton, A. Drodge. 2007. "The epidemiology of major joint contractures: a systematic review of the literature". *Clinical Orthopaedics and Related Research,* 456:22 - 9. doi: 10.1097/BLO.0b013e3180308456.

[10] Davoodi, P. and J. M. Fernandez, S. J. O. 2008. "Postburn sequelae in the pediatric patient: clinical presentations and treatment options". The *Journal of Craniofacial Surgery,* 19:1047 - 52. doi: 10.1097/SCS.0b013e318175f4df.

[11] Peck, M. and J. Molnar, D. Swart. 2009. "A global plan for burn prevention and care". *Bulletin of the World Health Organisation,* 87:802 - 3.

[12] Bazalinski, D. and J. Przybek-Mita, B. Baranska, P. Wiech. 2017. "Marjolin's ulcer in chronic wounds - review of available literature". *Contemporary Oncology, (Poznan, Poland)* 21:197 - 202. doi: 10.5114/wo.2017.70109.

[13] Yu, N. and X. Long, J. R. Lujan-Hernandez, K. Z. Hassan, M. Bai, Y. Wang, X. Wang, R. Zhao. 2013. "Marjolin's ulcer: a preventable malignancy arising from scars". *World Journal of Surgical Oncology,* 11:313. doi: 10.1186/1477-7819-11-313.

[14] Copcu, E. 2009. "Marjolin's ulcer: a preventable complication of burns?" *Plastic and Reconstructive Surgery,* 124:156e-64e. doi: 10.1097/PRS.0b013e3181a8082e.

[15] Malek, M. M. and P. O. Emanuel, C. M. Divino. 2007. "Malignant degeneration of pilonidal disease in an immunosuppressed patient: report of a case and review of the literature". *Diseases of the Colon and Rectum,* 50:1475 - 7. doi: 10.1007/s10350-007-0267-9.

[16] Chou, C. Y. and Z. Y. Huang, H. Y. Chiao, C. Y. Wang, Y. S. Sun, S. G. Chen, T. M. Chen, S. C. Chang. 2015. "Squamous cell carcinoma arising from a recurrent ischial pressure ulcer: a case report". *Ostomy Wound Manage,* 61:48 - 50.

[17] Eliassen, A. and F. Vandy, J. McHugh, P. K. Henke. 2013. "Marjolin's ulcer in a patient with chronic venous stasis". *Annals of Vascular Surgery,* 27:1182 e5-8. doi: 10.1016/j.avsg.2013.06.002.

[18] Alconchel, M. D. and C. Olivares, R. Alvarez. 1997. "Squamous cell carcinoma, malignant melanoma and malignant fibrous histiocytoma arising in burn scars". The *British Journal of Dermatology,* 137:793 - 8.

[19] Pekarek, B. and S. Buck, L. Osher. 2011. "A Comprehensive Review on Marjolin's Ulcers: Diagnosis and Treatment". The *Journal of the American College of Certified Wound Specialists,* 3:60 - 4. doi: 10.1016/j.jcws.2012.04.001.

[20] Lee, S. H. and M. S. Shin, H. S. Kim, W. S. Park, S. Y. Kim, J. J. Jang, K. J. Rhim, J. Jang, H. K. Lee, J. Y. Park, R. R. Oh, S. Y. Han, J. H. Lee, J. Y. Lee, N. J. Yoo. 2000. "Somatic mutations of Fas (Apo-1/CD95) gene in cutaneous squamous cell carcinoma arising from a burn scar". The *Journal of Investigative Dermatology,* 114:122 - 6. doi: 10.1046/j.1523-1747.2000.00819.x.

[21] Harland, D. L. and W. A. Robinson, W. A. Franklin. 1997. "Deletion of the p53 gene in a patient with aggressive burn scar carcinoma". The *Journal of Trauma,* 42:104 - 7.

[22] Kowal-Vern, A. and B. K. Criswell. 2005. "Burn scar neoplasms: a literature review and statistical analysis". *Burns,* 31:403 - 13. doi: 10.1016/j.burns.2005.02.015.

[23] Lee, M. A. and J. Yi, J. M. Chae. 2017. "Cutaneous osteosarcoma arising from a burn scar". *Skeletal Radiology,* 46:547 - 551. doi: 10.1007/s00256-016-2565-6.

[24] Ribero, S. and M. Grassi, V. Caliendo, D. Lauro, G. Macripo. 2012. "Melanoma arising on a scar 10 years after a burn: management and review of the literature". *Annals of Plastic Surgery,* 69:27 - 9. doi: 10.1097/SAP.0b013e318250f084.

[25] Gonzalez-Sixto, B. and C. De la Torre, R. Pardavila, M. L. Carpintero. 2008. "Leiomyosarcoma arising from scrofuloderma scar". *Clinical and Experimental Dermatology,* 33:776 - 8. doi: 10.1111/j.1365-2230.2008.02805.x.

[26] Ben, D. and L. Liu, B. Ma, Y. Li, Z. Xia. 2010. "Extramammary Paget's disease arising from a burn scar of right forearm: An uncommon case report". *Burns,* 36:e145 - 7. doi: 10.1016/j.burns.2008.11.006.

In: Cutaneous Scars: Biology, Clinics and Management ISBN: 978-1-53615-657-7
Editors: Berna Aksoy, Hasan Mete Aksoy et al. © 2019 Nova Science Publishers, Inc.

Chapter 16

COURSE AND PROGNOSIS

Ezgi Ozkur*
Department of Dermatology, Health Science University,
Sisli Etfal Training and Research Hospital,
Istanbul, Turkey

ABSTRACT

All wounds eventually heal with some degree of scar formation. However, the mechanisms that lead to a fine thin scar, an atrophic or hypertrophic scar, or a keloid are still poorly understood.

The proposed etiologic factors for scar course and prognosis include: genetic predisposition; depth, type, and location of the skin injury or wound; degree of tension; local infection or inflammation; and hormonal influences.

Keywords: course, prognosis

1. INTRODUCTION

Cutaneous scarring is inevitable following damage to more than 33.1% of the thickness of the skin [1]. In the United Kingdom, it is estimated that 23 million people have significant cutaneous scars [2].

Although most cutaneous scars are insignificant, people with exaggerated skin scarring may face physical and psychosocial consequences [3]. Understanding the *course*

*Corresponding Author's Email: ezgierdal@hotmail.com.

and *prognosis* of cutaneous scars will allow for a better understanding of scar reduction management.

2. Course of Scars

Conventional wound healing occurs in three phases: an inflammatory phase that encloses the injury and prevents infection, a proliferative phase for the formation of granulation tissue, and a remodeling (maturation) phase in which the erythema of the wound lightens and the scar mostly softens and flattens due to collagen synthesis and degradation, which was discussed in another chapter [4]. The final appearance is mostly influenced by the interval between wound occurence and 2 to 3 weeks following complete healing.

This time interval is when we can do most to prevent the development of pathologic scarring [5]. Once the scar has finally formed, it undergoes several macro- and microscopic changes during the maturation phase, which is completed after approximately 1 year [6].

3. Types of Scars

Clinically, scars can be divided into subtypes: normal, hypertrophic or keloid. Hypertrophic scars are defined as excessive tissue production that remains within the boundaries of the initial lesion. These can be divided into linear or widespread hypertrophic scars.

Linear scars usually result from surgery or trauma, whereas widespread hypertrophic scars can be a result of an extensive burns or soft tissue infections. Unlike hypertrophic scars, keloids extend beyond the boundaries of the initial injury. They have a low chance of spontaneous regression and a high chance of recurrence after treatment [7]. Keloids are described as minor or major depending on whether the scar extends less than or more than 0.5 cm beyond the border of the initial injury, respectively [8]. The scar classification system of the International Advisory Panel of Scar Management (IAPSM) is shown in Table 1. [9, 10].

4. Prognosis

There are many factors that could influence scar *prognosis* (Figure 1). The most frequent factors are listed below.

Table 1. International Advisory Panel of Scar Management classification of different types of scars

Scar type	Appearance	Characteristics
Mature	• Light-coloured • Flat	
Immature	• Red	• Slightly pruritic and painful • Can develop into a linear hypertrophic scar
Linear hypertrophic	• Rope-like appearance • Red • Raised • Confined to the border of the original injury	• Develops weeks after initial insult • May grow slowly
Widespread hypertrophic	• Widespread • Red • Raised • Confined to the border of the original injury	• Burns are the main cause
Minor keloid	• Raised • Extends <0.5cm beyond the border of the original injury	• Develops months to years after the event • Does not regress • High recurrence rate
Major keloid	• Large • Raised • Extends >0.5 cm beyond the border of the original injury	• Slightly pruritic and painful • Continues to grow • Does not regress • Very high recurrence rate

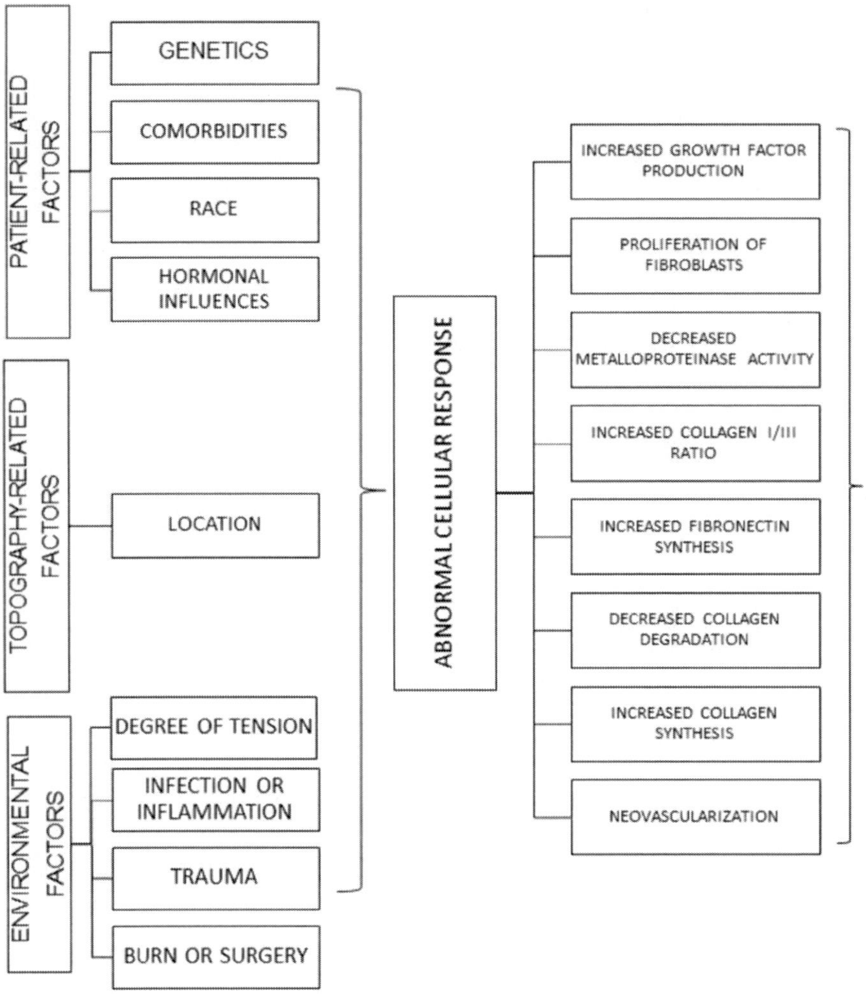

Figure 1. Factors that influence scar prognosis.

4.1. Ethnicity

It is reported in the literature that ethnic groups of darkly pigmented skin including Afro-Caribbeans, Asians, and Hispanics have a higher preponderance compared with Caucasians towards the development of keloid scars [11, 12].

4.2. Arterial and Venous Insufficiency

Increased venous pressure leads to localized edema with plasma extravazation. Fibrinogen leakage results in formation of a fibrin layer that reduces oxygen and nutrient diffusion, which can affect scar formation [13]. Also it is obvious that ischemic wounds heal poorly and have higher risk of infection in the presence of arterial insufficiency [14].

4.3. Endocrinologic Disease

The best-studied endocrinologic disease that affects scar formation is diabetes mellitus. However, other endocrinologic diseases may affect scar formation through altered expression of growth factors in wounds.

Patients with diabetes have impaired wound healing due to several mechanisms: neuropathy, decreased expression of the granulocyte-macrophage colony-stimulating factor (GM-CSF) receptor, platelet-derived growth factors (PDGFs), vascular endothelial growth factor (VEGF), epidermal growth factor (EGF), and insulin-like growth factor (IGF) in the wound, and impaired granulation tissue formation through deregulation of matrix metalloproteinases (MMP) [15, 16]. Other hormones such as thyroid-stimulating hormone (TSH) and growth hormone (GH) have also been associated with keloid formation based on the observation that acromegalics have increased susceptibility to develop keloids, which may be secondary to increased levels of TSH and GH [17]. Obesity leads to poor wound perfusion [18].

4.4. Infections

At the wound site, inflammatory infiltrates due to infection slow fibroblast proliferation. Also, sepsis causes systemic effects that also impair wound healing [19].

4.5. Malnutrition and Obesity

Wound dehiscence risk is increased in hypoproteinemia [20]. Vitamin C (ascorbic acid) deficiency results in arrest in fibroplasia due to scurvy [21]. Vitamin A (retinoic acid) has roles in fibroplasia, collagen synthesis, collagen crosslinking, and epithelization. Vitamin B6 (pyridoxine) deficiency impairs collagen cross-linking. Vitamin B1 and B2 deficiencies cause poor wound healing [21]. Zinc deficiency is associated with poor epithelization [22].

4.6. Treatments

Systemic and topical corticosteroids impair wound healing [23]. Also, radiation and chemotherapeutic agents retard wound healing [24]. In the *prognosis* of keloids, it is reported that incomplete surgical excision of keloids is correlated with increased risk of recurrence [25].

5. Prevention

The common belief is that the initiating event of keloid and hypertrophic scar formation is trauma, but the rest of the process remains uncertain. A combination of unchangeable factors such as biochemical factors, endocrinologic factors, and genetic factors are likely to be involved [26]; however, other additional factors can be prevented. Following surgery or trauma, the first priority should always be the prevention of abnormal scar formation [27]. Incision lines should be parallel to the relaxed skin tension lines. Other major components of scar prevention are: tension relief, hydration/taping/occlusion, and pressure garment therapy, which will be discussed in another chapter.

Conclusion

The mechanisms that lead to a fine thin normal scar, or a hypertrophic scar / keloid, or an atrophic scar are still poorly understood. The proposed factors for scar course and prognosis include: genetic predisposition; depth, type, and location of the skin injury or wound; degree of tension; local infection or inflammation; and hormonal influences. Following any cutaneous surgery or trauma, the first priority should always be the prevention of abnormal scar formation.

References

[1] Baker, Richard and Fulvio Urso-Baiarda, Claire Linge, Adriaan Grobbelaar. 2009. “Cutaneous scarring: a clinical review”. *Dermatology Research and Practice*, 2009:625376. doi: 10.1155/2009/625376.

[2] Thomas, D. W. and I. D. O'neill, K. G. Harding, J. P. Shepherd. 1995. “Cutaneous wound healing: a current perspective”. *Journal of Oral and Maxillofacial Surgery*, 53:442 - 447.

[3] Bayat, A. and D. A. McGrouther, M. W. J. Ferguson. 2003. “Skin scarring”. *BMJ,* 326(7380):88 - 92.

[4] Partridge, J. and N. Rumsey. 2003. “Skin scarring: new insights may make adjustment easier”. *BMJ,* 326 (7392):765.

[5] Mustoe, Thomas A. and Rodney D. Cooter, Michael H. Gold, F. D. Richard Hobbs, Albert-Adrien Ramelet, Peter G. Shakespeare, Maurizio Stella, Luc Teot, Fiona M. Wood, Ulrich E. Ziegler. 2002. “International clinical recommendations on scar management”. *Plastic and Reconstructive Surgery,* 110:560 - 71.

[6] Bond, Jeremy S. and Jonathan A. Duncan, Abdul Sattar, Adam Boanas, Tracey Mason, Sharon O'Kane, Mark W. J. Ferguson. 2008. “Maturation of the human scar: an observational study”. *Plastic and Reconstructive Surgery,* 121:1650 - 8. doi: 10.1097/PRS.0b013e31816a9f6f.

[7] Al-Shaqsi, Sultan and Taimoor Al-Bulushi. 2016. "Cutaneous Scar Prevention and Management: Overview of current therapies". *Sultan Qaboos University Medical Journal,* 16:e3 - 8. doi: 10.18295/squmj.2016.16.01.002.

[8] Arno, Anna I. and Gerd G. Gauglitz, Juan P. Barret, Marc G. Jeschke. 2014. "Up-to-date approach to manage keloids and hypertrophic scars: a useful guide". *Burns,* 40 (7):1255 - 66. doi: 10.1016/j.burns.2014.02.011.

[9] Gold, Michael H. and Brian Berman, Matteo T. Clementoni, Gerd G. Gauglitz, Foad Nahai, Crystal Murcia. 2014. Updated international clinical recommendations on scar management: part 1--evaluating the evidence. *Dermatologic Surgery,* 40:817 - 24. doi: 10.1111/dsu.0000000000000049.

[10] Gold, Michael H. and Michael McGuire, Thomas A. Mustoe, Aandrea Pusic, Mukta Sachdev, Jill Waibel, Crystal Murcia. 2014. "Updated international clinical recommendations on scar management: part 2--algorithms for scar prevention and treatment". *Dermatologic Surgery,* 40: 825 - 31. doi: 10.1111/dsu.0000000000000050.

[11] Santucci, M. and L. Borgognoni, U. M. Reali, G. Gabbiani. 2001. "Keloids and hypertrophic scars of Caucasians show distinctive morphologic and immunophenotypic profiles". *Virchows Archiv.,* 438:457 - 63.

[12] Alhady, Syed M. A. and K. Sivanantharajah. 1969. "Keloids in various races: a review of 175 cases". *Plastic and Reconstructive Surgery,* 44:564 - 6.

[13] Raju, Seshadri and Peter Neglen. 2009. "Clinical practice. Chronic venous insufficiency and varicose veins". The *New England Journal of Medicine,* 360(22):2319 - 27. doi: 10.1056/NEJMcp0802444.

[14] Sen, Chandan K. 2009. "Wound healing essentials: let there be oxygen". *Wound Repair and Regeneration,* 17:1 - 18. doi: 10.1111/j.1524-475X.2008.00436.x.

[15] Galkowska, Hanna and Urszula Wojewodzka, Waldemar L. Olszewski. 2006. "Chemokines, cytokines, and growth factors in keratinocytes and dermal

endothelial cells in the margin of chronic diabetic foot ulcers". *Wound Repair and Regeneration,* 14:558 - 565. Doi: 10.1111/j.1743-6109.2006.00155.x.
[16] Mishima, Yasuo and Ayako Kuyama, Atsuhiko Tada, Kiyoshi Takahashi, Tatsuji Ishioka, Masayoshi Kibata. 2001. "Relationship between serum tumor necrosis factor-alpha and insulin resistance in obese men with Type 2 diabetes mellitus". *Diabetes Research and Clinical Practice,* 52:119 - 23.
[17] Koonin, A. J. 1964. "The Aetiology of Keloids: A Review of the Literature and a New Hypothesis". *South African Medical Journal,* 38:913 - 6.
[18] Goodson 3rd, William H. and Thomas K. Hunt. 1979. "Deficient collagen formation by obese mice in a standard wound model". *American Journal of Surgery,* 138:692 - 4.
[19] Robson, M. C. and B. D. Stenberg, J. P. Heggers. 1990. "Wound healing alterations caused by infection". *Clinics in Plastic Surgery,* 17:485 - 92.
[20] Col, Cavit and Atilla Soran, Meltem Col. 1998. "Can postoperative abdominal wound dehiscence be predicted". The *Tokai Journal of Experimental and Clinical Medicine,* 23 (3):123 - 7.
[21] Rembe, Julian-Dario and Carolin Fromm-Dornieden, Ewa K. Stuermer. 2018. "Effects of Vitamin B Complex and Vitamin C on Human Skin Cells: Is the Perceived Effect Measurable?" *Advances in Skin and Wound Care,* 31:225 - 33. doi: 10.1097/01.ASW.0000531351.85866.d9.
[22] Lin, Pei-Hui and Matthew Sermersheim, Haichang Li, Peter H. U. Lee, Steven M. Steinberg, Jianjie Ma. 2017. "Zinc in Wound Healing Modulation". *Nutrients,* 10 (1). doi: 10.3390/nu10010016.
[23] Marks, J. G. and Jr., C. Cano, K. Leitzel, A. Lipton. 1983. "Inhibition of wound healing by topical steroids". The *Journal of Dermatologic Surgery and Oncology,* 9:819 - 21.
[24] Drake, D. B. and S. N. Oishi. 1995. "Wound healing considerations in chemotherapy and radiation therapy". *Clinics in Plastic Surgery,* 22:31 - 7.
[25] Tan, Kian T. and Nigam Shah, Susan A. Pritchard, Duncan A. McGrouther, Ardeshir Bayat. 2010. "The influence of surgical excision margins on keloid prognosis". *Annals of Plastic Surgery,* 64:55 - 8. doi: 10.1097/SAP.0b013e31819b6c3a.
[26] Brissett, Anthony E. and David A. Sherris. 2001. "Scar contractures, hypertrophic scars, and keloids". *Facial Plastic Surgery,* 17 (04):263 - 272.
[27] Monstrey, Stan and Esther Middelkoop, Jan J. Vranckx, Franco Bassetto, Ulrich E. Ziegler, Sylvie Meaume, Luc Teot. 2014. "Updated scar management practical guidelines: non-invasive and invasive measures". *Journal of Plastic, Reconstructive and Aesthetic Surgery,* 67:1017 - 25. doi: 10.1016/j.bjps.2014.04.011.

In: Cutaneous Scars: Biology, Clinics and Management ISBN: 978-1-53615-657-7
Editors: Berna Aksoy, Hasan Mete Aksoy et al. © 2019 Nova Science Publishers, Inc.

Chapter 17

PREVENTION OF ABNORMAL SCARRING

***Hilal Gokalp*[1] *and Zekayi Kutlubay*[2,*]**
Department of Dermatology,
[1]Faculty of Medicine, Istinye University, Istanbul, Turkey
[2]Cerrahpasa Faculty of Medicine, Istanbul University, Istanbul, Turkey

ABSTRACT

Abnormal scarring causes functional and cosmetic deformities, discomfort, and psychological stress. To date, there is unfortunately no treatment method to prevent scar formation completely. However, prevention of abnormal scar formation should always be the priority following a burn, surgery or trauma. Combination of therapies is the mainstay of current scar prevention strategy, including tension relief, hydration/taping/occlusion, and pressure garments. In this section, we will discuss all methods used for scar prevention.

Keywords: avotermin, bioflavonoids, botulinum toxin, curcumin, hydration, moist wound healing, nutraceuticals, occlusion, pressure garment therapy, prevention, silicone, sunscreen, taping, tension relief, TGF-β, zinc oxide

1. INTRODUCTION

Prevention of abnormal scar formation should always be the priority following a burn, surgery or trauma. However, we are unfortunately unable to fully prevent scar formation with any treatment method at present time. It is only possible to minimize scar

*Corresponding Author's Email: zekayikutlubay@hotmail.com.

development by using some preventive measures and suppressive treatments [1]. This process should be managed during or even before the surgery regarding surgical scars. For elective surgery, paying attention to the position and length of the incision, avoiding excessive tension, and making sure the incision line is parallel to relaxed skin tension lines are paramount [2].

The healing process in the skin begins as soon as skin integrity is disrupted. The primary aim during wound healing should be to restore skin integrity as quickly as possible [3]. The process is quite complex and can be divided into three main processes: inflammation, proliferation and remodeling [4]. These phases may vary depending on the developmental stage. Inflammation starts with disruptions in capillary blood vessels and induction of hemostatic cascade [5]. Inflammation is relatively less significant in the fetal skin, leading to wound healing that is considered excellent when compared to adults. The relative insignificance of the inflammation during the fetal period results in wound healing without scar development [6]. The second stage in healing process is proliferation, which begins at 4-5th day with fibroblast migration into the wound matrix [7]. Wound contraction begins around day 10-12, however it can be variable according to wound severity and patient [8]. The last stage in wound healing is the remodeling phase, which begins around 3 weeks. However, a scar can develop during proliferation and remodeling phases in the postnatal period [9]. Decreasing the intensity and duration of inflammation is known to minimize the scar risk [10]. Decreasing inflammation and ensuring rapid closure of the wound require debridement of the dead tissue and disinfection [1, 2].

2. Prevention of Abnormal Scarring

There are 3 major components of scar *prevention* after wound closure: tension relief, hydration/taping/occlusion, and pressure garments [11]. We will discuss all scar prevention methods in this section. The effectiveness of these methods should be evaluated every 4 to 8 weeks in general and preventive therapy discontinued or supported by additional interventions as necessary [1].

2.1. Tension Relief

The risk of excessive scarring is higher in high-tension areas such as the deltoid and the sternal region. Post-surgical *taping* for 3 months on average is recommended to decrease the mechanical stress in these areas [12]. The stress-shielding device developed by Gurtner et al. has also been shown to decrease mechanical stress and excessive scar formation in high-tension areas [13]. It is recommended to apply this device consisting of silicone polymer sheets and pressure-sensitive adhesive immediately after skin closure. A beneficial effect of *botulinum toxin* injections in decreasing tensile forces and scar development in post-surgical scars has been demonstrated when compared to placebo [14].

2.2. Moist Wound Healing (Wet Environment)

Moist wound healing plays a crucial role in preventing the development of abnormal scarring. It decreases the inflammatory reaction while optimizing tissue improvement, thus accelerating epithelization and shortening the wound healing duration [3, 15]. Many studies have compared the wet and dry environments in wound healing [3, 4, 15, 16]. A wet environment has been shown to accelerate reepithelization and the wound healing process and to decrease the risk of scar development [4, 16].

A wet environment has first been suggested by Winter et al. in the 1960s and has been improved in various studies afterwards. The most commonly used products to create a wet environment at present are moist dressings, hydrocolloids, and various foams, alginates and hydrogels [4, 17, 18]. A wet environment has also been shown to provide significant clinical advantages for split-thickness skin donor sites [19]. Water evaporates much more quickly from scar tissue and more than a year is required for water levels to reach the pre-wounding state [20].

2.3. Silicone-Based Products

Silicone-based products (i.e., gels, creams, ointments, sprays, oils, sheets and tapes) help prevent excessive scar formation by restoring the water barrier through *occlusion* and *hydration* of the stratum corneum [21, 22]. *Silicone* materials are polymers with a silicone-oxygen, or siloxane, backbone chain with additional methyl groups attached through silicone-carbon bonds, generating polydimethylsiloxane units [23, 24]. *Silicone* gel/sheets increase the hydration of the stratum corneum. They also provide the necessary hydration environment for wound healing by decreasing transepidermal fluid loss. This *hydration,* in turn, increases oxygen permeability [25]. Hypoxia-induced angiogenesis and tissue growth are decreased in the end [26, 27]. Topical *silicone* gels also provide a protective barrier against environmental contaminants [28, 29].

Another hypothesis is that temperature changes in the wound can play a role in scar development. Musgrave et al. have reported that *silicone* gel sheeting increases the temperature of the application area by 1.7°C compared to the surrounding tissue and reduces the amount of collagen within the scar tissue. This decrease in the collagen amount is thought to be by way of increased collagenase activity [30].

It is recommended to use *silicone*-based products after epithelization is completed. They need to be regularly used for at least a month for maximum effect. *Silicone* sheets should stay in the wound for at least 12 hours a day [24, 31]. Their use together with intralesional corticosteroid treatment provides a synergistic effect in patients with a high risk of scar development [24, 30].

2.4. Pressure Garment Therapy

Pressure Garment Therapy is another scarring *prevention* method used to normalize the cellular process using mechanical pressure [11, 32]. Its prophylactic use is recommended to suppress scar development, especially after large burns [1, 33]. A pressure of 15-25 mmHg has been shown to decrease capillary flow with a potential reduction in the risk of hypertrophic or keloid scar development [11, 33]. The mechanism of action is decreasing the oxygen and nutrient supply to the affected region. The decreased blood supply in the pressurized area decreases collagen production [34]. It also creates a *moist wound healing* environment, increases granulation tissue development, decreases edema, and stimulates angiogenesis [4]. In addition, it decreases the levels of matrix metalloproteinases (MMPs) and collagenase, thus regulating the wound microenvironment. All these support normal wound healing and the abnormal scarring risk is reduced [35]. However, *pressure garment therapy* is quite difficult both for the patient and the family. The patient is recommended to use the pressure garment clothes at least 22 hours a day. The recommended *pressure garment therapy* duration can be increased up to 18 months so that skin maturation is completed [36]. However, side effects such as altered bone growth, heat reactions, friction damage and skin breakdown together with its psychological effects decrease patient compliance [11].

2.5. Topical Zinc Oxide

Application of topical *zinc oxide* accelerates healing of wounds via epithelization predominantly. Lansdown et al. has shown that topical *zinc oxide* promotes healing of leg ulcers [37]. Adhesive tapes containing *zinc oxide* were used for the treatment of burns and other wounds [38, 39]. Application of *zinc oxide* tapes was shown to enhance development of granulation tissue in burn wounds [40]. Aksoy et al. also showed that once in a day application of 40% *zinc oxide* ointment decreased clinical scar hypertrophy scores significantly at 6th week in comparison with placebo [39]. Zinc sulfadiazine was also shown to be effective in the treatment of burns [41].

2.6. Transforming Growth Factor-β3

Transforming growth factor-β (TGF-β) isoforms play a key role in scar formation [42]. Recently, a significantly higher ratio of TGF-β3 to the other TGF-β isoforms has been shown to be associated with less scarring [43]. So, many experimental studies investigating the role of TGF-β have been accomplished. Collectively, data from these experimental studies suggest that TGF-β3 plays an important role at the end of the wound healing process and decreases connective tissue deposition [42, 44]. After these developments, an extensive program has been started and human recombinant TGF-β3 *(avotermin)* has been developed. Shah et al. have shown that intradermal injection of *avotermin* (50 - 100 ng/100 μL/linear cm of wound edge) to cutaneous incisional wounds significantly reduced scarring compared with controls in adult rats [45]. It was also shown to decrease scar formation following full-thickness skin incisions and avotermin is the first in a new class of prophylactic therapeutics in development for the improvement of scarring [43, 44].

2.7. Sunscreen

Human and animal studies have shown that ultraviolet radiation can cause scar pigmentation and further disrupt the scar appearance [44, 46]. Protection of the whole scar with a high sun protection factor (SPF >50) *sunscreen* product until the scar has matured is therefore recommended for all scar types [24, 47].

2.8. Drugs or Supplements

2.8.1. Protein Supplementation

Proteins are an important building block of the skin and therefore need to be supplemented in patients with large wound areas [4]. Abdel-Salam et al. have reported that whey (serum milk) protein has a beneficial effect on the wound healing process. Protein supplementation has been demonstrated to accelerate wound closure in diabetic patients with prolonged wound healing duration and also to decrease the levels of pro-inflammatory (IL-1β, IL-6, and TNF-α) and anti-inflammatory (IL-4 and IL-10) cytokine levels in the diabetic group to almost non-diabetic levels [48].

2.8.2. Nutraceuticals

The term "*nutraceutical*" combines two words – "nutrient" (a nourishing food component) and "pharmaceutical" (a medical drug). *Nutraceuticals* are believed to have effects on the immune system and to decrease the development risk of some disorders.

The *bioflavanoids* have been shown to accelerate wound healing by decreasing the levels of inflammatory cytokines, MMPs and Neutrophil Gelatinase-Associated Lipocalin (NGAL). Their use in patients with a risk of scar development and/or a wide wound area has therefore been considered [4, 49].

2.8.3. Curcumin

Curcumin, another supplement accelerating the wound healing process, has anti-inflammatory and antioxidant features [50]. The mechanism of action is decreasing inflammatory cytokine secretion and increasing anti-inflammatory cytokine levels. It has been shown to accelerate wound healing and decrease the scar development risk in diabetic patients, as it is observed with protein supplementation [51].

Conclusion

Many patients suffer psychological and physical trauma due to scarring. While current treatments for scarring have limited efficacy, current prevention methods acquire more important roles. Meticulous surgical techniques, wet environment, silicone products and pressure garments constitute the majority of prevention methods. However, topical zinc oxide, TGF-β3, protein supplementation and nutraceuticals can help prevent abnormal scarring.

References

[1] Middelkoop, Esther, and Stan Monstrey, Luc Téot, Jan-Jeroen Vranckx. 2011. *Scar Management: Practical Guidelines*. Elsene, Belgium: Maca-Cloetens.

[2] Bloemen, M. C., and W. M. van der Veer, M. M. Ulrich, P. P. van Zuijlen, F. B. Niessen, E. Middelkoop. 2009. "Prevention and curative management of hypertrophic scar formation." *Burns* 35:463–75. doi: 10.1016/j.burns.2008.07.016.

[3] Marini, L., and D. Odendaal, S. Smirnyi. 2017. "Importance of Scar Prevention and Treatment: An Approach from Wound Care Principles." *Dermatologic Surgery* 43:85–90. doi: 10.1097/DSS.0000000000001001.

[4] Rosique, R. G., and M. J. Rosique, J. A. Farina Junior. 2015. "Curbing Inflammation in Skin Wound Healing: A Review." *International Journal of Inflammation* 2015:316235. doi: 10.1155/2015/316235.

[5] Son, D., and A. Harijan. 2014. "Overview of surgical scar prevention and management." *Journal of Korean Medical Science* 29:751–7. doi: 10.3346/jkms.2014.29.6.751.

[6] Frantz, F. W., and D. A. Bettinger, J. H. Haynes, D. E. Johnson, K. M. Harvey, H. P. Dalton, D. R. Yager, R. F. Diegelmann, I. K. Cohen. 1993. "Biology of fetal repair:the presence of bacteria in fetal wounds induces an adult - like healingresponse." *Journal of Pediatric Surgery* 28:428–33.

[7] Almine, J. F., and S. G. Wise, A. S. Weiss. 2012. "Elastin signaling in wound repair." Birth Defects Research. Part C, Embryo Today. *Reviews* 96:248–57. doi: 10.1002/bdrc.21016.

[8] Bae, S. H., and Y. C. Bae, S. B. Nam, S. J. Choi. 2012. "A skin fixation method for decreasing the influence of wound contraction on wound healing in a rat model." *Archives of Plastic Surgery* 39:457–62. doi: 10.5999/aps.2012.39.5.457.

[9] Welshhans, J. L., and D. B. Hom. 2017. "Soft Tissue Principles to Minimize Scarring: An Overview." *Facial Plastic Surgery Clinics of North America* 25(1):1–13. doi: 10.1016/j.fsc.2016.08.002.

[10] Robson, M. C., and A. Barbul. 2006. "Guidelines for the best care of chronic wounds." *Wound Repair and Regeneration* 14:647–8. doi: 10.1111/j.1524-475X.2006.00173.x.

[11] Wiseman, J., and M. Simons, R. Kimble, R. Ware, S. McPhail, Z. Tyack. 2017. "Effectiveness of topical silicone gel and pressure garment therapy for burn scar prevention and management in children: study protocol for randomised controlled trial." *Trials* 18:72. doi: 10.1186/s13063-017-1820-z.

[12] Reiffel, R. S. 1995. "Prevention of hypertrophic scars by long-term paper tape application." *Plastic and Reconstructive Surgery* 96:1715–8.

[13] Gurtner, G. C., and R. H. Dauskardt, V. W. Wong, K. A. Bhatt, K. Wu, I. N. Vial, K. Padois, J. M. Korman, M. T. Longaker. 2011. "Improving cutaneous scar formation by controlling the mechanical environment: large animal and phase I studies." *Annals of Surgery* 254:217–25. doi: 10.1097/SLA.0b013e318220b159.

[14] Gassner, H. G., and D. A. Sherris, C. C. Otley. 2000. "Treatment of facial wounds with botulinum toxin A improves cosmetic outcome in primates." *Plastic and Reconstructive Surgery* 105:1948–53.

[15] Sussman, Carrie, and Barbara Bates-Jensen. 2007. *Wound Care: a collaborative practice manual for health professionals* Philadelphia: Wolters Kluwer Health/Lippincott Williams & Wilkins Health.

[16] Junker, J. P., and R. A. Kamel, E. J. Caterson, E. Eriksson. 2013. "Clinical Impact Upon Wound Healing and Inflammation in Moist, Wet, and Dry Environments." *Advances in Wound Care* (New Rochelle) 2:348–56. doi: 10.1089/wound.2012.0412.

[17] Carter, Kate. 2003. "Hydropolymer dressings in the management of wound exudate." *British Journal of Community Nursing* 8:10–6. doi: 10.12968/bjcn.2003.8.Sup3.11579.

[18] Fletcher, J. 2003. "The application of foam dressings." *Nursing Times* 31:59.

[19] Wiechula, R. 2003. "The use of moist wound-healing dressings in the management of split-thickness skin graft donor sites: a systematic review." *International Journal of Nursing Practice* 9:9–17.

[20] Suetake, T., and S. Sasai, Y. X. Zhen, T. Ohi, H. Tagami. 1996. "Functional analyses of the stratum corneum in scars. Sequential studies after injury and comparison among keloids, hypertrophic scars, and atrophic scars." *Archives of Dermatology* 132:1453–8.

[21] Arno, Anna I., and Gerd G. Gauglitz, Juan P. Barret, Marc G. Jeschke. 2014. "Up-to-date approach to manage keloids and hypertrophic scars: A useful guide." *Burns* 40:1255–66. doi: 10.1016/j.burns.2014.02.011.

[22] Mustoe, Thomas A. 2008. "Evolution of silicone therapy and mechanism of action in scar management." *Aesthetic Plastic Surgery* 32:82–92. doi: 10.1007/s00266-007-9030-9.

[23] Del Toro, Drew, and Raj Dedhia, Travis T. Tollefson. 2016. "Advances in scar management: prevention and management of hypertrophic scars and keloids." *Current Opinion in Otolaryngology & Head and Neck Surgery* 24:322–9. doi: 10.1097/MOO.0000000000000268.

[24] Chan, Kin Y., and Chee L. Lau, Syed M. Adeeb, Sathappan Somasundaram, Mohd Nasir-Zahari. 2005. "A randomized, placebo-controlled, double-blind, prospective clinical trial of silicone gel in prevention of hypertrophic scar development in median sternotomy wound." *Plastic and Reconstructive Surgery* 116:1013 – 1020.

[25] Mustoe, Thomas A., and Rodney D. Cooter, Michael H. Gold, F. D. Richard Hobbs, Albert-Adrien Ramelet, Peter G. Shakespeare, Maurizio Stella, Luc Téot, Fiona M. Wood, Ulrich E. Ziegler; International Advisory Panel on Scar Management. 2002. "International clinical recommendations on scar management." *Plastic and Reconstructive Surgery* 110:560–71.

[26] Gilman, T. H. 2003. "Silicone sheet for treatment and prevention of hypertrophic scar: a new proposal for the mechanism of efficacy." *Wound Repair and Regeneration* 11:235–6.

[27] Knighton, D. R., and I. A. Silver, T. K. Hunt. 1981. "Regulation of wound-healing angiogenesis-effect of oxygen gradients and inspired oxygen concentration." *Surgery* 90:262–70.

[28] Puri, Neerja, and Ashutosh Talwar. 2009 "The efficacy of silicone gel for the treatment of hypertrophic scars and keloids." *Journal of Cutaneous and Aesthetic Surgery* 2:104–6. doi: 10.4103/0974-2077.58527.

[29] Mustoe, Thomas A. 2008. "Evolution of silicone therapy and mechanism of action in scar management." *Aesthetic Plastic Surgery* 32:82–92.

[30] Musgrave, Melinda A., and Nisha Umraw, Joel S. Fish, Manuel Gomez, Robert C. Cartotto. 2002 "The effect of silicone gel sheets on perfusion of hypertrophic burn scars." The *Journal of Burn Care & Rehabilitation* 23:208–14.

[31] Signorini, Massimo, and Matteo T. Clementoni. 2007. "Clinical evaluation of a new self-drying silicone gel in the treatment of scars: A preliminary report." *Aesthetic Plastic Surgery* 31:183–7. doi: 10.1007/s00266-005-0122-0.

[32] Mokos, Zrinka B., and Anamaria Jović, Lovorka Grgurević, Ivo Dumić-Čule, Kresimir Kostović, Romana Čeović, Branca Marinović. 2017. "Current Therapeutic Approach to Hypertrophic Scars." *Frontiers in Medicine* (Lausanne). 4:83. doi: 10.3389/fmed.2017.00083.

[33] Engrav, L. H., and D. M. Heimbach, F. P. Rivara, M. L. Moore, J. Wang, G. J. Carrougher, B. Costa, S. Numhom, J. Calderon, N. S. Gibran. 2010. "12-Year within- wound study of the effectiveness of custom pressure garment therapy." *Burns* 36:975–83. doi: 10.1016/j.burns.2010.04.014.

[34] Atiyeh, B. S., and C. A. Amm, K. A. El Musa. 2003. "Improved scar quality following primary and secondary healing of cutaneous wounds." *Aesthetic Plastic Surgery* 27:411–7.

[35] Mouës, Chantal M., and Albert W. van Toorenenbergen, Freerk Heule, Wim C. Hop, Steven E. Hovius. 2008. "The role of topical negative pressure in wound repair: expression of biochemical markers in woundfluid during wound healing." *Wound Repairand Regeneration* 16:488–94. doi: 10.1111/j.1524-475X. 2008.00395.x.

[36] Anzarut, Alexander, and Jarret Olson, Prabhjyot Singh, Brian H. Rowe, Edward E. Tredget. 2009. "The effectiveness of pressure garment therapy for the prevention of abnormal scarring after burn injury: a meta-analysis." *Journal of Plastic, Reconstructive & Aesthetic Surgery* 62:77–84. doi: 10.1016/j.bjps.2007.10.052.

[37] Lansdown, Alan B. G., and Ursula Mirastschijski, Nicky Stubbs, Elizabeth Scanlon, Magnus S. Agren. 2007. "Zinc in wound healing: theoretical, experimental, and clinical aspects." *Wound Repair and Regeneration* 15:2–16. doi: 10.1111/j.1524-475X.2006.00179.x.

[38] Hughes, G., and N. R. McLean. 1988. "Zinc oxide tape: a useful dressing for the recalcitrant finger-tip and soft-tissue injury." *Archives of Emergency Medicine* 5:223–7.

[39] Aksoy, Berna, and Nilgun Atakan, H. Mete Aksoy, Gaya G. Tezel, Nurten Renda, H. Asuman Ozkara, Evren Onder. 2010. "Effectiveness of topical zinc oxide application on hypertrophicscar development in rabbits." *Burns* 36:1027–35. doi: 10.1016/j.burns.2010.01.020.

[40] Hallmans, G. 1978. "Healing of experimentally induced burn wounds: a comparative study of the healing of exposed burn wounds and burn wounds covered with adhesive zinc-tape and a scanning electron microscopic study of the microvasculature of wound healing in the rabbit ear." *Scandinavian Journal of Plastic and Reconstructive Surgery* 12:105–9.

[41] Lee, A. R., and W. H. Huang. 1995. "Zinc sulphadiazines: novel topical antimicrobial agents for burns." The *Journal of Pharmacy and Pharmacology* 47:503–9.

[42] Bush, Jim, and Karen So, Tracey Mason, Nick L. Occleston, Sharon O'Kane, Mark W. J. Ferguson. 2010. "Therapies with emerging evidence of efficacy: avotermin forthe improvement of scarring." *Dermatology Research and Practice* 2010. doi: 10.1155/2010/690613.

[43] Schrementi, Megan E., and Ahalia M. Ferreira, Chad Zender, Luisa A. DiPietro. 2008. "Site specific production of TGF-beta in oral mucosal and cutaneous wounds." *Wound Repair and Regeneration* 16:80–6. doi: 10.1111/j.1524-475X.2007.00320.x.

[44] Monstrey, Stan, and Esther Middelkoop, Jan J. Vranckx, Franco Bassetto, Ulrich E. Ziegler, Sylvie Meaume, Luc Téot. 2014. "Updated scar management practical guidelines: non-invasive and invasive measures." *Journal of Plastic, Reconstructive & Aesthetic Surgery* 67:1017–25. doi: 10.1016/j.bjps.2014.04.011.

[45] Shah, M., and D. M. Foreman, M. W. J. Ferguson. 1995. "Neutralisation of TGF-β1 and TGF-β2 or exogenous addition of TGF-β3 to cutaneous rat wounds reduces scarring." *Journal of Cell Science* 108:985–1002.

[46] Due, Eva, and Kristian Rossen, Lars T. Sorensen, Anette Kliem, Tonny Karlsmark, Merete Haedersdal. 2007. "Effect of UV irradiation on cutaneous cicatrices: a randomized, controlled trial with clinical, skin reflectance, histological, immunohistochemical and biochemical evaluations." *Acta Dermato-Venereologica* 87:27–32. doi: 10.2340/00015555-0154.

[47] Al-Shaqsi, Sultan, and Taimor Al-Bulushi. 2016. "Cutaneous Scar Prevention and Management: Overview of current therapies." *Sultan Qaboos University Medical Journal* 16:3–8. doi: 10.18295/squmj.2016.16.01.002.

[48] Abdel-Salam, Bahaa K. 2014. "Modulatory effect of whey proteins in some cytokines involved in wound healing in male diabetic albino rats." *Inflammation* 37:1616–22. doi: 10.1007/s10753-014-9888-z.

[49] Serra, Raffaele, and Raffaele Grande, Lucia Butrico, Gianluca Buffone, Francesco G. Caliò, Aida Squillace, Barbara A. Rizzo, Mafalda Massara, Francesco Spinelli, Alessia G. Ferrarese, Giovanni de Caridi, Luca Gallelli, Stefano de Franciscis. 2016. "Effects of a new nutraceutical substance on clinical and molecular parameters in patients with chronic venous ulceration." *International Wound Journal* 13:88–96. doi: 10.1111/iwj.12240.

[50] Kant, Vinay, and Anu Gopal, Nitya N. Pathak, Pawan Kumar, Surendra K. Tandan, Dinesh Kumar. 2014. "Antioxidant and anti-inflammatory potential of curcumin accelerated the cutaneous wound healing in streptozotocin-induced diabetic rats." *International Immunopharmacology* 20:322–30. doi: 10.1016/j.intimp.2014.03.009.

[51] Jagetia, Ganesh C., and Golgod K. Rajanikant. 2012. "Acceleration of wound repair by curcumin inthe excision wound of mice exposed to differentdoses of fractionated γ radiation. "*International Wound Journal* 9:76–92. doi: 10.1111/j.1742-481X.2011.00848.x.

In: Cutaneous Scars: Biology, Clinics and Management ISBN: 978-1-53615-657-7
Editors: Berna Aksoy, Hasan Mete Aksoy et al. © 2019 Nova Science Publishers, Inc.

Chapter 18

BIOPHYSICAL THERAPEUTICS

Zeynep Topkarci*

Department of Dermatology, Health Science University,
Bakirkoy Dr Sadi Konuk Training and Research Hospital, Istanbul, Turkey

ABSTRACT

Hypertrophic scars and keloids are all examples of abnormal response to cutaneous wound healing and can be associated with physical and psychological distress. Numerous treatment options exist, but there is still no single proven best treatment or combination of treatments. Biophysical treatment modalities including pressure therapy, silicone sheets and gel formulations, massage therapy, cryotherapy, adhesive tape support, radiofrequency, skin tension and electrical stimulation are effective and safe procedures for the management of hypertrophic scars and keloids but further large-sample clinical trials are required.

Keywords: hypertrophic scar, keloid, pressure therapy, silicone sheets, silicone gel, massage therapy, cryotherapy, adhesive tape support, radiofrequency, skin tension, electrical stimulation

1. INTRODUCTION

Hypertrophic scars and *keloids* are defined as abnormal scarring of the skin in certain individuals and anatomic sites [1].

---

*Corresponding Author's Email: ztopkarci@yahoo.com.

Patients with *keloids* or *hypertrophic scars* have severe impairment of quality of life because of aesthetic, functional, and social impairments. Proliferative scar related symptoms may include itching, stiffness, scar contractures, tenderness and pain [2].

A wide variety of treatments have been advocated for proliferative scars but none of these treatments has been adequately evaluated in high-quality studies and the optimal treatment method has not been established [3]. The current chapter will focus on the biophysical treatment modalities including *pressure therapy, silicone sheets* and gel formulations, *massage therapy, cryotherapy, adhesive tape support, radiofrequency, skin tension* and *electrical stimulation* for managing *hypertrophic scars* and *keloids.*

2. Pressure Therapy

Pressure therapy is usually performed with pressure garments, bandages, or devices for special locations. Pressure garments still represent the current first-line prophylactic therapy for *hypertrophic scars* especially after burns, although there is not any scientific evidence [4, 5].

The mechanism of action is through the reduction of collagen synthesis by several mechanisms; occlusion of small blood vessels resulting in a decreased blood, oxygen and nutrients delivery to the scar, matrix metalloprotease-28 (MMP-28) downregulation and increase of prostaglandin-E2 (PGE2) which activates collagenase [6]. The optimal amount of pressure must exceed the inherent capillary pressure without diminishing the peripheral blood circulation. The arterial capillary closure pressure is 25 mmHg, so pressures above 24 mmHg are required to overcome the capillary pressure. At least 15 mm Hg pressure is required to accelerate maturation, however maceration and paresthesia can occur at pressures above 40 mm Hg. [7]. So, the ideal pressure is between 20 to 40 mmHg and should be maintained for 12 to 24 hours per day for 6 to 12 months [5-7].

Application area is one of the most important factors that determines the efficacy of *pressure therapy* [8]. As good clinical response correlate with higher pressures [9-11], joints and trunk usually show pressures lower than 10 mmHg and the response to therapy is poor; in areas with medium response such as thighs, calves, and arms show mean pressures of 20.5 mmHg with higher clinical response to treatment [8].

A prospective trial investigating the influence of two different levels of pressure on burn scars showed that pressure garments that deliver a pressure of at least 15 mmHg pressure tend to accelerate scar maturation [12].

Also, balloon-compression wear has been described for keloid and *hypertrophic scars* in complicated surfaces such as chest area. Using air as a compression source, the garment has a greater compression force than the sponge or supporter and it is easy to wear and does not require tape fixation [13].

In a meta-analysis that included 6 randomized clinical trials, with 316 burn patients, *pressure therapy* appeared to improve scar height, although there was no difference in the global scar scores between the pressure garment therapy and control groups [14].

An auricular keloid after ear-piercing is a serious cosmetic problem. In observational studies of ear keloids, it has been shown that custom-made pressure devices may be beneficial to reduce post-surgical recurrence risk [15-18]. Several types of pressure earrings are available. Zimmer splints are cheap, easily moulded to fit the patient's ear and can be worn as earrings [15]. In another study, 88 patients who had undergone surgery for ear keloids were treated with custom-made pressure clips for 12 hours a day for 6 to 18 months and they had a recurrence rate of 29.5%. There were not any severe side effects observed after the therapy [19].

There are many problems associated with the use of pressure garments. The least of these is poor patient compliance due to problems with comfort, appearance and movement [5, 20, 21]. The heat and sweat disturbance is also a handicap especially in hot weather. Swelling, eczema, redness and pruritus have been reported on the extremities caused by pressure garments. Excessive friction, blistering, ulceration and scarring can occur as a consequence of high pressure and development of moisture in hot air and these side effects will lead to interruption of treatment [5, 21, 22].

Pressure-related skeletal and dental deformities can be seen in growing children and adults. In some recent studies, it has been shown that the pressure exerted by tight-fitting garments can adversely affect normal physiological balance [5, 23].

3. Silicone Sheets and Gel Formulations (Occlusive Dressings)

Silicone products are recommended as the "gold standard" option for the prevention and treatment of keloids and *hypertrophic scars* and available for the past 30 years. Silicones have been manufactured in various forms such as creams, oil or gel with additives such as Vitamin E, cushions or sheets, in combination with other dressing types, and as custom-made silicon applications. *Silicone gel* sheeting is soft, self-adhesive and semiocclusive [24, 25].

Although the exact mechanism of action of silicone products is unknown, occlusion and hydration of the stratum corneum are the major mechanisms [25]. *Silicone sheets* decrease evaporation of water from the skin and increase hydration of the stratum corneum. The reduction in transepidermal water loss reduces the stimulation of keratinocytes, and as a result, cytokine production stops and dermal fibroblasts cannot be activated [26-28]. The impact of occlusion is shown with a study in which silicone cream containing 20% silicone oil and occlusive dressing has a greater improvement in scars than silicone cream covered with gauze [29].

Temperature alteration may be another mechanism of action of silicone products in *hypertrophic scars* and *keloids.* Surface temperature of the scar increased significantly following gel application, which can increase collagenase activity leading to collagen breakdown [30]. Also, a negative static electric field between the silicone product and the skin may cause realignment of collagen, resulting in involution of hypertrophic and keloid scars [31, 32].

In one study, *silicone gel* was found to be responsible for increased basic fibroblast growth factor (bFGF) levels in normal and fetal dermal fibroblasts. An increase in bFGF levels in fibroblasts leads to reduction in collagen production [33].

Another investigation indicated that silicone sheeting may act by down-regulating the production of the fibrogenic cytokine, transforming growth factor β2, by fibroblasts [34].

Silicone sheets are applied within 2 to 3 weeks after the complete epithelialization and wound healing. The sheet should be cut to fit the size of the scar, placed on top of the scar, taped into place and left for 12 to 24 hours per day, for 2 to 6 months. The sheet should be replaced every 10 to 14 days, and need to be washed daily with mild soap and water to prevent side effects such as rashes and infections. *Silicone gels* should be applied twice daily for 3 to 6 months [35].

Silicone gel sheeting should not be used on open wounds and some dermatological conditions such as acne and psoriasis which disrupt the integrity of the skin. Common problems with silicone sheeting include local skin reactions, such as maceration, pruritus, folliculitis and bad smell of the gel [36]. Complications are reported to increase when silicone therapy is combined with *pressure therapy* [37]. Silicone products are not painful and can be used in children [38].

Silicone materials do not have any effect on mature *keloids* and *hypertrophic scars* [24].

A systematic review that included 20 trials involving a total of 873 patients compared adhesive *silicone gel* sheeting with non-silicone dressing, other silicone products, laser therapy, triamcinolone acetonide injection, topical onion extract, *pressure therapy*, and no therapy. *Silicone gel* sheeting was shown to reduce the incidence of hypertrophic scarring in patients prone to scarring, this form of therapy also produced a statistically significant reduction in scar thickness and color improvement when compared with no treatment. However, many of the included studies are of poor quality and are highly susceptible to bias. There was a weak evidence for the benefit of *silicone gel* sheeting in preventing and treating *hypertrophic scars* and *keloids* [24].

Fluid *silicone gel* formulation is an alternative to *silicone sheets* for use on large and visible areas such as face and hands. Silicone topical elastomer gel Dermatix® is a Food and Drug Administration (FDA)-registered substantial equivalent to *silicone gel* sheeting for the prevention and management of *hypertrophic scars* and *keloids.* In the study of

Chernoff et al., it has been shown that better resolution and improvement of scars are possible with Dermatix® treatment or the combined use of Dermatix® and *silicone gel* sheeting than with *silicone gel* sheeting alone. Both Dermatix® and *silicone gel* sheeting reduced symptoms of itching and irritation. However, Dermatix® treatment was favored with regard to patient acceptability. Safety profile was favorable and in contrast with *silicone gel* sheeting, Dermatix® caused no skin breakdown [39].

Combinations of therapies can be used, particularly in anatomic areas which do not respond well to *silicone sheeting* because of difficulty to maintain gel contact with the skin (e.g., chin, breast, clavicle, neck, and face). The most common combination is that of a silicone silastic sheet, gel sheet, or pad with a classical pressure garment (Figure 1) [37]. One of these combination methods for treating scars is the inflatable silicone inserts in which the pressure on the scar can be adjusted by means of a pump. The system is indicated for the treatment of scars or keloids in concave areas (presternal, axillary, subclavicular) or in soft tissue parts of the face and neck [37]. However, a randomized controlled trial with intra-individual comparison showed no added beneficial effect when applying silicone underneath the pressure garment in burn *hypertrophic scars* [40]. In another study, Vitamin E was added to *silicone gel* and found to be beneficial but there is no controlled study about its efficacy [41].

In a recent retrospective pilot study to determine the effectiveness of topical scar-reducing treatments and patients' compliance, there were significant differences in efficacy scores between treatment groups and control group. Additionally efficacy scores were significantly higher in *silicone gel,* onion extract gel, and combined treatments in comparison to silicone sheet, ($p < 0.05$). Patient satisfaction scores were significantly higher in *silicone gel,* onion extract gel, and combined treatments in comparison to silicone sheet and control group ($p < 0.05$). However, the patients reported that the silicone sheet and combined therapies were significantly more difficult to apply than the *silicone gel* and onion extract gel ($p < 0.05$) [42].

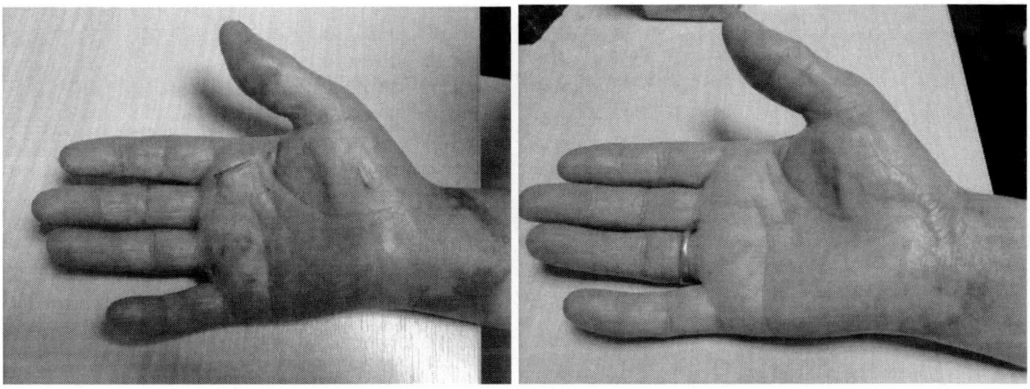

Figure 1. Third degree burn scar located on hand a) before and b) after 4 months use of silicone sheet under pressure garment therapy (Courtesy of Berna Aksoy, MD).

There is limited data about the efficacy, so larger randomized clinical trials with higher number of patients are needed to confirm the efficacy of silicone based products in the treatment and prevention of hypertrophic and keloid scars.

4. Massage Therapy

Massage therapy is a standard therapy in the treatment of scars and burns in rehabilitation centers. It can be manual or mechanical (i.e., compressed air, threadlike showers, vacuum therapy, etc.) [43]. The exact mechanism of action is unknown, but massage may be effective through its ability to affect matrix remodeling and fibroblast apoptosis [44]. In addition, *massage therapy* produced an elevation of beta endorphins, resulted in decreased urinary cortisol and increased serotonin and dopamin levels [45, 46].

Scar massage with creams and oils can help to improve relationship with the patient, reveals patients' anxiety and improves their mood and mental status, reduces scar-related pain and itching, hydrates the skin and increases scar pliability, however, there is not any scientific evidence [47, 48]. Only reduction of pain and itching has been documented in studies investigating adult patients [47].

There are several options of moisturising creams and oils for *massage therapy* to help reduce scaring. The emolient should be nonirritating and free of any sensitizers. One of them is Medline Remedy® Phytoplex™, which contains 24% silicone with additonal botanical oils with antioxidant and anti-inflammatory properties, and no fragrance or parabens [49].

In a review of Shin et al. 10 publications including 144 patients who received scar massage were examined. Time to treatment onset ranged from after suture removal to longer than 2 years. Treatment protocols ranged from 10 minutes twice daily to 30 minutes twice weekly. Treatment duration varied from one treatment to 6 months. According to this review, scar massage is anectodally effective but the scientific data in the literature is limited, and its efficacy appears to be greater in postsurgical scars than in posttraumatic or postburn scars [44].

Mechanical massage techniques include compressed air, thread like showers, and vacuum massage but none of them has been validated [43]. Vacuum massage is a non-invasive mechanical massage technique performed with a mechanical device that lifts the skin by means of suction, creates a skin fold and mobilizes that skin fold. It has been frequently used to treat traumatic or burn scars [50].

Nineteen articles were examined in a review about the physical and physiological effects of vacuum massage. Improvement of the tissue hardness and the elasticity of the skin were the most frequently reported physical effects. One of the reported physiological effects was an increased number of fibroblasts and collagen fibers accompanied by an alteration of fibroblast phenotype and collagen orientation. Vacuum massage may release the mechanical tension associated with scar retraction and thus induces apoptosis of myofibroblasts. Information about the reduction of pain and itch secondary to vacuum massage was little and the technique has not been validated [50].

Contraindications for *massage therapy* are cutaneous fragility, open wounds, infection, pain, and inflammation. Complications of the *massage therapy* are inflammation, cutaneous lesions, epithelial breakdown, and infection [43]. Further large-sampled clinical trials are required to prove the effectiveness of this therapy.

5. CRYOTHERAPY

Cryotherapy can be administered as spray, contact or intra-lesional for the treatment of *hypertrophic scars* and *keloids.* It can be used either alone or in combination with other therapies although combination therapy is more effective. It has been proven to reduce the volume of keloid by vascular damage and ischemic cell death leading to reduction in blood supply and tissue necrosis. Better results can be achieved for early keloids which are more vascular than older lesions. *Cryotherapy* has total or partial success after at least three sessions of 20-30 seconds. Each session is applied once monthly and 3 to 6 treatments are often needed. To reduce pain, local anesthesia is recommended [51, 52].

A combination of *cryotherapy* and intra-lesional steroids has been described as the most common traditional therapy for *hypertrophic scars* and *keloids* and the combination has a synergistic effect. *Cryotherapy* should be performed prior to injections, as it softens the keloid and makes the injections easier [52, 53].

Hirshowitz and colleagues, combined contact cryosurgery with intra-lesional corticosteroid injections and approximately 70% of the treated cases showed improvement of their keloids [54].

The most effective *cryotherapy* method is intra-lesional *cryotherapy* (ILC). ILC is able to reach the deeper dermis with a better protection of the superficial epithelial layer and concentrate the cold temperature within the lesion more than spray therapy. It is a better form of scar treatment than external *cryotherapy* in which multiple sessions are required to achieve visible and sustained results [55, 56].

Har-Shai and colleagues developed an intra-lesional cryo-probe device with disposable cryo-needles connected to a canister of liquid nitrogen. The intra-lesional cryosurgery was performed under local anesthesia. The probe is inserted directly into the scarred tissue leading to a deep freeze from inside. After the *hypertrophic scar* or *keloid* has been completely frozen, the cryo-probe is defrosted and withdrawn. Depending on the keloid size, the freezing time may vary; 10 to 30 second freeze-thaw cycle can be used and if necessary it may be repeated up to three times per treatment session.

Treatments can be repeated at two to six week intervals until response occurs. There was an approximately 67.4% reduction of scar volume at the end of the 18-month follow-up period after a single intra-lesional treatment. Additional improvements were noted in hardness, elevation and redness as well as itching, pain, and tenderness [57].

A multicenter prospective trial consisting of a patient population of different Fitzpatrick skin phototypes (I through VI) demonstrated that intra-lesional *cryotherapy* has a favorable effect on the reduction of the scar volume, and relieving complaints of pain and pruritus. However, the device failed to achieve complete scar clearance in all cases; recurring scars and persistent hypopigmentation were higher in incidence in Fitzpatrick type V and VI patients than Fitzpatrick type I and II patients [58].

In a retrospective study, intra-lesional cryosurgery was used as monotherapy or combined with the application of topical *silicone gel* sheeting for comparison. The combined therapy showed better results with regard to keloid hardness, pain, and discomfort. The results of this study support the use of combination therapy consisting of intra-lesional cryosurgery followed by the application of *silicone gel* sheeting to treat refractory *keloids* [59].

Cryotherapy can also be used for small based and earlobe keloids as postoperative combination treatment after the initial treatment with surgical excision. Surgical excision followed by immediate freezing of the open wound was performed in one study of 66 patients with 97 large ear *keloids*. After a median follow-up time of 12 months, 36% of lesions recurred and required further treatment [60].

Most frequent side effects are local pain during freezing or shortly after treatment, hypopigmentation or hyperpigmentation. Freezing temperatures are different for individual cell types ranging from -4 to -7°C for melanocytes, and -30 to -35°C for fibroblasts. As a result of melanocyte hypersensitivity to cold temperatures, hypopigmentation can be seen in this therapy [61, 62].

According to Har-Shai et al. thermal insulation of the skin surface during the intra-lesional cryosurgery technique may provide a better survival environment for melanocytes compared with that of the contact method, thus producing lower incidence of permanent hypopigmentation. As a result, keloids of darker/black-colored skin exhibit less depigmentation following intra-lesional cryosurgery when compared with the contact method [62].

Recurrence rates after intra-lesional *cryotherapy* are reported to be in the range of 0% and 24% in the literature [63].

6. Adhesive Tape Support

Tension plays a major pathophysiologic role in hypertrophic scar formation. Surgical scars are sensitive to *skin tension* after suture removal. Longitudinal stretching of wounds appears to be the stimulus for hypertrophic scarring. The exact mechanism of microporous paper tape is unknown. It is able to reduce tension by controlling or eliminating stretching forces [64, 65].

Paper tape is a noninvasive, inexpensive method for the prevention of hypertrophic scarring. It is inflexible, microporous and semiocclusive [64].

In a randomized controlled trial, microporous paper tape was compared with no intervention and shown to be a convenient and effective way to reduce both the scar volume and incidence of hypertrophic scar formation in women undergoing cesarean section [64].

Hydration is another mechanism of paper tape. The production of collagen, and glycosaminoglycan by fibroblasts is reduced in well hydrated tissues. Paper tape is also thought to reduce the risk of abnormal scar formation by mimicking the stratum corneum and reducing evaporative losses from the wound [66]. In a study comparing Micropore paper tape and Blenderm plastic tape (3M, St. Paul, MN, USA), areas treated with Blenderm that provide better hydration were less red and less hypertrophic than areas treated with Micropore. However, the difference was not significant, suggesting that hydration is not the main mechanism of action of reduction of scarring with *adhesive tape support* [67].

It is necessary to use microporous hypoallergenic paper tape to fresh surgical incisions with an appropriate adhesive, beginning at 2 weeks and used for at least 12 weeks after surgery. It has been reported to be effective in controlling scar tension, eliminating stretching forces, and preventing hypertrophic scarring [64]. Elastic composite tape can be used for scars on mobile surfaces such as joints [68, 69].

Individuals with a higher risk of developing *hypertrophic scars* are advised to use paper strips for a longer period of time, beginning at 2 weeks until the scar maturation. It can be used continuously for 4 to 7 days, even during bathing [64]. However, this treatment appears to be less effective than more conventional treatments such as *silicone gel,* but may be used as a preventive treatment for low-risk patients. It is not effective and practical for plaque-like scars after deep burns [68, 69].

Adverse reactions are few and mainly involve a localized red rash under the tape. These reactions are transient, and resolve without medical intervention [64].

7. Other Treatments

7.1. ThermaCool TC Radiofrequency

Thermage *radiofrequency* instruments were used for *hypertrophic scars* based on the hypothesis that they could do collagen remodeling. In a single center, open-label, pilot study with ThermaCool (ThermaCoolTM System, Thermage, Inc., Hayward, CA), no difference was observed with the control group in terms of clinical and histopathological recovery. Differences in collagen morphology were detected in some subjects. Increased collagen production (type III > type I) was observed, appeared to peak between 6 and 10 weeks posttreatment and did not return to baseline even after 12 weeks [70]. Further studies should be done to evaluate the collagen effects of this device and to optimize its therapeutic potential.

7.2. Skin Tension Offloading Device

Tension is one of the most important factors in the development of wide and *hypertrophic scars* [71]. Embrace Advanced Scar Therapy device is a tension offloading device and reduce mechanical forces on surgical incisions.

In a randomized controlled trial to evaluate abdominoplasty scar appearance following postoperative treatment with the embrace Advanced Scar Therapy device, embrace treatment was applied to half of the abdominoplasty incision, while control treatment (surgeon's optimal care methods) was performed on the other half. Mean visual analogue scale score for embrace-treated scars was significantly improved compared with control at follow-up period of 12 months. This may represent an important therapy in the future for the prevention of keloids and *hypertrophic scars*. These results demonstrate that the embrace device significantly reduces scarring following abdominoplasty surgery [72].

7.3. Electrical Stimulation

Electrical stimulation (ES) is a promising area of development in the management of abnormal skin scarring. Various forms of ES have shown to have clinical benefit in the treatment of abnormal raised dermal scarring. These include low-intensity direct current (LIDC), low-intensity pulsed direct current (LIPDC), high-voltage pulsed current (HVPC) and transcutaneous electrical nerve stimulation (TENS) [73, 74].

Perry et al. demonstrated the utility of a non-invasive ES namely degenerate waveform, based on the Fenzian electrical biofeedback system, in the treatment of skin scarring. The study resulted in a clinically and statistically significant ($P < 0.05$) reduction of symptoms and scar scores. Individuals with keloid scars showed the greatest pain relief; those with hypertrophic scars had the best improved itch symptoms, while scar score reduction was better achieved in hypertrophic and surgical scar cases. However, patient age and the number of problematic scars present affect the response to biofeedback ES [75].

Fenzian biofeedback ES treatment system delivers a low-intensity transcutaneous ES current to specific skin areas. It has been shown to reduce the symptoms of pain, pruritus and inflammation in patients with raised cutaneous scars. A range of patients with varying skin types (I–VI) were included and this modality effectively controlled their symptoms [76].

Sebastian et al. investigated the effect of photodynamic treatment (PDT) on keloid fibroblasts with or without ES and showed that ES enhanced the cytotoxic effects of PDT and could be used as a combination therapy. However, further studies with long-term follow-up and histologic evidence may provide more information on this treatment in the management of abnormal skin scars [77].

Conclusion

Keloids and hypertrophic scars present potential cosmetic and functional problems for patients. It is more important to prevent hypertrophic scars than to treat them. The exact timing of the hypertrophic scar or keloid treatment is when the scar is immature and the overlying epithelium is intact.

Silicone-based therapies are the best option for the prevention and initial management of abnormal scarring. For unresponsive lesions, combination therapy (pressure therapy, cryotherapy, intra-lesional steroid, electric stimulation, photodynamic treatment, laser treatment, surgical treatment) can be effective.

As a result, there are multiple medical and surgical therapies for the treatment of keloids and hypertrophic scars. However, data on the efficacy of these treatments is still limited. A better understanding of the pathogenesis will allow the development of newer and more targeted therapies in the future.

References

[1] English, R. S., and P. D. Shenefelt. 1999. "Keloids and hypertrophic scars." *Dermatologic Surgery* 25:631–8.

[2] Bock, Oliver, and Gerhard Schmid-Ott, Peter Malewski, Ulrich Mrowietz. 2006. "Quality of life of patients with keloid and hypertrophic scarring." *Archives of Dermatological Research* 297:433–8. doi: 10.1007/s00403-006-0651-7.

[3] Gauglitz, Gerd G. 2013. "Management of keloids and hypertrophic scars: current and emerging options." *Clinical, Cosmetic and Investigational Dermatology* 6:103–14. doi: 10.2147/CCID.S35252.

[4] Atiyeh, Bishara S. 2007. "Nonsurgical management of hypertrophic scars: evidence-based therapies, standard practices, and emerging methods." *Aesthetic Plastic Surgery* 31:468–92. doi: 10.1007/s00266-006-0253-y.

[5] Macintyre, Lisa, and Margot Baird. 2006. "Pressure garments for use in the treatment of hypertrophic scars: a review of the problems associated with their use." *Burns* 32:10–5. doi: 10.1016/j.burns.2004.06.018.

[6] Reno, F., and P. Grazianetti, M. Cannas. 2001. "Effects of mechanical compression on hypertrophic scars: prostaglandin E2 release." *Burns* 27:215–8.

[7] Reid, W. H., and J. H. Evangs, R. S. Naismith, A. E. Tully, S. Sherwin. 1987. "Hypertrophic scarring and pressure therapy." *Burns* 13:829–32.

[8] Giele, H., and K. Liddiard, K. Booth, F. Wood. 1998. "Anatomical variations in pressures generated by pressure garments." *Plastic and Reconstructive Surgery* 101:399.

[9] Leung, P. C., and M. Ng. 1980. "Pressure therapy for hypertrophic scars resulting from burns." *Burns* 6:244.

[10] Rose, M. P., and E. A. Deitch. 1985. "The clinical use of a tubular compression bandage, Tubigrip, for burn-scar therapy: A critical analysis." *Burns* 12:58.

[11] Cheng, J. C. Y., and J. H. Evans, K. S. Leung, J. A. Clark, T. T. Choy, P. C. Leung. 1984. "Pressure therapy in the treatment of postburn hypertrophic scar: A clinical look into its usefulness and fallacies by pressure monitoring." *Burns* 10:154.

[12] Van den Kerckhove, Eric, and Karel Stappaerts, Steffen Fieuws, Jan Laperre, Patrick Massage, Mieke Flour, Willy Boeckx. 2005. "The assessment of erythema and thickness on burn related scars during pressure garment therapy as a preventive measure for hypertrophic scarring." *Burns* 31:696. doi: 10.1016/j.burns.2005.04.014

[13] Kosaka, Masaaki, and Hiroshi Kamiishi. 2001. "New concept of balloon-compression wear for the treatment of keloids and hypertrophic scars." *Plastic and Reconstructive Surgery* 108:1454.

[14] Anzarut, Alexander, and Jarret Olson, Prabhjyot Singh, Brian H. Rowe, Edward E. Tredget. 2009. "The effectiveness of pressure garment therapy for the prevention of abnormal scarring after burn injury: a meta-analysis." *Journal of Plastic, Reconstructive & Aesthetic Surgery* 62:77. doi: 10.1016/j.bjps.2007.10.052.

[15] Russell, R., and N. Horlock, D. Gault. 2001. "Zimmer splintage: a simple effective treatment for keloids following ear-piercing." *British Journal of Plastic Surgery* 54:509. doi: 10.1054/bjps.2001.3649.

[16] Bran, Gregor M., and Jörn Brom, Karl Hörmann, Boris A. Stuck. 2012. "Auricular keloids: combined therapy with a new pressure device." *Archives of Facial Plastic Surgery* 14:20-6. doi: 10.1001/archfacial.2011.57.

[17] Park, Tae H., and Sang W. Seo, June-Kyu Kim, Choong H. Chang. 2011."Outcomes of surgical excision with pressure therapy using magnets and

identification of risk factors for recurrent keloids." *Plastic and Reconstructive Surgery* 128:431-9. doi: 10.1097/PRS.0b013e31821e7006.

[18] Park, Tae H., Ji H. Park, June-Kyu Kim, Sang W. Seo, Dong K. Rah, Choong H. Chang. 2013. "Analysis of 15 cases of auricular keloids following conchal cartilage grafts in an asian population." *Aesthetic Plastic Surgery* 37:102-5. doi: 10.1007/s00266-012-9998-7.

[19] Tanaydin, V., and J. Beugels, A. Piatkowski, C. Colla, E. van den Kerckhove, G. C. Hugenholtz, R. R. van der Hulst. 2016. "Efficacy of custom-made pressure clips for ear keloid treatment after surgical excision." *Journal of Plastic, Reconstructive & Aesthetic Surgery* 69:115–21. doi: 10.1016/j.bjps.2015.09.013.

[20] Johnson, J., and B. Greenspan, D. Gorga, W. Nagler, C. Goodwin. 1994. "Compliance with pressure garment use in burn rehabilitation." The *Journal of Burn Care & Rehabilitation* 15:181.

[21] Stewart, Rene, and Anil M. Bhagwanjee, Yoliswa Mbakaza, Tabisa Binase. 2000. "Pressure garment adherence in adult patients with burn injuries: An analysis of patient and clinician perceptions." The *American Journal of Occupational Therapy* 54:598.

[22] Brown, Cary A. 2001. "A comparison of the outcomes of two clinical audits of burn pressure garment satisfaction and compliance in Saudi Arabia". *Burns* 27:342.

[23] Harumi, Morooka, and Nakahashi Miyuki, Morooka Hideo, Kitamura Kiyokazu. 2001. "Effects of clothing pressure exerted on a trunk on heart rate, blood pressure, skin blood flow, and respiratory function." *Journal of Textile Machinery Society of Japan* 54:57.

[24] O'Brien, Lisa, and Abhay Pandit. 2006. "Silicon gel sheeting for preventing and treating hypertrophic and keloid scars." The *Cochrane Database of Systematic Reviews* (1):CD003826. doi: 10.1002/14651858.CD003826.pub2.

[25] Mustoe, Thomas A. 2008. "Evolution of silicone therapy and mechanism of action in scar management". *Aesthetic Plastic Surgery* 32:82-92. doi: 10.1007/s00266-007-9030-9.

[26] Quinn, K. J., and J. H. Evans, J. M. Courtney, J. D. Gaylor, W. H. Reid. 1985. "Non-pressure treatment of hypertrophic scars." *Burns, Including Thermal Injury* 12:102-8.

[27] Gilman, T. H. 2003. "Silicone sheet for treatment and prevention of hypertrophic scar: a new proposal for the mechanism of efficacy." *Wound Repair and Regeneration* 11: 235-6.

[28] Branagan, M., and D. H. Chenery, S. Nicholson. 2000. "Use of infrared attenuated total reflectance spectroscopy for the in vivo measurement of hydration level and silicone distribution in the stratum corneum following skin coverage by polymeric dressings." *Skin Pharmacology and Applied Skin Physiology* 13:157-64. doi: 10.1159/000029921.

[29] Sawada, Y., and K. Sone. 1990. "Treatment of scars and keloids with a cream containing silicone oil." *British Journal of Plastic Surgery* 43:683-8.

[30] Musgrave, Melinda A., and Nisha Umraw, Joel S. Fish, Manuel Gomez, Robert C. Cartotto. 2002. "The effect of silicone gel sheets on perfusion of hypertrophic burn scars." The *Journal of Burn Care & Rehabilitation* 23:208-14.

[31] Har-Shai, Y., and E. Lindenbaum, M. Tendler, A. Gamliel-Lazarovich, L. Feitelberg, B. Hirshowitz. 1999. "Negatively charged static electricity stimulation as a possible mechanism for enhancing the involution of hypertrophic and keloid scars." The *Israel Medical Association Journal* 1:203-5.

[32] Hirshowitz, Bernard, and Ella Lindenbaum, Yaron Har-Shai, Lev Feitelberg, Mark Tendler, Deganit Katz. 1998. "Static-electric field induction by a silicone cushion for the treatment of hypertrophic and keloid scars." *Plastic and Reconstructive Surgery* 101:1173-83.

[33] Hanasono, Matthew M., and Joanne Lum, Lisa A. Carroll, Anthony A. Mikulec, R. James Koch. 2004. "The effect of silicone gel on basic fibroblast growth factor levels in fibroblast cell culture." *Archives of Facial Plastic Surgery* 6:88-93. Doi: 10.1001/archfaci.6.2.88

[34] Kuhn, M. A., and M. R. Moffit, P. D. Smith, W. G. Lyle, F. Ko, D. D. Meltzer, M. C. Robson. 2001. "Silicone sheeting decreases fibroblast activity and downregulates TGFbeta2 in hypertrophic scar model." *International Journal of Surgical Investigation* 2:467-74.

[35] Nast, Alexander, and Sabine Eming, Joachim Fluhr, Klaus Fritz, Gerd Gauglitz, Silvia Hohenleutner, Renato G. Panizzon, Günther Sebastian, Birte Sporbeck, Josef Koller. 2012. "German S2k guidelines for the therapy of pathological scars (hypertrophic scars and keloids)." *Journal der Deutschen Dermatologicshen Gesselschaft* 10:747-62. doi: 10.1111/j.1610-0387.2012.08012.x.

[36] Nedelec, Bernadette, and Alissa Carter, Lisa Forbes, Shu-Chuan C. Hsu, Margaret McMahon, Ingrid Parry, Colleen M. Ryan, Michael A. Serghiou, Jeffrey C. Schneider, Patricia A. Sharp, Ana de Oliveira, Jill Boruff. 2015. "Practice guidelines for the application of nonsilicone or silicone gels and gel sheets after burn injury." *Journal of Burn Care & Research* 36:345-74. doi: 10.1097/BCR.0000000000000124.

[37] Van den Kerckhove, Eric, and Karel Stappaerts, Willy Boeckx, Bert Van den Hof, Stan Monstrey, Alain Van der Kelen, Jan De Cubber. 2001 "Silicones in the rehabilitation of burns: A review and overview." *Burns* 27:205-14.

[38] Berman, Brian, and Martha H. Viera, Sadegh Amini, Ran Huo, Isaac S. Jones. 2008. "Prevention and management of hypertrophic scars and keloids after burns in children." The *Journal of Craniofacial Surgery* 19:989-1006. doi: 10.1097/SCS. 0b013e318175f3a7.

[39] Chernoff, W. Gregory, and Harvey Cramer, Stephanie Su-Huang. 2007. "The efficacy of topical silicone gel elastomers in the treatment of hypertrophic scars, keloid scars, and post-laser exfoliation erythema." *Aesthetic Plastic Surgery* 31:495- 500. doi: 10.1007/s00266-006-0218-1.

[40] Steinstraesser, Lars, and Eva Flak, Bernd Witte, Andrej Ring, Daniel Tilkorn, Jörg Hauser, Stefan Langer, Hans-Ulrich Steinau, Sammy Al-Benna. 2011. "Pressure garment therapy alone and in combination with silicone for the prevention of hypertrophic scarring: randomized controlled tiral with intraindividual comparison." *Plastic and Reconstructive Surgery* 128:306e–13e. doi: 10.1097/PRS.0b013e3182268c69.

[41] Palmieri, Beniamino, and Glauco Gozzi, Gaspare Palmieri. 1995. "Vitamin E added silicone gel sheets for treatment of hypertrophic scars and keloids." *International Journal of Dermatology* 34:506-9.

[42] Aksoy, H. Mete, and Berna Aksoy, Asli Tatlıparmak, Emel Çalıkoğlu. 2018. "The effectiveness of topical scar-reducing therapies administered for scarring due to burns and other causes: A retrospective pilot clinical research." *Gulhane Medical Journal* 60:139-44. doi: 10.26657/gulhane.00039.

[43] Roques, C. 2002. "Massage applied to scars." *Wound Repair and Regeneration* 10:126–8.

[44] Shin, Thuzar M., and Jeremy S. Bordeaux. 2012. "The role of massage in scar management: a literature review." *Dermatologic Surgery* 38:414–23. doi: 10.1111/ j.1524-4725.2011.02201.x.

[45] Kaada, Birger, and Ove Torsteinbo.1989." Increase of plasma beta-endorphins in connective tissue massage." *General Pharmacology* 20:487-9.

[46] Field, T., and N. Grizzle, F. Scafidi, S. Schanberg. 1996. "Massage and relaxation therapies' effects on depressed adolescent mothers." *Adolescence* 31:903-11.

[47] Field, T., and M. Peck, M. Hernandez-Rief, S. Krugman, I. Burman, L. Ozment-Schenk. 2000. "Postburn itching: pain, and psychological symptoms are reduced with massage therapy." The *Journal of Burn Care & Rehabilitation* 21:189–93.

[48] Patino, O., and C. Novick, A. Merlo, F. Benaim. 1999. "Massage in hypertrophic scars." The *Journal of Burn Care & Rehabilitation* 20:268–71.

[49] Romay, C., and J. Arnesto, D. Remirez, R. Gonzalez, N. Ledon, I. Garcia. 1998. "Antioxidant and anti-inflammatory properties of C-phycocyanin from blue-green algae." *Inflammation Research* 47:36-41. doi: 10.1007/s000110050256.

[50] Moortgat, Peter, and Mieke Anthonissen, Jill Meirte, Ulrike Van Daele, Koen Maertens. 2016. "The physical and physiological effects of vacuum massage on the different skin layers: a current status of the literature." *Burns & Trauma* 4:34. doi: 10.1186/s41038-016-0053-9.

[51] Zouboulis, C. C., and C. E Orfanos. 1990. "Cryosurgical treatment of hypertrophic scars and keloids." *Hautarzt* 41:683–8.

[52] Leventhal, Douglas, and Maxwell Furr, David Reiter. 2006. "Treatment of keloids and hypertrophic scars: a meta-analysis and review of the literature." *Archives of Facial Plastic Surgery* 8:362-8. doi: 10.1001/archfaci.8.6.362

[53] Layton, A. M., and J. Yip, W. J. Cunliffe. 1994. "A comparison of intralesional triamcinolone and cryosurgery in the treatment of acne keloids." The *British Journal of Dermatology* 130:498–501.

[54] Hirshowitz, B., and D. Lerner, A. R. Moscona. 1982."Treatment of keloid scars by combined cryosurgery and intralesional corticosteroids." *Aesthetic Plastic Surgery* 6:153–8.

[55] Love, P. B., and R. V. Kundu. 2013. "Keloids: an update on medical and surgical treatments". *Journal of Drugs in Dermatology* 12(4):403–9.

[56] Har-Shai, Yaron, and Wifred Brown, Daniel Labbé, Anne Dompmartin, Irina Goldine, Tamir Gil, Issa Mettanes, Norbert Pallua. 2008. "Intralesional cryosurgery for the treatment of hypertrophic scars and keloids following aesthetic surgery: the results of a prospective observational study." The *International Journal of Lower Extremity Wounds* 7(3):169–175. doi:10.1177/1534734608322813.

[57] Har-Shai, Y., and E. Sabo, E. Rohde, M. Hyams, C. Assaf, C. C. Zouboulis. 2006. "Intralesional cryosurgery enhances the involution of recalcitrant auricular keloids: a new clinical approach supported by experimental studies." *Wound Repair and Regeneration* 14:18–27. doi: 10.1111/j.1743-6109.2005.00084.x.

[58] van Leeuwen, Michiel C., and Martijn B. van der Wal, Anne-Eva Bulstra, Francisca Galindo-Garre, Jonneke Molier, Paul P. van Zuijlen, Paul A. van Leeuwen, Frank B. Niessen. 2015. "Intralesional cryotherapy for treatment of keloid scars: a prospective study." *Plastic and Reconstructive Surgery* 135:580–9. doi: 10.1097/PRS.0000000000000911.

[59] Stromps, Jan-Philipp, and Sebastian Dunda, Ron-Julius Eppstein, Denis Babic, Yaron Har-Shai, Norbert Pallua. 2014. "Intralesional cryosurgery combined with topical silicone gel sheeting for the treatment of refractory keloids." *Dermatologic Surgery* 40:996-1003. doi: 10.1097/01.DSS.0000452627.91586.cc.

[60] Litrowski, N., and M. C. Boullie, D. Dehesdin, A. De Barros, P. Joly. 2014." Treatment of earlobe keloids by surgical excision and cryosurgery." *Journal of the European Academy of Dermatology and Venereology* 28:1324. doi: 10.1111/jdv.12282.

[61] Rusciani, L., and G. Rossi, R. Bono. 1993. "Use of cryotherapy in the treatment of keloids." The *Journal of Dermatologic Surgery and Oncology* 19:529–34.

[62] Har-Shai, Y., and E. Dujovny, E. Rohde, C. C. Zouboulis. 2007. "Effect of skin surface temperature on skin pigmentation during contact and intralesional cryosurgery of keloids." *Journal of the European Academy of Dermatology and Venereology* 21:191-8. doi: 10.1111/j.1468-3083.2006.01890.x.

[63] Zouboulis, Christos C., and Ulrike Blume, Petra Büttner, Constantin E. Orfanos. 1993. "Outcomes of cryosurgery in keloids and hypertrophic scars. A prospective consecutive trial of case series. "*Archives of Dermatology* 129:1146-51.

[64] Atkinson, Jo-An M., and Kryss T. McKenna, Adrian G. Barnett, David J. McGrath, Michael Rudd. 2005. "A randomized, controlled trial to determine the efficacy of paper tape in preventing hypertrophic scar formation in surgical incision that traverse Langer's skin tension lines." *Plastic and Reconstructive Surgery* 116:1648–56.

[65] Curtis, A. S., and G. M. Seehar. 1978. "The control of cell division by tension or diffusion." *Nature* 274:52–3.

[66] Chang, Chih-Cheng, and Yea-Fhey Kuo, Hsien-Ching Chiu, Jia-Luen Lee, Tak-Wah Wong, Shiou-Howa Jee. 1995. "Hydration, not silicone, modulates the effects of keratinocytes on fibroblasts." The *Journal of Surgical Research* 59:705–11. doi: 10.1006/jsre.1995.1227.

[67] Sawada, Y., and S. Urushidate, Y. Nihei. 1998. "Hydration and occlusive treatment of a sutured wound." *Annals of Plastic Surgery* 41:508-12.

[68] Mustoe, Thomas A., and Rodney D. Cooter, Michael H. Gold, F. D. Richard Hobbs, Albert-Adrien Ramelet, Peter G. Shakespeare, Maurizio Stella, Luc Téot, Fiona M. Wood, Ulrich E. Ziegler. 2002. "International clinical recommendations on scar management." *Plastic and Reconstructive Surgery* 110:560-71.

[69] Reiffel, R. S. 1995. "Prevention of hypertrophic scars by long-term paper tape application." *Plastic and Reconstructive Surgery* 96:1715-8.

[70] Meshkinpour, Azin, and Peyman Ghasri, Karl Pope, Julia G. Lyubovitsky, Juha Risteli, Tatiana B. Krasieva, Kristen M. Kelly. 2005. "Treatment of hypertrophic scars and keloids with a radiofrequency device: A study of collagen effects." *Lasers in Surgery and Medicine* 37:343-9. doi: 10.1002/lsm.20268.

[71] Wong, Victor W., and Kristine C. Rustad, Satoshi Akaishi, Michael Sorkin, Jason P. Glotzbach, Michael Januszyk, Emily R. Nelson, Kemal Levi, Josemaria Paterno, Ivan N. Vial, Anna A. Kuang, Michael T. Longaker, Geoffrey C. Gurtner. 2012. "Focal adhesion kinase links mechanical force to skin fibrosis via inflammatory signaling." *Nature Medicine* 18:148–52. doi: 10.1038/nm.2574.

[72] Longaker, Michael T., and Rod J. Rohrich, Lauren Greenberg, Heather Furnas, Robert Wald, Vivek Bansal, Hisham Seify, Anthony Tran, Jane Weston, Joshua M. Korman, Rodney Chan, David Kaufman, Vipul R. Dev, Joseph A. Mele, Michael Januszyk, Christy Cowley, Peggy McLaughlin, Bill Beasley, Geoffrey C. Gurtner. 2014. "A randomized controlled trial of the embrace advanced scar therapy device to reduce incisional scar formation." *Plastic and Reconstructive Surgery* 134:536–46. doi: 10.1097/PRS.0000000000000417.

[73] Baker, L. L., and S. Rubayi, F. Villar, S. K. Demuth. 1996. "Effect of electrical stimulation on chronic wound healing: a meta-analysis." *Wound Repair and Regeneration* 4:21–8.

[74] Junger, M., and D. Zuder, A. Steins, M. Hahn, T. Klyscz. 1997. "Treatment of venous ulcers with low frequency pulsed current (Dermapulse): effects on cutaneous microstimulation." *Der Hautartz* 18:879–903.

[75] Perry, D., and J. Colthurst, P. Giddings, D. A. McGrouther, J. Morris, A. Bayat. 2010. "Treatment of symptomatic abnormal skin scars with electrical stimulation." *Journal of Wound Care* 19:447–53. Doi: 10.12968/jowc.2010.19.10.79092.

[76] Ud-Din, S., and P. Giddings, J. Colthurst, S. Whiteside, J. Morris, A. Bayat. 2013. "Significant reduction of symptoms of scarring with electrical stimulation: evaluated with subjective and objective assessment tools." *Wounds* 25:212–24.

[77] Sebastian, Anil, and Ernest Allan, Donald Allan, James Colthurst, Ardeshir Bayat. 2011. "Addition of novel degenerate electrical waveform stimulation with photodynamic therapy significantly enhances its cytotoxic effect in keloid fibroblasts: first report of a potential combination therapy." *Journal of Dermatological Science* 64:174–84. doi: 10.1016/j.jdermsci.2011.08.012.

In: Cutaneous Scars: Biology, Clinics and Management ISBN: 978-1-53615-657-7
Editors: Berna Aksoy, Hasan Mete Aksoy et al. © 2019 Nova Science Publishers, Inc.

Chapter 19

TOPICAL MEDICAL TREATMENTS

Sevil Savas Erdogan*
Department of Dermatology,
Sultan Abdulhamit Han Training and Research Hospital, Istanbul, Turkey

ABSTRACT

Many wounds heal with asymptomatic scars, but some lead to an abnormal scar formation. Both the severity of inflammation and type of immune response lead to excessive scarring. Scars take many forms, depending on the size and severity, type of initiating injury, and anatomical location. The approach to the treatment program and its goals should be set for each individual patient. There are numerous treatment modalities that are discussed in other chapters. The following chapter aims to describe the topical medical treatments including imiquimod cream, mitomycin C, vitamin derivatives, herbal extracts, moist exposed burn ointment (MEBO), topical corticosteroids and others that are used in the management and treatment of scars.

Keywords: allium cepa, aloe vera, calcipotriol, captopril, centella asiatica, corticosteroids, Gotu kola, herbal extracts, imiquimod, mitomycin C, moist exposed burn ointment, onion extract, tacrolimus, tamoxifen, tranilast, tretinoin, vitamin

1. INTRODUCTION

The wound healing process is a complex and carefully organized physiological reaction to traumatic skin injury, consisting of three overlapping phases. An early

*Corresponding Author's Email: doktorsevilsavas@gmail.com.

inflammatory cascade occurs immediately after injury, subsequently resulting in scar development [1]. In the inflammatory phase, macrophages secrete inflammatory mediators while neutrophils destroy bacteria and debris through phagocytosis. The proliferative phase includes angiogenesis, collagen accumulation, formation of granulation tissue, epithelization, fibroblast proliferation and migration with extracellular matrix (ECM) formation, and wound contraction. Collagen synthesis and lysis in the process of remodeling may last two years after the occurrence of the injury. There is a sophisticated interaction between cells that modulates growth factors, cytokines, extracellular matrix components, and collagen metabolism [2]. Growth factors, such as tumor necrosis factor (TNF), platelet-derived growth factor (PDGF), transforming growth factor (TGF), basic fibroblast growth factor (bFGF), vascular endothelial growth factor (VEGF), insulin-like growth factor, and keratinocyte growth factor, and cytokines play an important role in inflammatory and remodeling phases [3-6]. Myofibroblasts help initiate wound contraction. After the wound is closed, abundant ECM is disrupted and immature type III collagen is transformed into mature type I collagen, and thus the immature scar is transformed into a final mature scar [7].

Many wounds heal with asymptomatic scars, but some lead to abnormal scar formation. Thus, the transformation of a fibrin clot into scar tissue requires a delicate balance between ECM protein deposition and degradation, and when this is disturbed, abnormalities occur in the scars. A healing wound is filled intensively with inflammatory cells that secrete fibrogenic factors such as transforming growth factor (TGF)-β1 and β2. This environment increases the accumulation of ECM. As recent evidence suggests, both the severity of inflammation and type of immune response lead to excess scarring [8]. Scars take many forms, depending on the size and severity, type of injury, and anatomical location. Scars can be classified as mature, immature, linear hypertrophic (e.g., surgical/traumatic), widespread hypertrophic (e.g., burns), minor and major keloid, and atrophic scars. Many of these scar types may be associated with various symptoms, such as pruritus and pain [9]. When assessing scars, their size, contour, color, height (thickness), surface area, surface texture, pliability, location, and subjective symptoms, such as itching and pain, as well as the patient's feelings should be taken into account. It has been indicated that this subjective component of the patients is as important as the objective features and may be very effective in determining the patient's quality of life [10, 11]. Scar scales are used to assess the severity of the clinical and patient perspectives [12]. These include the Vancouver Scar Scale (VSS), Visual Analog Scale (VAS), Manchester Scar Scale, and Patient and Observer Scar Assessment Scale (POSAS) [13]. For routine clinical practice, at minimum, the evaluation of size, thickness, symptom severity (e.g., pain, itching), and patient concerns should be considered. Choosing a treatment modality is based on a careful evaluation of the scar characteristics.

The approach to the treatment program and its goals should be set for each individual patient based upon scar evaluation, the patient's characteristics, and expectations in the process of reducing the scar volume, minimizing subjective symptoms, and improving function and aesthetic appearance. The advancement of technology has allowed for the development of more specific and localized therapies. There are numerous treatment modalities, including intralesional corticosteroid injections, pressure therapy, surgical revision, radiation therapy, topical silicone gel, and laser therapy. The following sections describe and assess the topical treatments of imiquimod cream, mitomycin C, vitamin derivatives, herbal extracts, moist exposed burn ointment (MEBO), and topical corticosteroids that are used in the management and treatment of scars.

2. Imiquimod

Imiquimod 5% cream is an immune response modifier that induces interferon to increase collagen degradation and also modifies apoptotic genes [14]. It has been reported that *topical imiquimod* decreases the recurrence rate of excised keloids [15-17]. A randomized, double-blind, placebo-controlled trial of *imiquimod* 5% cream in the prevention of hypertrophic scarring after breast surgery reported a better scar quality than control groups (no treatment and treatment with petrolatum) [18]. In addition, in small, non-randomized studies, there is some evidence that the use of *topical imiquimod* cream decreases the rate of keloid recurrence after surgical excision, especially on or near the earlobe [16, 19-21]. However, in one study, this success was not seen in truncal keloids, with a reported high rate of recurrence after surgical excision and *imiquimod* therapy [22]. This study suggests that *imiquimod* 5% cream is not effective in preventing recurrence of trunkal keloids after surgical excision. Furthermore, in a prospective, double-blind, placebo-controlled study, there was no significant reduction in keloid relapse rates when using *imiquimod* versus placebo after keloid excision [23].

Although there is no approved indication for the use of *imiquimod* 5% cream, there is some support for night time administration to the surgical incision site, two to three weeks after keloid excision, and this can be continued for two months when tolerated by the patient [24]. *Imiquimod* has local skin side effects such as erythema, edema, ulceration, desquamation and hypopigmentation, which have been observed in more than 75% of patients and can produce flu-like symptoms, such as headache, myalgia, fatigue, fever and diarrhea and these symptoms can be seen in 1% to 2% of patients [18, 25]. Due to these side effects, the use of *topical imiquimod* in scar prevention and treatment is limited; therefore, additional studies are necessary to further characterize the success rate and side-effect profile.

3. Mitomycin C

Mitomycin C is an antibiotic chemotherapeutic agent used topically or intravenously. It is isolated from Streptomyces species and inhibit DNA synthesis and hence cell proliferation [26]. It is used to prevent recurrence after keloid scar excision; however, there is limited research concerning the effect of *mitomycin C*. In a small case series study, keloid relapse was not observed at 6 to 24 months of follow-up after surgical excision and *topical mitomycin C* treatment [27]. In a series of two patients, triple therapy with excision, application of *mitomycin C*, and radiotherapy proved effective in the treatment of keloids and no recurrence was observed during two-year follow-up [26]. A different investigation showed *topical* application of *mitomycin C* following shave excision was safe and effective for the treatment of keloids and hypertrophic scars. However, intralesional *mitomycin C* treatment resulted in bullae, necrosis, and ulcer in keloids and hypertrophic scars [28]. Overall, there is lack of qualified evidence to advise on the use of *mitomycin C* for scar management.

4. Vitamin Derivatives

Vitamins have been used in *topical* cosmeceuticals and moisturizers for decades to help improve skin structure and for anti-oxidant properties. They are thought to help prevent UV damage to the skin.

4.1. Vitamin E

Vitamin E is a family of basic micronutrients with antioxidant activity consisting of tocopherol and tocotrienols. *Vitamin* E affects wound healing and scar formation positively by inhibiting collagen synthesis and reducing both fibroblast proliferation and inflammation [29, 30]. The use of *vitamin* E in the treatment of scars is recommended by clinicians, but there are only limited studies that show that *vitamin* E has a beneficial effect on scars [31].

In a study with 80 patients, hypertrophic scars and keloids were treated with *vitamin* E added silicone gel sheets (SGS) and SGS without *vitamin* E. The improvement in the group treated with combined *vitamin* E and SGS was better and this was statistically significant when compared with the improvement in the group treated with SGS alone [32]. In a large prospective randomized single-blind study, pre- and post-surgery use of *vitamin E* was evaluated in children. The authors concluded that after six months, the treated wounds had better appearance with less problematic scarring than the placebo group [33]. In another randomized controlled trial (RCT), the application of a silicone and *vitamin E* combination lotion showed significant improvement in scar induration, pigmentation and erythema compared to placebo, and it was more effective than the placebo in the management of hypertrophic scars and keloids [34]. In a double-blind study of patients undergoing surgery, the effectiveness of improving the scar appearance of a regular emollient was compared with an emollient containing *vitamin E* [35]. In this study, topical *vitamin E* did not affect or worsen the cosmetic appearance of scars; however, of the patients studied, 33% developed a contact dermatitis from *vitamin E*. In a recent prospective, randomized, double-blind study on 122 patients with surgical scars less than two weeks old, topical tocotrienol administered twice a day for six weeks showed no significant difference in the treatment and placebo groups [36].

Therefore, despite its popularity, the available evidence suggests that *vitamin* E is not effective in scar prevention. Due to the lack of sufficient scientific evidence, regular use of *topical vitamin E* for management and prevention of scars is not recommended. In addition, the use of this agent may cause potentially harmful effects, such as contact dermatitis [25].

4.2. Topical Vitamin A

Topical and systemic retinoids have been investigated for their potential effects on cutaneous wound healing. *Topical vitamin* A in the form of 0.05% retinoic acid has been used as superficial peeling agent and may improve scar features. Softening and smoothing of the scars and a decrease in itching complaints have been observed [37]. In another study by Panabiere-Castaings, 11 subjects were treated with 0.05% *tretinoin* nightly for 12 weeks, and a significant decrease in height and size of scars was reported, however two subjects discontinued the study due to irritant contact dermatitis [38]. In a study comparing *topical tretinoin* cream and silicone gel with the control group in the treatment of scars; silicone gel and *tretinoin* cream successfully prevented hypertrophic scar and keloid development and had beneficial effects on final scar appearance compared to the control group [39].

A randomised controlled trial using a porcine model evaluated the effects of perioperative *topical tretinoin* on the healing of excisional wounds and survival of full-thickness skin grafts. In the excisional areas, *topical tretinoin* had neither positive nor negative effects on wound healing or the appearance of the final scar. Impaired wound healing, larger graft necrosis, and poorer graft survival were observed in topical tretinoin-treated skin grafts [40]. Overall, the available data indicate that topical retinoids have significant benefits partially in the treatment of scars.

4.3. Topical Vitamin D

Calcipotriol is a synthetic *vitamin* D derivative commonly used in the treatment of psoriasis. It has anti-inflammatory properties and ability to induce keratinocyte terminal differentiation, decrease keratinocyte proliferation, and decrease the number of Langerhans cells and their function. Due to these properties, it was assumed that it could reduce the risk of hypertrophic scar. However, a randomized double-blind placebo controlled trial of the application of *topical vitamin* D (*calcipotriol*) twice daily for three months following a bilateral reduction mammoplasty concluded that there was no effect in reducing hypertrophic scar formation with calcipotriol use compared to control after 12-month follow-up period [41].

5. Herbal Extracts

A number of *herbal extracts*, which are the basis of traditional medicine, have been used as natural products in a variety of wound healing and cosmetic formulations. Most are used in combination with other therapeutic agents. They are added to creams and dressings to improve wound healing and scar appearance. These include extract from plants including *Allium cepa* (*onion extract*), *Centella asiatica* (madecassol, madecassic acid), and *Aloe vera*. Despite the fact that the use of *herbal extracts* is recommended, their efficacy has not been proven by studies [42, 43].

5.1. Onion Extract

Allium cepa (*onion extract*) is used as a *topical* agent to reduce scar formation, and it has both bactericidal and anti-inflammatory properties. Flavonoids (quercetin and kaempferol) in *onion extract* play a major role in decreasing scar formation by inhibiting fibroblast proliferation and collagen production [44]. Onion extract was essentially used for treating full and partial thickness burns; however, this extract has been investigated for use in the treatment of hypertrophic scars and keloids and also in healing wounds. Mederma® is the American formulation of 10% *onion extract* and 1% allantoin, while Contractubex® is the European formulation and additionally contains 50 U/g heparin.

In a randomized controlled trial, *onion extract* was found to improve scar height and itchiness but not erythema, elasticity, and overall appearance, compared to a placebo [45]. In another randomised controlled trial, the use of *onion extract* gel in pediatric median sternotomies resulted in less hypertrophic scarring than the placebo [46]. On the other hand, Chung et al. did not observe any difference between *onion extract* gel and moisturizer in preventing hypertrophic scars after surgery [47]. Also in another study, the silicone gel sheet combined with *onion extract* reduced itching and improved pigmentation compared to a silicone gel sheet and a placebo ointment but no difference was observed in terms of scar flexibility or height [48]. The benefit of the combination of intralesional triamcinolone and *onion extract* gel for the treatment of hypertrophic scars and keloids has been reported to be statistically significant compared to monotherapy with triamcinolone alone [49]. However, in a comparative study, *onion extract* was not found to be as effective as the silicone-based products in treating burn hypertrophic scars [50].

Although *onion extract* may have beneficial effects on scars, its clinical efficacy in scar prevention and treatment has not been fully proven [51]. According to German guidelines on scarring, creams containing *onion extract* can be considered as additional treatment for active hypertrophic scars and for postoperative prophylaxis of scarring [52].

Topical application should usually be performed several times daily with mild massage of the scar tissue. In old and stiff scars, the application should be given under occlusion. In order to prevent the scarring of open wounds, treatment should be initiated after the complete epithelization of the wound. Treatment usually continues over several weeks to months (Figure 1) [52].

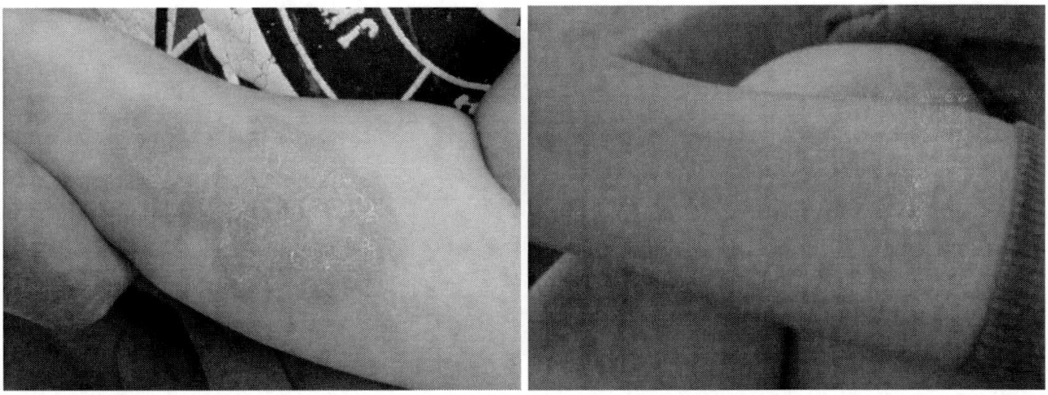

a) b)

Figure 1. Second degree burn scar a) before and b) 5 years after 3.5 months of regular onion extract gel (Contractubex®) application with massage (Courtesy of Berna Aksoy, MD).

5.2. *Aloe vera*

Aloe vera has been used in traditional medicine for centuries; however, there is inadequate literature on its use for wound healing and especially for the prevention of scar formation. A systematic review concluded that there is confusion in terms of the clinical evidence for the benefits of using *Aloe vera* in the treatment of acute and chronic wounds. Moreover the precise outcome of the improvement of the wound healing rate or the quality of the produced scar was insufficient. This is due to the lack of high quality studies and use of different treatment regimens and evaluation criteria [53].

5.3. *Centella asiatica*

Centella asiatica, which is also commonly known as *Gotu kola* and originated from Asia, is a small herbal plant that grows in soil in which water is trapped. This plant is used in traditional as well as western medicine [54]. The active compounds of C. asiatica responsible for wound healing and prevention of hypertrophic scars are pentacyclic triterpenes, including asiaticoside and madecassoside. An in vitro study demonstrated that asiaticoside decreased fibroblast proliferation and reduced the expression of both TGF-β 1 and TGF-β 2 at the transcriptional and translational level [55]. The other active composition, madecassoside, is related to inhibition of the migration of fibroblasts obtained from keloids [56]. An animal model showed an effective outcome in hypertrophic scar reduction [57].

A randomised controlled trial involving 23 patients who underwent a split-thickness skin graft (STSG) operation revealed that Centella cream improved scar outcomes compared with placebo. The Centella cream significantly improved the pigmentation parameter of Vancouver scar scale (VSS) and had comparative total VSS scores between 4 and 12 weeks in comparison with that of the placebo group. The effect of Centella cream on scar development may provide better pigmentation [58].

5.4. Moist Exposed Burn Ointment

Moist Exposed Burn Ointment (MEBO) is a burn ointment with a U.S.-patented formulation. ß-sitosterol is the active ingredient and this burn ointment contains six *herbal extracts*. Similar to silicone gel, it is believed that it reduces vascular activity by increasing tissue moisture, and thus it prevents vascular hyperplasia and scar hypertrophy [59].

MEBO is often used for burns. Its effects on scar quality and wound healing were evaluated in two prospective studies [60, 61]. In one of these studies, MEBO was compared with an antibiotic ointment and no topical therapy in patients with traumatic and surgical facial wounds. It was concluded that MEBO had significantly better results after a follow-up period of up to six months [60]. In three clinical comparative prospective studies, MEBO use was associated with an improvement in primary and secondary wound healing. Additionally, improvement in scar quality, earlier anatomical healing and faster functional healing have been demonstrated [61].

6. Topical Corticosteroids

The therapeutic effects of *corticosteroids* are mainly due to their suppressive effects on the inflammatory process in the wound. The other effects are decreased collagen and glycosaminoglycan synthesis, inhibition of fibroblast growth, as well as increased collagen degradation and fibroblast degeneration [1, 62]. One study has demonstrated that *corticosteroids* alter the expression of multiple genes and play an important role in tissue remodeling and scar formation by suppressing the expression of TGF-β 1 and 2 and MMP1, -2, -9, and -10 and collagens in fibroblasts and keratinocytes [63].

Intralesional injections of *corticosteroids* have been a mainstay of treatment for keloids and hypertrophic scars. However, intralesional *corticosteroid* injection may not be easily tolerated by patients especially in the pediatric population because it is usually a painful procedure [64]. There is no consensus on topically administered *corticosteroids.* Topical absorption through the intact epidermis into deep dermis is limited, and studies have shown no reduction in post-burn scarring from the use of *topical corticosteroids* [65].

Purely topical use of *corticosteroids* is not recommended for the prophylaxis or treatment of scarring as a cream or ointment [52]. They may have utility in reduction of scar pruritus and in obtaining color change through glucocorticoid-mediated vasoconstriction. So they can be used as adjuvant therapy for symptoms, such as pain or itching.

7. Other Topical Therapeutic Options

Tacrolimus has multiple potential therapeutic targets for treatment of keloids. It has been shown to block TGF-β/Smad signaling pathway in vitro in keloidal fibroblasts by down-regulating TGF-β receptors, leading to reduced keloidal fibroblast proliferation, migration, and collagen production [66]. *Tacrolimus* is also known to bind the Gli-1 oncogene, which may have a role in keloid pathogenesis [67]. In a study by Berman and colleagues, 11 subjects were treated with *tacrolimus* 0.1% ointment twice daily for 12 weeks, and though statistical significance was not achieved, most subjects did experience decreased induration, tenderness, erythema, and pruritus [68]. However, further research is needed to characterize the role of *tacrolimus* in the prevention and treatment of keloids and hypertrophic scars.

Tamoxifen has been successfully used for treatment of retroperitoneal fibrosis and desmoid tumors, thus, it plays a role as an antifibrotic agent [69, 70]. Tamoxifen has been shown to inhibit cultured keloidal fibroblast proliferation and the contraction of collagen lattices [71]. Also, it has been shown to decrease TGF-β1 production in cultured keloidal fibroblasts [72]. In a prospective study by Ruiz and colleagues, 46 burn patients with hypertrophic scars were treated with *topical tamoxifen* citrate (0.1%). The patients were followed up for 6 months and since there was improvement in all scars, the treatment was considered successful [73]. More studies are needed to determine the potential efficacy of this medication.

The local renin-angiotensin system is also known to play a role in the control of collagen biosynthesis and wound healing. It has been reported that angiotensin-converting enzyme inhibitors (ACEIs) improve the fibrotic processes in the heart, lung, liver, and kidneys [74-76]. Recent studies have shown that ACEIs inhibit scar formation by suppressing both TGF-β1/SMAD2/3 and TGF-β1/TAK1 pathways, and this may have clinical utility in the future [77, 78]. Ardekani et al. reported the first successfully treated human case with *topical captopril* [79]. Randomised controlled trials are needed to evaluate the clinical efficacy and side effects of *topical captopril* as a novel, effective, safe and easy to use treatment against hypertrophic scar and keloid formation.

Tranilast (N-[3, 4-dimethoxycinnamoyl] anthranilic acid) has been shown to be effective as an antiallergic and suppress collagen synthesis in fibroblasts by limiting the action of TGF-β1, thus inhibiting scar contracture [80, 81]. In a recent prospective double-blind, split-scar study, *topical tranilast* 8% gel provided significantly better post-caesarian section scar cosmesis and user satisfaction compared with placebo [82]. However, further studies are required to compare the efficacy of *tranilast* with other modalities and to assess the possible advantages of combination therapies.

Recombinant Human Transforming Growth Factor—Beta 1 (rhTGF-β1) when applied topically to porcine second intention wounds has been shown to enhance wound healing and strength and increase blood flow [83].

Platelet rich plasma (PRP) can be used as a topical gel to make scars better or can be combined with other modalities like nonablative fractional laser, erbium or CO2 resurfacing. PRP gel applications are reported to provide significant improvements in clinical appearance of acne scars. PRP gel use also leads to faster resolution of erythema, edema and shorter recovery times following laser resurfacing [84].

8. Options for Treatment of Scars

Topical treatment options and their effects are summarized in Table 1; therapeutic options for fresh surgical scars and hypertrophic scars are summarized in Table 2 and that for keloids are summarized in Table 3.

Table 1. Topical treatment options and their effects

Topical treatment	Mechanism of action	Effect
Imiquimod 5% cream	Induces local synthesis of cytokines and interferon to increase collagen degradation Modifies apoptotic genes	Decreases the recurrence of excised keloid Prevents hypertrophic scars and keloids
Mitomycin C	Inhibits fibroblast proliferation and DNA synthesis and proliferation	Prevents recurrence after keloid and hypertrophic scar excision
Vitamin E	Inhibits collagen synthesis Reduces both fibroblast proliferation and inflammation	May improve scar appearance Hydration and moisturization Contact dermatitis in >30% of patients
Vitamin A	Reduces collagen synthesis Inhibits matrix metalloproteinases (MMPs)	May prevent hypertrophic scars and keloids May improve scar appearance
Onion extract	Anti-inflammatory properties Inhibits fibroblast proliferation and collagen production	May prevent hypertrophic scar development May improve cosmetic appearance of scars
Centella asiatica	Decreases fibroblast proliferation Reduces the expression of both TGF-β 1 and TGF-β 2	May provide better pigmentation
Moist Exposed Burn Ointment	Reduces vascular activity Prevents vascular hyperplasia and scar hypertrophy	May improve scar quality May improve cosmetic appearance of scars

Table 2. Therapeutic options for fresh surgical scars and hypertrophic scars [24, 44, 52, 85]

Scar type	First-line therapy	Second-line therapy	Other options
Fresh surgical scars	-Silicone-based products (at least 1 month) or onion extract-containing preparations (at least 3 month) after epithelization	-Concurrent intralesional corticosteroid injections -PDL for persistent erythema	
Immature or erythematous hypertrophic scars	-Silicone-based products, hypoallergenic paper tape, and onion extract-containing preparations	If persistent erythema >1 month, manage as a linear hypertrophic scar	-PDL or fractional laser therapy
Linear/small hypertrophic scars	-Silicone-based products -Intralesional injection of corticosteroid and/or 5-FU	-PDL or fractional laser therapy -Pressure therapy	-Surgical excision + postoperative silicone-based products -If tension present: surgical relief of tension by Z-, W-plasty For larger scars: -Skin graft or local flaps For severe scars: Surgical excision plus -Intralesional corticosteroid -Intralesional 5-FU + corticosteroid -Bleomycin or mitomycin C
Extensive hypertrophic scars/Hypertrophic burn scars	-Acute treatment at a specialty burn unit After epithelization and wound stabilization -Silicone-based products ± pressure therapy or onion-extract containing preparations	If erythema occurs, laser therapy should be initiated as soon as possible -Fractional laser therapy and vascular laser therapy	Combination or alternative therapies -Silicone gel sheeting, pressure therapy, massage/physical therapy, corticosteroids, surgical relief of tension, excision, skin graft or local flaps, laser therapy, hydrocolloid dressings, antihistamines

Table 3. Therapeutic options for keloids [24, 44, 52, 85]

Scar type	First-line therapy	Second-line therapy	Other options
Minor keloids	-Silicone-based products + monthly intralesional corticosteroid injections -Contact or intralesional cryotherapy	-Combination of intralesional corticosteroid and/or cryotherapy with pressure -5-FU + intralesional corticosteroids -Fractional laser therapy or PDL	Surgery with adjuvant therapy -Silicone-based products or intralesional corticosteroids or both -Anti-tension therapy -Radiotherapy -Chemotherapeutic agents (bleomycin, mitomycin C, imiquimod)
Major keloids	-Intralesional corticosteroid ± adjuvant cryotherapy -Intralesional 5-FU + corticosteroid	-Fractional laser therapy or PDL	

CONCLUSION

Many wounds heal with asymptomatic scars, but some lead to abnormal scar formation. The approach to the scar prevention or treatment program and its goals should be set individually for each patient. There are numerous topical medical treatment modalities available.

The use of topical imiquimod in scar prevention and treatment is limited and controversial. Although there are some promising reports, there is lack of qualified evidence to advise the use of mitomycin C for scar management. Despite its popularity, the available evidence suggests that vitamin E is not effective in scar prevention even it may cause potentially harmful effects, such as contact dermatitis. Available data indicates that topical retinoids have partially significant benefits in the treatment of scars. There was no effect of topical vitamin D analogues in reducing hypertrophic scar formation compared to control. Despite the use of herbal extracts has been recommended, their efficacy has not been proven by evidence based studies. There are promising preliminary results but further studies are required to evaluate the efficacy of tacrolimus, tamoxifen, captopril and tranilast.

Therefore, additional studies are necessary to further characterize the efficacy, potential for combined use and side-effect profiles of these *topical* medical therapeutics.

REFERENCES

[1] Reish, Richard G. and Elof Eriksson. 2008. "Scar treatments: preclinical and clinical studies." *Journal of the American College of Surgeons* 206:719-30. doi:10.1016/j.jamcollsurg.2007.11.022.

[2] Rockwell, W. B., and I. K. Cohen, H. P. Ehrlich. 1989. "Keloids and hypertrophic scars: A comprehensive review." *Plastic and Reconstructive Surgery* 84: 827-37.

[3] Niessen, Frank B., and Monique P. Andriessen, Joost Schalkwijk, Lidia Visser, Wim Timens. 2001. "Keratinocyte-derived growth factors play a role in the formation of hypertrophic scars." *The Journal of Pathology* 194:207-16. doi:10.1002/path.853.

[4] Pierce, G. F., and J. E. Tarpley, D. Yanagihara, T. A. Mustoe, G. M. Fox, A. Thomason. 1992. "Platelet-derived growth factor (BB homodimer), transforming growth factor-beta 1, and basic fibroblast growth factor in dermal wound healing. Neovessel and matrix formation and cessation of repair." *American Journal of Pathology* 140:1375-88.

[5] Pierce, G. F., and J. Vande Berg, R. Rudolph, J. Tarpley, T. A. Mustoe. 1991. "Platelet-derived growth factor-BB and transforming growth factor beta 1 selectively modulate glycosaminoglycans, collagen, and myofibroblasts in excisional wounds." *American Journal of Pathology* 138:629-46.

[6] Singer, Adam J. and Richard A. Clark. 1999. "Cutaneous wound healing." The *New England Journal of Medicine* 341:738-46. doi:10.1056/nejm19990902 3411006.

[7] Slemp, Alison E. and Richard E. Kirschner. 2006. "Keloids and scars: A review of keloids and scars, their pathogenesis, risk factors, and management." *Current Opinion in Pediatrics* 18:396-402. doi:10.1097/01.mop.0000236389.41462.ef.

[8] Brown, J. J. and A. Bayat. 2009. "Genetic susceptibility to raised dermal scarring." The *British Journal of Dermatology* 161:8-18. doi:10.1111/j.1365-2133.2009. 09258.x.

[9] Mustoe, Thomas A., and Rodney D. Cooter, Michael H. Gold, F. D. Richard Hobbs, Albert-Adrien Ramelet, Peter G. Shakespeare, Maurizio Stella, Luc Teot, Fiona M. Wood, Ulrich E. Ziegler. 2002. "International clinical recommendations on scar management." *Plastic and Reconstructive Surgery* 110:560-71.

[10] Collins, Lindsey K., and Thomas J. Knackstedt, Pamela Ganger, Emily Scherer, Faramarz H. Samie. 2017. "Applying a Visual Assessment Tool to Facial Linear Scars." *Facial Plastic Surgery* 33:97-101. doi:10.1055/s-0036-1597684.

[11] Powers, P. S., and S. Sarkar, D. B. Goldgof, C. W. Cruse, L. V. Tsap. 1999. "Scar assessment: current problems and future solutions." The *Journal of Burn Care & Rehabilitation* 20:54-60.

[12] Durani, Piyush, and D. A. McGrouther, M. W. J. Ferguson. 2009. "Current scales for assessing human scarring: a review." *Journal of Plastic, Reconstructive & Aesthetic Surgery* 62:713-20. doi:10.1016/j.bjps.2009.01.080.

[13] Roques, C. and Luc Teot. 2007. "A critical analysis of measurements used to assess and manage scars." The *International Journal of Lower Extremity Wounds* 6:249-53. doi:10.1177/1534734607308249.

[14] Jacob, S. E., and B. Berman, M. Nassiri, V. Vincek. 2003. "Topical application of imiquimod 5% cream to keloids alters expression genes associated with apoptosis." The *British Journal of Dermatology* 149:S62-5.

[15] Anzarut, Alexander, and Jarret Olson, Prabhjyot Singh, Brian H. Rowe, Edward E. Tredget. 2009. "The effectiveness of pressure garment therapy for the prevention of abnormal scarring after burn injury: a meta-analysis." *Journal of Plastic, Reconstructive & Aesthetic Surgery* 62:77-84. doi:10.1016/j.bjps.2007.10.052.

[16] Berman, B. and J. Kaufman. 2002. "Pilot study of the effect of postoperative imiquimod 5% cream on the recurrence rate of excised keloids." *Journal of the American Academy of Dermatology* 47: S209-11.

[17] Malhotra, A. K., and S. Gupta, B. K. Khaitan, V. K. Sharma. 2007. "Imiquimod 5% cream for the prevention of recurrence after excision of presternal keloids." *Dermatology* 215:63-5. doi:10.1159/000102036.

[18] Prado, Arturo, and Patricio Andrades, Susana Benitez, Miguel Umana. 2005. "Scar management after breast surgery: preliminary results of a prospective, randomized, and double-blind clinical study with aldara cream 5% (imiquimod)." *Plastic and Reconstructive Surgery* 115:966-72.

[19] Chuangsuwanich, A. and S. Gunjittisomram. 2007. "The efficacy of 5% imiquimod cream in the prevention of recurrence of excised keloids." *Journal of the Medical Association of Thailand* 90:1363-7.

[20] Martin-Garcia, Rafael F. 2005. "Imiquimod: an effective alternative for the treatment of invasive cutaneous squamous cell carcinoma." *Dermatologic Surgery* 31:371-4.

[21] Stashower, Mitchell E. 2006. "Successful treatment of earlobe keloids with imiquimod after tangential shave excision." *Dermatologic Surgery* 32:380-6. doi:10.1111/j.1524-4725.2006.32077.x.

[22] Cacao, Fernanda M., and Vanessa Tanaka, Maria C. Messina. 2009. "Failure of imiquimod 5% cream to prevent recurrence of surgically excised trunk keloids." *Dermatologic Surgery* 35:629-33.

[23] Berman, B., and C. Harrison-Balestra, O. A. Perez, M. Viera, A. Villa, D. Zell, C. Ramirez. 2009. "Treatment of keloid scars post-shave excision with imiquimod 5% cream: A prospective, double-blind, placebo-controlled pilot study." *Journal of Drugs in Dermatology* 8:455-8.

[24] Gold, Michael H., and Michael McGuire, Thomas A. Mustoe, Andrea Pusic, Mukta Sachdev, Jill Waibel, Crystal Murcia. 2014. "Updated international clinical recommendations on scar management: part 2--algorithms for scar prevention and treatment." *Dermatologic Surgery* 40:825-31. doi:10.1111/dsu.0000000000000050.

[25] Foo, Chong W. and Payam Tristani-Firouzi. 2011. "Topical modalities for treatment and prevention of postsurgical hypertrophic scars." *Facial Plastic Surgery Clinics of North America* 19:551-7. doi:10.1016/j.fsc.2011.06.008.

[26] Willett, Matthew, and Kent Handfield, Jason Marquart. 2014. "Multimodal keloid therapy with excision, application of mitomycin C, and radiotherapy." *Dermatologic Surgery* 40:480-2. doi:10.1111/dsu.12423.

[27] Gupta, M. and T. Narang. 2011. "Role of mitomycin C in reducing keloid recurrence: patient series and literature review." The *Journal of Laryngology and Otology* 125:297-300. doi:10.1017/s0022215110002045.

[28] Seo, S. H. and H. W. Sung. 2012. "Treatment of keloids and hypertrophic scars using topical and intralesional mitomycin C." *Journal of the European Academy of Dermatology and Venereology* 26:634-8, doi:10.1111/j.1468-3083.2011.04140.x.

[29] Ehrlich, H. P., and H. Tarver, T. K. Hunt. 1972. "Inhibitory effects of vitamin E on collagen synthesis and wound repair." *Annals of Surgery* 175:235-40.

[30] Musalmah, Mazlan, and Abd H. Fairuz, Mat T. Gapor, Wan Z. W. Ngah. 2002. "Effect of vitamin E on plasma malondialdehyde, antioxidant enzyme levels and the rates of wound closures during wound healing in normal and diabetic rats." *Asia Pacific Journal of Clinical Nutrition* 11:S448-51.

[31] Curran, John N., and Miranda Crealey, Gaitri Sadadcharam, Gareth Fitzpatrick, Margaret O'Donnell. 2006. "Vitamin E: patterns of understanding, use, and prescription by health professionals and students at a university teaching hospital." *Plastic and Reconstructive Surgery* 118:248-52, doi:10.1097/01.prs.0000221306.86450.c5.

[32] Palmieri, B., and G. Gozzi, G. Palmieri. 1995. "Vitamin E added silicone gel sheets for treatment of hypertrophic scars and keloids." *International Journal of Dermatology* 34:506-9.

[33] Zampieri, Nicola, and Veronica Zuin, Roberto Burro, Alberto Ottolenghi, Francesco S. Camoglio. 2010. "A prospective study in children: Pre- and post-surgery use of vitamin E in surgical incisions." *Journal of Plastic, Reconstructive & Aesthetic Surgery* 63:1474-8. doi:10.1016/j.bjps.2009.08.018.

[34] Perez, O. A., and M. H. Viera, J. K. Patel, S. Konda, S. Amini, R. Huo, D. Zell, S. Tadicherla, B. Berman. 2010. "A comparative study evaluating the tolerability and efficacy of two topical therapies for the treatment of keloids and hypertrophic scars." *Journal of Drugs in Dermatology* 9:514-8.

[35] Baumann, L. S. and J. Spencer. 1999. "The effects of topical vitamin E on the cosmetic appearance of scars." *Dermatologic Surgery* 25:311-5.

[36] Khoo, T. L., and A. S. Halim, Z. Zakaria, A. Z. Mat Saad, L. Y. Wu, H. Y. Lau. 2011. "A prospective, randomised, double-blinded trial to study the efficacy of topical tocotrienol in the prevention of hypertrophic scars." *Journal of Plastic, Reconstructive & Aesthetic Surgery* 64:e137-45. doi:10.1016/j.bjps.2010.08.029.

[37] Janssen de Limpens, A. M. 1980. "The local treatment of hypertrophic scars and keloids with topical retinoic acid." The *British Journal of Dermatology* 103:319-23.

[38] Panabiere-Castaings, M. H. 1988. "Retinoic acid in the treatment of keloids." The *Journal of Dermatologic Surgery and Oncology* 14:1275-6.

[39] Kwon, S. Y., and S. D. Park, K. Park. 2014. "Comparative effect of topical silicone gel and topical tretinoin cream for the prevention of hypertrophic scar and keloid formation and the improvement of scars." *Journal of the European Academy of Dermatology and Venereology* 28:1025-33. doi:10.1111/jdv.12242.

[40] Otley, Clark C., and Scott M. Gayner, Iftikhar Ahmed, Eric J. Moore, Randal K. Roenigk, David A. Sherris. 1999. "Preoperative and postoperative topical tretinoin on high-tension excisional wounds and full-thickness skin grafts in a porcine model: A pilot study." *Dermatologic Surgery* 25:716-21.

[41] van der Veer, Willem M., and Xander E. Jacobs, Ingmar E. Waardenburg, Magda M. Ulrich, Frank B. Niessen. 2009. "Topical calcipotriol for preventive treatment of hypertrophic scars: A randomized, double-blind, placebo-controlled trial." *Archives of Dermatology* 145:1269-75. doi:10.1001/archdermatol.2009.237.

[42] Jackson, Brooke A. and Andrea J. Shelton. 1999. "Pilot study evaluating topical onion extract as treatment for postsurgical scars." *Dermatologic Surgery* 25:267-9.

[43] Widgerow, A. D., and L. A. Chait, R. Stals, P. J. Stals. 2000. "New innovations in scar management." *Aesthetic Plastic Surgery* 24:227-34.

[44] Gauglitz, Gerd G. 2013. "Management of keloids and hypertrophic scars: current and emerging options." *Clinical, Cosmetic and Investigational Dermatology* 6:103-14. doi:10.2147/ccid.s35252.

[45] Chanprapaph, Kumurtnart, and Somsak Tanrattanakorn, Penpun Wattanakrai, Pranee Wongkitisophon, Vasanop Vachiramon. 2012. "Effectiveness of onion extract gel on surgical scars in asians." *Dermatol Research and Practice* 2012:212945. doi:10.1155/2012/212945.

[46] Wananukul, S., and S. Chatpreodprai, D. Peongsujarit, P. Lertsapcharoen. 2013. "A prospective placebo-controlled study on the efficacy of onion extract in silicone derivative gel for the prevention of hypertrophic scar and keloid in median sternotomy wound in pediatric patients." *Journal of Medical Association of Thailand* 96:1428-33.

[47] Chung, Vinh Q., and Larisa Kelley, Diego Marra, Sbrian B. Jiang. 2006. "Onion extract gel versus petrolatum emollient on new surgical scars: prospective double-blinded study." *Dermatologic Surgery* 32:193-7.

[48] Jenwitheesuk, Kamonwan, and Palakorn Surakunprapha, Kriansgsak Jenwitheesuk, Chusak Kuptarnond, Sompop Prathanee, Worawit Intanoo. 2012. "Role of silicone derivative plus onion extract gel in presternal hypertrophic scar protection: a prospective randomized, double blinded, controlled trial." *International Wound Journal* 9:397-402. doi:10.1111/j.1742-481X.2011.00898.x.

[49] Koc, Erol, and Ercan Arca, Baris Surucu, Zafer Kurumlu. 2008. "An open, randomized, controlled, comparative study of the combined effect of intralesional

triamcinolone acetonide and onion extract gel and intralesional triamcinolone acetonide alone in the treatment of hypertrophic scars and keloids." *Dermatologic Surgery* 34:1507-14. doi:10.1111/j.1524-4725.2008.34314.x.

[50] Karagoz, Huseyin, and Fuat Yuksel, Ersin Ulkur, Rahmi Evinc. 2009. "Comparison of efficacy of silicone gel, silicone gel sheeting, and topical onion extract including heparin and allantoin for the treatment of postburn hypertrophic scars." *Burns* 35:1097-103. doi:10.1016/j.burns.2009.06.206.

[51] Khansa, Ibrahim, and Bridget Harrison, Jeffrey E. Janis. 2016. "Evidence-Based Scar Management: How to Improve Results with Technique and Technology." *Plastic and Reconstructive Surgery* 138:165s-78s. doi:10.1097/prs.000000000 0002647.

[52] Nast, Alexander, and Sabine Eming, Joachim Fluhr, Klaus Fritz, Gerd Gauglitz, Silvia Hohenleutner, Renato G. Panizzon, Günther Sebastian, Birte Sporbeck, Josef Koller. 2012. "German S2k guidelines for the therapy of pathological scars (hypertrophic scars and keloids)." *Journal der Deutschen Dermatologischen Gesselschaft* 10:747-62. doi:10.1111/j.1610-0387.2012.08012.x.

[53] Dat, Anthony D., and Flora Poon, Kim B. Pham, Jenny Doust. 2012. "Aloe vera for treating acute and chronic wounds." The *Cochrane Database of Systematic Reviews* 2: Cd008762. doi:10.1002/14651858.CD008762.pub2.

[54] Bylka, Wieslawa, and Paulina Znajdek-Awizen, Elzbieta Studzinska-Sroka, Malgorzata Brzezinska. 2013. "Centella asiatica in cosmetology." *Postepy Dermatologii i Alergologii* 30:46-9. doi:10.5114/pdia.2013.33378.

[55] Tang, Bing, and Bin Zhu, Yueying Liang, Liangkuan Bi, Zhicheng Hu, Bin Chen, Kai Zhang, Jiayuan Zhu. 2011. "Asiaticoside suppresses collagen expression and TGF-beta/Smad signaling through inducing Smad7 and inhibiting TGF-betaRI and TGF-betaRII in keloid fibroblasts." *Archives of Dermatological Research* 303:563-72. doi:10.1007/s00403-010-1114-8.

[56] Song, Jie, and Huan Xu, Qian Lu, Zhao Xu, Difei Bian, Yufeng Xia, Zhifeng Wei, Zhunan Gong, Yue Dai. 2012. "Madecassoside suppresses migration of fibroblasts from keloids: involvement of p38 kinase and PI3K signaling pathways." *Burns* 38:677-84. doi:10.1016/j.burns.2011.12.017.

[57] Ju-Lin, Xie, and Qi Shao-Hai, Li Tian-Zeng, Huang Bin, Tang Jing-Ming, Xu Ying-Bin, Liu Xu-Sheng, Shu Bin, Liang Hui-Zhen, Huang Yong. 2009. "Effect of asiaticoside on hypertrophic scar in the rabbit ear model." *Journal of Cutaneous Pathology* 36:234-9. doi:10.1111/j.1600-0560.2008.01015.x.

[58] Jenwitheesuk, Kamonwan, and Porntip Rojsanga, Bowornsilp Chowchuen, Palakorn Surakunprapha. 2018. "A Prospective Randomized, Controlled, Double-Blind Trial of the Efficacy Using Centella Cream for Scar Improvement." *Evidence-Based Complementary and Alternative Medicine* 2018:9525624. doi:10.1155/2018/9525624.

[59] Liu, Austin, and Ronald L. Moy, David M. Ozog. 2011. “Current methods employed in the prevention and minimization of surgical scars.” *Dermatologic Surgery* 37:1740-6. doi:10.1111/j.1524-4725.2011.02166.x.

[60] Atiyeh, Bishara S., and John Ioannovich, Christian A. Al-Amm, Kusai A. El-Musa, Ruwayda Dham. 2002. “Improving scar quality: a prospective clinical study.” *Aesthetic Plastic Surgery* 26:470-6. doi:10.1007/s00266-002-2019-5.

[61] Atiyeh, Bishara S., and Christian A. Amm, Kusai A. El Musa. 2003. “Improved scar quality following primary and secondary healing of cutaneous wounds.” *Aesthetic Plastic Surgery* 27:411-7. doi:10.1007/s00266-003-3049-3.

[62] Boyadjiev, C., and E. Popchristova, J. Mazgalova. 1995. “Histomorphologic changes in keloids treated with Kenacort.” The *Journal of Trauma* 38:299-302.

[63] Stojadinovic, Olivera, and Brian Lee, Constantinos Vouthounis, Sasa Vukelic, Irena Pastar, Miroslav Blumenberg, Harald Brem, Marjana Tomic-Canic. 2007. “Novel genomic effects of glucocorticoids in epidermal keratinocytes: inhibition of apoptosis, interferon-gamma pathway, and wound healing along with promotion of terminal differentiation.” The *Journal of Biological Chemistry* 282:4021-34. doi:10.1074/jbc.M606262200.

[64] Block, Lisa, and Ankush Gosain, Timothy W. King. 2015. “Emerging Therapies for Scar Prevention.” *Advances in Wound Care (New Rochelle)* 4:607-14. doi:10.1089/wound.2015.0646.

[65] Leventhal, Doouglas, and Maxwell Furr, David Reiter. 2006. “Treatment of keloids and hypertrophic scars: a meta-analysis and review of the literature.” *Archives of Facial Plastic Surgery* 8:362-8. doi:10.1001/archfaci.8.6.362.

[66] Wu, C. S., and P. H. Wu, A. H. Fang, C. C. Lan. 2012. “FK506 inhibits the enhancing effects of transforming growth factor (TGF)-beta1 on collagen expression and TGF-beta/Smad signalling in keloid fibroblasts: implication for new therapeutic approach.” The *British Journal of Dermatology* 167:532-41. doi:10.1111/j.1365-2133.2012.11023.x.

[67] Kim, Amy, and Josh DiCarlo, Cynthia Cohen, Calvin McCall, Darlene Johnson, Barbara McAlpine, Anthony G. Quinn, Elizabeth R. McLaughlin, Jack L. Arbiser. 2001. “Are keloids really “gli-loids?: High-level expression of gli-1 oncogene in keloids.” *Journal of the American Academy of Dermatology* 45:707-11. doi:10.1067/mjd.2001.117736.

[68] Berman, B., and V. Poochareon, A. M. Villa. 2005. “An open-label pilot study to evaluate the safety and tolerability of tacrolimus ointment 0.1% for the treatment of keloids.” *Cosmetic Dermatology* 18:399-404.

[69] Clark, C. P., and D. Vanderpool, J. T. Preskitt. 1991. “The response of retroperitoneal fibrosis to tamoxifen.” *Surgery* 109:502-6.

[70] Kinzbrunner, B., and S. Ritter, J. Domingo, C. J. Rosenthal. 1983. “Remission of rapidly growing desmoid tumors after tamoxifen therapy.” *Cancer* 52:2201-4.

[71] Hu, D., and M. A. Hughes, G. W. Cherry. 1998. "Topical tamoxifen--a potential therapeutic regime in treating excessive dermal scarring?" *British Journal of Plastic Surgery* 51:462-9.

[72] Mikulec, A. A., and M. M. Hanasono, J. Lum, J. M. Kadleck, M. Kita, R. J. Koch. 2001. "Effect of tamoxifen on transforming growth factor beta1 production by keloid and fetal fibroblasts." *Archives of Facial Plastic Surgery* 3:111-4.

[73] Pasquetti, A. F., and W. M. Mota, M. R. Santos, H. L. F. Brito. 2010. "Tamoxifen as treatment to keloids and hypertrophic scars." *Revista Brasileira de Cirurgia Plástico* 25:372-78.

[74] Abbas, G., and M. G. Silveira, K. D. Lindor. 2011. "Hepatic fibrosis and the renin-angiotensin system." *American Journal of Therapeutics* 18:e202-8. doi:10.1097/MJT.0b013e3181df8df5.

[75] Brilla, C. G., and H. Rupp, B. Maisch. 2003. "Effects of ACE inhibition versus non-ACE inhibitor antihypertensive treatment on myocardial fibrosis in patients with arterial hypertension. Retrospective analysis of 120 patients with left ventricular endomyocardial biopsies." *Herz* 28:744-53. doi:10.1007/s00059-003-2524-6.

[76] Mohammadi-Karakani, Ali, and Mahmoud Ghazi-Khansari, Masoud Sotoudeh. 2006. "Lisinopril ameliorates paraquat-induced lung fibrosis." *Clinica Chimica Acta* 367:170-4. doi:10.1016/j.cca.2005.12.012.

[77] Fang, Qing-Qing, and Xiao-Feng Wang, Wan-Yi Zhao, Shi-Li Ding, Bang-Hui Shi, Ying Xia, Hu Yang, Li-Hong Wu, Cai-Yun Li, Wei-Qiang Tan. 2018. "Angiotensin-converting enzyme inhibitor reduces scar formation by inhibiting both canonical and noncanonical TGF-beta1 pathways." *Scientific Reports* 8:3332. doi:10.1038/s41598-018-21600-w.

[78] Tan, W. Q., and Q. Q. Fang, X. Z. Shen, J. F. Giani, T. V. Zhao, P. Shi, L. Y. Zhang, Z. Khan, Y. Li, L. Li, J. H. Xu, E. A. Bernstein, K. E. Bernstein. 2018. "Angiotensin-converting enzyme inhibitor works as a scar formation inhibitor by down-regulating Smad and TGF-beta-activated kinase 1 (TAK1) pathways in mice." *British Journal of Pharmacology* 175:4239-52. doi:10.1111/bph.14489.

[79] Ardekani, Gholamreza S., and Shahin Aghaei, Mohammad H. Nemati, Farhad Handjani, Behrooz Kasraee. 2009. "Treatment of a postburn keloid scar with topical captopril: report of the first case." *Plastic and Reconstructive Surgery* 123:112e-13e. doi:10.1097/PRS.0b013e31819a34db.

[80] Suzawa, H., and S. Kikuchi, N. Arai, A. Koda. 1992. "The mechanism involved in the inhibitory action of tranilast on collagen biosynthesis of keloid fibroblasts." *Japanese Journal of Pharmacology* 60:91-6.

[81] Yamada, H., and S. Tajima, T. Nishikawa, S. Murad, S. R. Pinnell. 1994. "Tranilast, a selective inhibitor of collagen synthesis in human skin fibroblasts." *Journal of Biochemistry* 116:892-7.

[82] Kohavi, Libi, and Eli Sprecher, Eyal Zur, Ofir Artzi. 2017. "The Effect of Tranilast 8% Liposomal Gel Versus Placebo on Post-Cesarean Surgical Scars: A Prospective Double-Blind Split-Scar Study." *Dermatologic Surgery* 43:1157-63. doi:10.1097/dss.0000000000001140.

[83] Beck, L. Steven, and Theresa L. Chen, Philip Mikalauski Arthur J. Ammann.1990. 'Recombinant Human Transforming Growth Factor—Beta 1 (rhTGF-β1) Enhances Healing and Strength of Granulation Skin Wounds.' *Growth Factors* 3 :267-75.

[84] Leo, Michael S., and Alur S. Kumar, Raj Kirit, Rajyalaxmi Konathan, Raja K Sivamani. 2015. 'Systematic review of the use of platelet-rich plasma in aesthetic dermatology.' *Journal of Cosmetic Dermatology* 14 :315-23.

[85] Poetschke, Julian and Gerd G. Gauglitz. 2016. "Current options for the treatment of pathological scarring." *Journal der Deutschen Dermatologischen Gessault* 14:467-77, doi:10.1111/ddg.13027.

In: Cutaneous Scars: Biology, Clinics and Management ISBN: 978-1-53615-657-7
Editors: Berna Aksoy, Hasan Mete Aksoy et al. © 2019 Nova Science Publishers, Inc.

Chapter 20

INTRALESIONAL TREATMENTS

Asli Hapa[*]
Dermatology Clinic, University of Health Sciences,
Bozyaka Training and Research Hospital, Izmir, Turkey

ABSTRACT

Although many intralesional therapies for keloids and hypertrophic scars are currently available, randomized controlled studies are still needed to assess new treatment modalities. In this chapter, we will review the intralesional treatments especially for keloids and hypertrophic scars.

Keywords: intralesional, bleomycin, corticosteroid, cryotherapy, 5-fluorouracil, interferon, platelet rich plasma, verapamil, botulinum toxin A

1. INTRODUCTION

There are many treatment modalities currently in use for keloids and hypertrophic scars. Intralesional injection treatments are the most preferrred treatment modalities demonstrating promising results. However, there is still no consensus regarding which intralesional agents are optimal for the treatment. This section will focus on available literature on this subject and summarize the possible intralesional treatment strategies for especially hypertrophic scars and keloids.

[*]Corresponding Author's Email: draltaykan@yahoo.com.

2. CORTICOSTEROIDS

Intralesional corticosteroid injection is the most frequently used modality and the most commonly used corticosteroid is the depot preparation of triamcinolone acetonide. The concentration of the triamcinolone acetonide depends on the size and site of the lesion. It is used in a concentration of 10-20 mg/ml tough it can be used up to 40 mg/ml for bigger lesions. It is typically injected into the mid-dermis to avoid atrophy. Injections are repeated in 3 to 4 weeks periodically depending on the size of lesions as well as the clinical response (Figures 1 and 2) [1].

The effects of corticosteroids are primarily due to their anti-inflammatory properties affecting wound healing, reduction in collagen and glycosaminoglycan synthesis, and the inhibiton of fibroblast growth. In addition, triamcinolone has been shown to inhibit transforming growth factor (TGF)-β1 expression and to induce apoptosis in fibroblasts [2].

The most common side effects of the corticosteroid intralesional injections are the pain during execution of treatment, atrophy of the skin, and dyspigmentation.

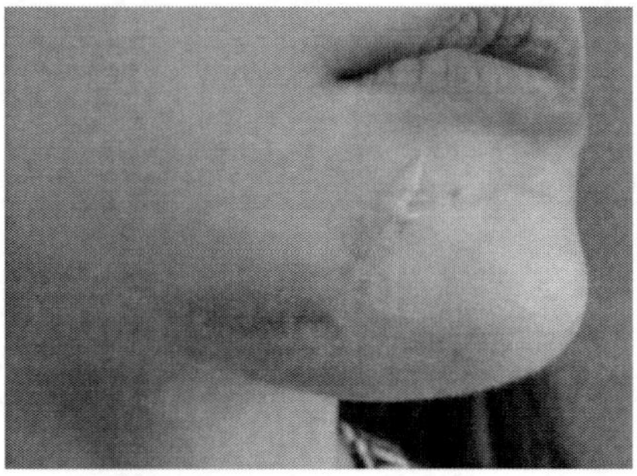

Figure 1. A sutured hypertrophic scar after trauma on the chin of 12-year old girl (Same patient in part 3 chapter 3, Figure 2.2) (Courtesy of Berna Aksoy, MD).

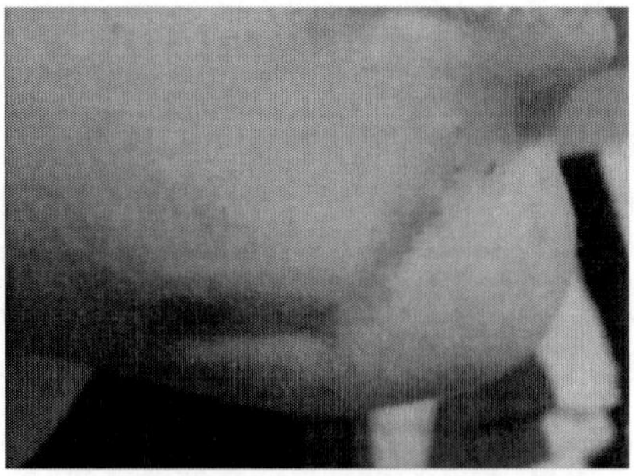

Figure 2. After a 4 month treatment with 4 intralesional injections of triamcinolone (1 session at a dose of 20 mg/ml - 3 sessions at a dose of 10 mg/ml) (Courtesy of Berna Aksoy, MD).

3. CRYOTHERAPY

For decades, liquid nitrogen has been applied externally to freeze and destruct keloids and its use has been associated with side effects such as blistering, hypopigmentation and delayed healing. To solve these problems, Weshahy was the first who attempted intralesional cryotherapy with needles [3]. Afterwards, Zouboulis et al. found that only small number of keloids showed 50% reduction with a modified device [4]. However, Har-Shai et al. found 68% reduction in scar volume 18 months after one treatment [5].

In a systematic review, intralesional cryotherapy is suggested to be a promising treatment in terms of reduction in volume, pain and pruritus. However, it is also stated that complete scar eradication is not achieved and scar recurrence is seen [6].

4. 5-FLUOROURACIL

5-fluorouracil is an anti-neplastic agent known to inhibit transforming growth factor-beta as well as fibroblast proliferation [7]. 5-fluorouracil (5-FU) was used in treatment of keloids alone or in combination with triamcinolone acetonide and/or excision in the literature. Kontochristopoulos et al. treated 20 patients with only intralesional injections of 5-FU (50 mg/ml) once weekly for 7 weeks, they observed 50% improvement in 85% of the patients [8]. Sharma et al. treated small keloids with 5-FU alone versus 5-FU in combination with corticosteroids and found better results in the combination group [9]. In a study by Khare and Patil, excision combined with 5-FU injections revealed excellent results with up to 98% success rate [10].

Ulceration, hyperpigmentation, atrophy, erythema, tissue sloughing, swelling, pain, moulting and telangiectasia are the most commonly reported complications which have been reported to disappear quickly [11].

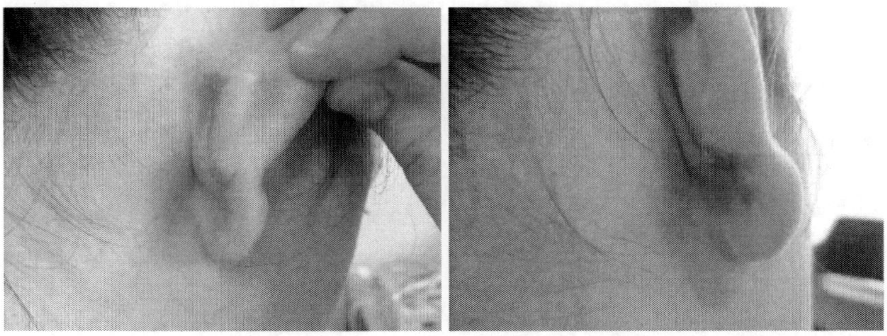

Figure 3. Earlobe keloid a) before and b) after 5 injections (every 2 weeks) of 5-FU combined with triamcinolone revealed decrease in size and volume of keloid with postinflammatory hyperpigmentation (Courtesy of Berna Aksoy, MD).

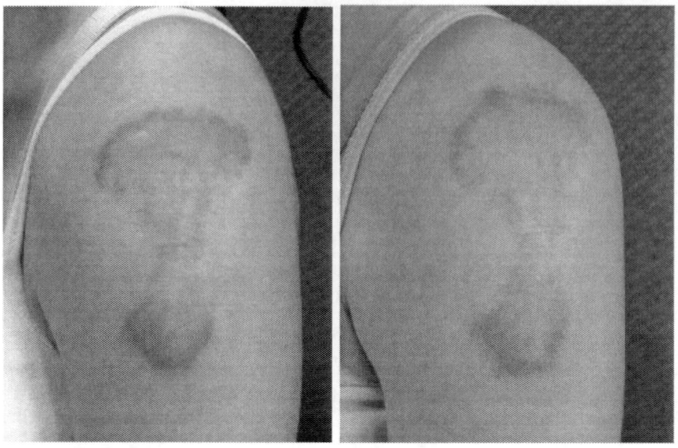

Figure 4. Deltoid area keloid a) before and b) after 3 injections (every 2 weeks) of 5-FU combined with triamcinolone revealed postinflammatory hyperpigmentation and resolution of keloid (Courtesy of Berna Aksoy, MD).

Based on a systematic review about intralesional 5-FU, 5-FU is recommended to be combined with triamcinolone acetonide at a dosage of 4:45 mg/ml (triamcinolone:5-FU) until a satisfactory result is reached. It is likely that approximately 8 injections are needed (Figures 3 and 4) [12].

5. Bleomycin

The main mode of action of bleomycin is inhibition of DNA, RNA and protein synthesis. It is commonly used for the treatment of hypertrophic scars and keloids by performing either intralesional injections or by multiple punctures with a 22 gauge needle [13]. Espena et al., administered bleomycin through multiple punctures [14]. The maximum bleomycin dose applied was 2 ml/cm2 with a concentration of 1.5 IU/ml. Substantial improvement occured in 100% of the lesions after 1-5 sessions with 2 recurrences at one year follow-up period [14]. Saray and Guleç treated 15 keloids with intralesional multiple jet injections of 0.1 ml bleomycin (1.5 IU/ml) applied to each lesion [15]. This treatment resulted in complete flattening in 73 % of the lesions. The most common side effects were small ulcerations that heal in 10 days and hyperpigmentation that resolves after one-year follow-up period [15].

6. Interferon

Interferon (IFN) is widely known to decrease the synthesis of collagen I and III. IFN-alpha 2b is also known to increase collagenase production. In vivo, IFN-α2b injections are used at a dose of 1.5 million IU twice daily over 4 days or three times weekly for excessive scarring [16]. IFN-γ has also been shown to be effective in treatment of keloids and hypertrophic scars with variable treatment protocols such as 0.01-0.1 mg 3 times a week for 3 weeks or a weekly maximal dose of 0.05 mg for 10 weeks [17]. The most important side effect was the occurrence of flu-like symptoms which can be prevented with pretreatment use of 500 mg acetaminophen.

7. Verapamil

Verapamil is a calcium channel blocker antiarrhythmic agent that alters fibroblast shape and inhibits synthesis of extracellular matrix molecules. In light of this knowledge, Lawrence found that excision of keloids followed by pressure dressings and intralesional injection of verapamil resulted in 55 % reduction in size [18]. A single-blind, parallel group study demostrated that efficacy of verapamil was comparable to that of triamcinolone in the treatment of keloids [19].

8. Botulinum Toxin Type A

Botulinum toxin A has been used for the treatment of keloids intralesionally by Zhibo et al. at a concentration of 35 U/ml, with total dose varying from 70 to 140 U per session, at 3 month intervals for a maxium of 9 months with promising results [20]. Xiao et al. also studied botulinum toxin A intralesionally at a dose of 2.5 U/cm3 per lesion at 1 month intervals for 3 months with succesful results [21]. No serious adverse reactions have been reported in the above mentioned studies as well.

9. Autologous Platelet Rich Plasma

Platelet rich plasma (PRP) is an autologous centrifuged solution of patient's own plasma that contains 4 to 7 times the baseline concentration of platelets. It has been used widely for various dermatological conditions including wound healing and scarring. PRP can be used as injectable or topical agent to make scars better or can be combined with other modalities like fat grafting, nonablative fractional laser, erbium or CO2 resurfacing. PRP injections are reported to prolong fat graft survival in scar revisions and provide significant improvements in clinical appearance and/or Manchester scar scale assessments in traumatic and acne scars. PRP injections also leads to faster resolution of erythema, edema; decrease of melanin index and shorter recovery times following laser resurfacing [22].

10. Other Promising Treatments

miRNAs are a class of small, non-coding RNAs that modify gene expression by binding to target messenger RNA (mRNA) and are involved in skin fibrosis. miRNAs are involved at each level of the TGF-beta pathway in skin fibrosis. Development of miRNA-targeted therapies for the management of skin fibrosis may be done by two approaches: increasing the expression of anti-fibrotic miRNAs or reducing the expression of profibrotic miRNAs. In the treatment of cutaneous fibrosis, anti-fibrotic miRNAs may be upregulated by using mimics or viral vectors. Efficacy of let-7a mimic was successfully tested in vivo in a mouse model of bleomycin-induced skin fibrosis by intraperitoneal injection. miRNA expression can be increased with the use of lentiviral, adenoviral, or adeno-associated viral vectors with built-in miRNA precursor constructs and has been tested in liver, lung and cardiac fibrosis. On the contrary, profibrotic miRNAs may be downregulated by administering anti-miRNAs, sponges, erasers and masks and has been successfully tested in other organ system models. miRNA modulators have the potential to contribute significantly to the treatment of cutaneous fibrosis and needs further investigations [23]. Antisense oligonucleotides targeting TGF-β have been shown to inhibit in vivo scarring and improve surgical outcome in animal conjunctival scarring and rabbit glaucoma models when applied subconjunctivally [24].

Transforming Growth Factors (TGF) are important in fibrosis and hypertrophic scarring. Anti-TGF-β1, 2, and 3 monoclonal antibodies are demonstrated to decrease scar hypertrophy when applied intradermally to rabbit ear wounds after one week of healing [25].

Human recombinant transforming growth factor beta 3 (avotermin) is the first in a new class of therapeutics to prophylactically improve cutaneous scar appearance [26]. Intradermal avotermin (in concentrations 0.25 to 500 ng/100 μL per linear cm wound margin) was administered to both margins of 1 cm, full-thickness skin incisions in healthy men and women in comparison to placebo or standard wound care. Avotermin significantly improved total scar scores, and collagen orientation versus placebo and side effects were similar for avotermin and control wounds [27]. Further studies have confirmed that avotermin reduces scarring when administered once or twice to the approximated margins of acute skin incisions or following scar revision surgery [28,29].

Interleukin 10 is an anti-inflammatory cytokine and involved in fetal scarless healing. A lentiviral vector expressing IL-10 was injected at the adult in vivo wound site 48 hours before wounding. These adult wounds demonstrated decreased inflammation, decreased quantities of all proinflammatory mediators, lack of abnormal collagen deposition, and restoration of normal dermal architecture and hence leading to regenerative adult wound healing [30].

CONCLUSION

Although different treatment options with promising results were reported in the literature, there is no accepted treatment totally curable for keloids and hypertrophic scars. Further investigations are still needed for novel modalities.

REFERENCES

[1] Gupta, Somesh, and V. K. Sharma. 2011. 'Standard guidelines of care:Keloids and hypertrofic scars.' *Indian Journal of Dermatology, Venereology and Leprology* 11:94-100. doi: 10.4103/0378-6323.74968.

[2] Boyadjiev, C., and E. Popchristova, J. Masgalova. 1995. 'Histomorphological changes in keloids treated with Kenacort.' *Journal of Trauma* 38:299-302.

[3] Weshahy, A. H. 1993. 'Intralesional cryosurgery. A new technique using cryoneedles.' The *Journal of Dermatologic Surgery and Oncology* 19:123-26.

[4] Zouboulis, Christos C., and Alina D. Rosenberger, Thomas Forster, Gisela Beller, Martina Kratzsch, Dieter Felsenberg. 2004. 'Modification of a device and its application for intralesional cryosurgery of old recalcitrant keloids.' *Archives of Dermatology* 140:1293-94.

[5] Har-Shai, Y., and E. Sabo, E. Rohde, M. Hyams, C. Assaf, C. C. Zouboulis. 2006. 'Intralesional cryosurgery enhances the involution of recalcitrant auricular keloids: a new clinical approach supported by experimental studies.' *Wound Repair and Regeneration* 14:18-27. Doi: 10.1111/j.1743-6109.2005.00084.x.

[6] Van Leeuwen, Michiel C. E., and Anne E. J. Bulstra, Johannes C. F. Ket, Marco J. P. F. Ritt, Van Paul A. M. Leeuwen, Frank B. Niessen. 2015. 'Intralesional cryotherapy for the treatment of keloid scars: evaluating effectiveness.' *Plastic and Reconstructive Surgery. Global Open* 3:e437. doi: 10.1097/GOX.0000000000000348.

[7] Huang, L., and Y. P. Wong, Y. J. Cai, I. Lung, C. S. Leung, A. Burd. 2010. 'Low-dose 5-fluorouracil induces cell cycle G2 arrest and apoptosis in keloid fibroblasts.' The *British Journal of Dermatology* 163:1181-85. doi: 10.1111/j.1365-2133.2010.09939.x.

[8] Kontrochristopoulos, George, and Christina Stefanaki, Antonios Panagiotopoulos, Kalliopi Stefanaki, Theodoros Argyrakos, Athanasios Petridis, Andreas Katsambas. 2005. 'Intralesional 5-Fluorouracil in the treatment of keloids: an open clinical and histopathological study.' *Journal of the American Academy of Dermatology* 52:474-79. Doi: 10.1016/j.jaad.2004.09.018.

[9] Sharma, Saurabh, and Roopam Bassi, Amid Gupta. 2012. 'Treatment of small keloids with intralesional 5-fluorouracil alone vs. intralesional triamcinolone

acetonide with 5-fluorouracil.' *Journal of Pakistan Association of Dermatologists* 22:35-40.

[10] Khare, Nishant, and Surendra B. Patil. 2012. 'A novel approach for the management of ear keloids:results of excision combined with 5-fluorouracil injection.' *Journal of Plastic, Reconstructive and Aesthetic Surgery* 65:e315-17. doi: 10.1016/j.bjps.2012.04.021.

[11] Apikian, Martine, and Greg Goodman. 2004. 'Intralesional 5-fluorouracil in the treatment of keloid scars.' The *Australasian Journal of Dermatology* 45:140-43. DOI: 10.1111/j.1440-0960.2004.00072.x.

[12] Bijlard, Eveline, and Sanne Stentenpool, Frank B. Niessen. 2015. 'Intralesional 5-fluorouracil in keloid treatment: a systemic review.' *Acta Dermato-Venereologica* 95:778-82. doi: 10.2340/00015555-2106.

[13] Bodokh, I., and P. Brun. 1996. 'Treatment of keloid with intralesional bleomycin.' *Annales de Dermatologie et de Venereologie* 123:791-94.

[14] Espana, Agustin, and Teresa Solona, Emilio Quintanilla. 2001. 'Bleomycin in the treatment of keloids and hypertrophic scars by multiple needle punctures.' *Dermatologic Surgery* 27:23-7.

[15] Saray, Yasemin, and A. Tülin Güleç. 2005. 'Treatment of keloids and hypertrophic scars with dermojet injections of bleomycin: a preliminary study.' *International Journal of Dermatology* 44:777-84. Doi: 10.1111/j.1365-4632.2005.02633.x.

[16] Mutalik, Sharad. 2005. 'Treatment of keloids and hypertrophic scars.' *Indian Journal of Dermatology, Venereology and Leprology* 71:3-8.

[17] Larrabee Jr, Wayne F., and Charles A. East, Howard S. Jaffe, Carol Stephenson, Karen E. Peterson. 1990. 'Intralesional interferon gamma treatment for keloids and hypertrophic scars.' *Archives of Otolaryngology - Head & Neck Surgery* 116:1159-62.

[18] Lawrence, W. T. 1996. 'Treatment of earlobe keloids with surgery plus adjuvant intralesional verapamil and pressure earrings.' *Annals of Plastic Surgery* 37:167-69.

[19] Shanthi, F. X. Margaret, and Kalpana Ernest, Prema Dhanraj. 2008. 'Comparison of intralesional verapamil with intralesional triamcinolone in the treatment of hypertrophics scars and keloids.' *Indian Journal of Dermatology, Venereology and Leprology* 74:343-48.

[20] Zhibo, Xiao, and Zhang Miaobo. 2009. 'Intralesional botulinum toxin type A injection as a new treatment measure for keloids.' *Plastic and Reconstructive Surgery* 124:275-77. doi: 10.1097/PRS.0b013e3181b98ee7.

[21] Xiao, Zhibo, and Fengmin Zhang, Ziwei Cui. 2009. 'Treatment of hypertrophic scars with intralesional botulinum toxin type A injections:a preliminary report.' *Aesthetic Plastic Surgery* 33:409-12. doi: 10.1007/s00266-009-9334-z.

[22] Leo, Michael S., and Alur S. Kumar, Raj Kirit, Rajyalaxmi Konathan, Raja K Sivamani. 2015. 'Systematic review of the use of platelet-rich plasma in aesthetic dermatology.' *Journal of Cosmetic Dermatology* 14:315-23.

[23] Babalola, Olubukola, and Andrew Mamalis, Hadar Lev-Tov, Jared Jagdeo. 2013. 'The role of microRNAs in skin fibrosis.' *Archives of Dermatological Research* 305;763–76. Doi: 10.1007/s00403-013-1410-1.

[24] Cordeiro, M. F., and A. Mead, R. R. Ali, R. A. Alexander, S. Murray, C. Chen, C. York-Defalco, N. M. Dean, G. S. Schultz, P. T. Khaw. 2003. 'Novel antisense oligonucleotides targeting TGF-β inhibit in vivo scarring and improve surgical outcome.' *Gene Therapy* 10;59–71.

[25] Lu, Leonard, and Alexandrina S. Saulis, W. Robert Liu, Nakshatra K. Roy Jerome D. Chao Steven Ledbetter, Thomas A. Mustoe. 2005. 'The Temporal Effects of Anti-TGF-β1, 2, and 3 Monoclonal Antibody on Wound Healing and Hypertrophic Scar Formation.' *Journal of the American College of Surgeons* 201:391-7. Doi: 10.1016/j.jamcollsurg.2005.03.032.

[26] Occleston, Nick L., and Sharon O'Kane, Hugh G. Laverty, Mark Cooper, David Fairlamb, Tracey Mason, Jim A. Bush, Mark W. J. Ferguson. 2011. 'Discovery and development of avotermin (recombinant human transforming growth factor beta 3): A new class of prophylactic therapeutic for the improvement of scarring.' *Wound Repair and Regeneration* 19;s38-s48. Doi: 10.1111/j.1524-475X.2011. 00711.x.

[27] Ferguson, Mark W. J., and Jonathan Duncan, Jeremy Bond, James Bush, Piyush Durani, Karen So, Lisa Taylor, Jonquille Chantrey, Tracey Mason, Gaynor James, Hugh Laverty, Nick L. Occleston, Abdul Sattar, Anna Ludlow, Sharon O'Kane. 2009. 'Prophylactic administration of avotermin for improvement of skin scarring: three double-blind, placebo-controlled, phase I/II studies.' The *Lancet* 373(9671):1264-74. Doi: 10.1016/S0140-6736(09)60322-6.

[28] Bush, James, and Jonathan Duncan, Jeremy Bond, Piyush Durani, Karen So, Tracey Mason, Sharon O'Kane, Mark W. J.Ferguson. 2010. 'Scar-Improving Efficacy of Avotermin Administered into the Wound Margins of Skin Incisions as Evaluated by a Randomized, Double-Blind, Placebo-Controlled, Phase II Clinical Trial.' *Plastic and Reconstructive Surgery* 126:1604-1615. doi: 10.1097/PRS.0b013e3181ef8e66.

[29] So, Karen, and Duncan McGrouther, James Bush, Piyush Durani, Lisa Taylor, Gaynor Skotny, Tracey Mason, Anthony Metcalfe, Sharon O'Kane, Mark W. J. Ferguson. 2011. 'Avotermin for Scar Improvement following Scar Revision Surgery: A Randomized, Double-Blind, Within-Patient, Placebo-Controlled, Phase II Clinical Trial.' *Plastic and Reconstructive Surgery* 128:163-172. doi: 10.1097/PRS.0b013e318217429b.

[30] Peranteau, William H., and Liping Zhang, Nidal Muvarak, Andrea T. Badillo, Antoneta Radu, Philip W. Zoltick, Kenneth W. Liechty. 2008. 'IL-10 Overexpression Decreases Inflammatory Mediators and Promotes Regenerative Healing in an Adult Model of Scar Formation.' *Journal of Investigative Dermatology* 128:1852-60. Doi: 10.1038/sj.jid.5701232.

In: Cutaneous Scars: Biology, Clinics and Management ISBN: 978-1-53615-657-7
Editors: Berna Aksoy, Hasan Mete Aksoy et al. © 2019 Nova Science Publishers, Inc.

Chapter 21

SYSTEMIC MEDICAL TREATMENTS

Sibel Dogan*
Department of Dermatology and Venereology,
Faculty of Medicine, Hacettepe University, Ankara, Turkey

ABSTRACT

Scar tissue is the final result of wound healing process where the injured area of the skin is replaced by fibrotic tissue. Keloids and hypertrophic scars are caused by excessive fibroproliferation that arise after any cutaneous injury to the skin's deeper parts involving the dermis. Disseminated keloids and hypertrophic scars may occur and generate a challenging medical condition which cause serious psychological burden in patients due to their cosmetic disfigurement. These lesions may even lead to functional limitations and sometimes intractable pruritus. Herein, systemic medical treatment of cutaneous scars regarding keloids and hypertrophic scars will be reviewed.

Keywords: colchicine, dietary, doxorubicin, interferon (IFN), methotrexate, penicillamine, pentoxifylline, sirolimus, tamoxifen, tranilast, vitamins

1. INTRODUCTION

Scarring after an injury to the skin is accepted as a physiologic response. Scar tissue is the final result of wound healing process where the injured area of the skin is replaced by fibrotic tissue and extracellular matrix deposition. Keloids and hypertrophic scars are caused by excessive fibroproliferation that arise after any cutaneous injury to the skin's

*Corresponding Author's Email: sibel.dogan@hacettepe.edu.tr.

deeper parts involving the dermis. Although scarring is the end of wound healing process, the scar tissue will never be as strong as the skin's previous healthy state [1]. Disseminated keloids and hypertrophic scars may occur and generate a challenging medical condition which cause serious psychological burden in patients due to cosmetic disfigurement. These lesions may even lead to functional limitations including joint contractures and intractable pruritus [2]. Both conditions are formed by local fibroblast proliferation and collagen overproduction at the injury site [3, 4]. The basic difference between hypertrophic scars and keloids is that keloids extend beyond the borders of the primary injury that typically involves the adjacent skin whereas hypertrophic scars are mainly confined to the site of injury [5].

Many treatment modalities have been used to treat hypertrophic scars and keloids. These include intralesional corticosteroids, intralesional 5-fluoruracil, silicone gel sheets, pressure therapy, cryotherapy, excision, postoperative radiation therapy and laser therapy which are reviewed in detail in other sections of this book thus will not be discussed within this chapter [1-5].

Systemic medical therapy of hypertrophic scars and keloids include off-label usage of conservative cytostatic medical treatments which have only been reported in case reports or small case series and are not widely used at the present time. In addition, there are other substances (growth factors, interleukins, antisense oligonucleotides blocking fibrogenic factors) that play a particular role in wound healing, fibrosis, collagen overproduction and degradation and they have been proved experimentally in animal models and may be promising treatment options for the future [1, 3].

2. Systemic Medical Treatments of Cutaneous Scarring

2.1. Medical Treatments Used for Hypertrophic Scars and Keloids

2.1.1. Methotrexate

Methotrexate is a folate antagonist and is used as an antineoplastic compound for the treatment of various cancers. Through its supressive effects on inflammatory cells and by changing adenosine levels via interaction with adenosine A2 receptors, methotrexate is widely used for the treatment inflammatory disorders including psoriasis and rheumatoid arthritis [6-7].

In a case report by Onwukwe, treatment of keloids with oral or intramuscular methotrexate with a dosage of 15 to 20 mg at 4 day intervals for 1 to 2 weeks before scar tissue excision led to delayed healing of excised keloid wounds and reduced their recurrence. In this report, methotrexate was continued after surgery until keloid resolution [6, 8]. In another case series report consisting of patients who developed keloids after reconstruction of syndactyly; two children treated with adjunctive methotrexate experienced successful treatment of their keloids with near-normal healing and recurrences were not observed after 4 years of follow-up [6,9].

2.1.2. Pentoxifylline

Pentoxifylline is a methylxanthine derivative that inhibits phosphodiesterase. It is widely used in peripheral vascular diseases due to its effects on blood components; pentoxifylline improves blood flow by increasing erythrocyte and leukocyte flexibility and inhibits platelet aggregation [1, 6]. It is also known to have immunomodulatory effects such as cytokine production stimulation, increasing IL-10 and thereby decreasing IL-6 [6]. In a study by Berman et al, where fibroblasts from the skin of patients with keloids, scleroderma and morphea were cultured in vitro, pentoxiflyline resulted in reduction in fibroblast proliferation. Fibroblast cultures also showed 95% reduced amounts of collagen and glucosaminoglycan content depending on the concentration of pentoxifylline. Similar inhibition of fibronectin production by keloid and scleroderma fibroblasts was also achieved [10]. In another in vitro study, pentoxifylline was shown to modify collagen lattice model contraction and expression of collagen types I and III by fibroblasts derived from post-burn hypertrophic scars [11].

In clinical observations, oral administration of 400 mg of pentoxifylline 2 to 3 times daily in 3 patients was reported to reduce pain and pruritus caused by keloids but symptoms re-occured in 2 of the patients after cessation of therapy [12]. In an animal model study simulating accidental acute localized overexposure to gamma irradiation in human, pigs were irradiated. They were investigated for changes in the density of palpated block of fibrotic scar tissue and dimensions of their projected cutaneous surface. Significant softening and shrinking of fibrosis were noted 13 weeks following treatment in the pigs that were given pentoxifylline and alpha-tocopherol. Complete normal muscle and subcutaneous tissue surrounding the residual scar tissue were achieved histologically [13].

2.1.3. Colchicine and Penicillamine

Peacock et al. have suggested that induction of lathyrism, which is production of poorly cross-linked collagen in healing wounds, can decrease scar tissue formation because poorly cross-linked collagen is more susceptible to digestion by tissue collagenases than normally cross-linked collagen [14]. Colchicine is a lysil oxidase inhibitor and stimulates tissue collagenase activity [6, 14]. In their study ten patients with massive keloids, resistant to conventional therapy by excision, grafting, and/or intralesional injection of steroids, were treated by excising the keloid, grafting the defect, inducing lathyrism with beta aminopropionitrile fumurate or penicillamine and administering colchicine. Patients were followed for 18 months to five years and they did not develop recurrent keloids while undergoing treatment [14]. Patients who were treated succesfully for plantar keloids were prescribed oral colchicine and additional topical treatment regimens [15]. There are contradictory reports regarding effectiveness and non-effectiveness of single use of d-penicillamine in keloid therapy [6, 16, 17].

2.1.4. Tranilast

Tranilast is a histamine receptor (H1) antagonist known for its vasoprotectant, analgesic and anti-inflammatory properties [6, 18]. Tranilast inhibits synthesis of type I and III collagen and inhibits the stimulatory effect of transforming growth factor-beta1 (TGF-β1) on collagen synthesis in scleroderma and keloid fibroblasts in vitro [19, 20]. The commercial drug containing tranilast (1000 mg capsule) is approved for the indication of hypertrophic scar treatment in Japan and Korea [6, 18].

2.1.5. Interferons

In hypertrophic scar tissues, it was found that IL-4 mRNA was increased whereas interferon gamma (IFN-γ) mRNA was reduced compared with normal skin and mature scar [1,6]. T helper 2 (Th2) fibrogenic cytokines in tissues may be the cause of development of fibrosis in the skin. Increased CD3(+) and CD4(+) cells were present and were coexpressed with the fibrogenic cytokine TGF-β. These findings suggest that fibrosis in the skin is associated with a polarized Th2 systemic response leading to increased T cells. [1, 6, 21]. The beneficial effect of IFNs when used intralesionally is well-established in the management of scars [1-6]. IFN-α2b is known to improve scar by supressing fibroblast functions. The efficacy of systemic subcutaneous administration of IFN on scar tissue components is demonstrated in clinical studies. In one study, two groups of patients underwent serial tissue biopsies; first group included six burn patients and second patient group included hypertrophic scar patients treated with systemic IFN-α2b. Scar tissue obtained from the patients who received systemic IFN-α2b showed a general reduction in total number of fibroblasts and myofibroblasts associated with a significant increase in the percentage of apoptotic cells compared with normal dermis from the same patient [22]. Significant reduction of fibrocytes in hypertrophic scar tissue obtained from patients after treatment with systemic IFN-α2b was also shown by a study by Wang et al. [23]. IFN-α2b was shown to abolish fibrocyte differentiation from peripheral blood mononuclear cells (PBMCs) in vitro in a dose-dependent fashion. In addition, IFN-α2b was shown to inhibit proliferation of fibrocytes and reduce TGF-mediated -smooth muscle actin expression in fibrocytes. In a subsequent clinical study, improvement of hypertrophic scar tissue after systemic IFN-α2b treatment was found to be associated with a significant reduction in angiogenesis in scar tissue [24]. IFN-α2b suppressed the proliferation of human umbilical vein endothelial cells (HUVECs) in a dose-dependent manner and inhibited vascular endothelial growth factor (VEGF) induced cell proliferation and tube formation by using HUVECs. These findings may be the result of VEGF receptor expression blockage [24].

2.2. Systemic Medical Treatments with Potential Inhibitory Properties on Scarring

2.2.1. Sirolimus

Sirolimus is a macrolide inhibitor of the mammalian target of rapamycin (mTOR) pathway which regulates cell growth and proliferation [1, 6, 25]. mTOR is also a regulator of type I collagen expression and is elevated in keloidal tissue [25]. Sirolimus decreases expression of collagen and alpha-smooth muscle actin in cultured normal and keloidal fibroblasts and inhibits extracellular matrix deposition. Sirolimus reduces collagen I and III overexpression by keloidal fibroblasts. [1, 6, 26, 27]. Sirolimus also inhibits platelet derived growth factor (PDGF), which is known to increase synthesis of extracellular matrix, and PDGF-induced vascular smooth muscle cell proliferation and collagen synthesis [28, 29]. However systemic administration of sirolimus has not yet been studied in the treatment of hypertrophic scars or keloids in clinical trials.

2.2.2. Tamoxifen Citrate

Tamoxifen is a selective estrogen receptor modulator treatment used for breast cancer. It has also been successfully used for treatment of desmoid tumors and retroperitoneal fibrosis, confirming its antifibrotic properties [1, 6, 30, 31]. Tamoxifen's mechanisms of action include RNA transcription alterations, decrease in cellular proliferation, delay in cell cycle by arrest of cells in G1 phase, and interfering with multiple growth factors, including TGF-β [1, 6, 32] This agent has been shown to inhibit proliferation of cultured keloidal fibroblasts, and contraction of collagen lattices and to decrease TGF-β1 production [33, 34]. Although afimoxifene gel is under investigation for keloidal scarring and other fibrotic disorders; phase II trials for treatment of keloidal scarring regarding this topical agent have not yet been reported and systemic tamoxifen has not yet been studied in the treatment of hypertrophic scars or keloids in clinical trials [1, 6, 18].

2.2.3. Doxorubicin

Doxorubicin is an anthracycline antineoplastic agent which is known for its side effect of poor wound healing that is caused by impaired collagen biosynthesis [1, 35]. In vitro, doxorubicin has been shown to reduce synthesis of hydroxyproline and reduce fibroblast proliferation through inhibition of prolidase activity. Prolidase is an enzyme which is important in freeing proline for collagen re-synthesis and its deficiency leads to chronic ulcers of the skin [1, 35, 36]. In a study by Sasaki and colleagues, clinical therapeutic levels of doxorubicin inhibited triple-helical conformation of collagen in vitro [36]. However systemic doxorubicin has not yet been studied in the treatment of hypertrophic scars or keloids in clinical trials.

2.3. Systemic Dietary Treatments for Potential Beneficial Effects on Wound Healing and Scarring

Malnourishment is an important risk factor for delayed wound healing, infections, and pressure ulcers which may also lead to abnormal scar tissue formation. Deficiencies in essential dietary elements along with certain vitamins can disrupt the normal physiological process of wound healing [1, 6, 37]. Fibroblast proliferation and collagen formation may decrease and this leads to atrophic or delayed scar formation depending on the degree of impairment of nutritional status of the host. Disregularities in immune cell functions may cause susceptibility to secondary infections and an excessive response of suppuration and granulation tissue formation. Angiogenesis may also be affected in severe deficiencies of micronutrients and vitamins which are crucial cofactors of certain enzymes responsible for wound healing [37].

A general caloric intake of 25-30 kcal/kg/day for optimal wound healing is suggested by The Wound Healing Society and the American Society for Parenteral and Enteral Nutrition [37,38]. This may differ depending on the general status and age of the patient and the amount of healing tissue. Burn patients are accepted as a specific subcategory and should be assessed carefully in experienced tertiary centers regarding their increased loss of protein and other essential micronutrients.

Multivitamin supplementation is recommended for patients with large wounds [37-40]. Vitamin C is a cofactor for collagen synthesis and deposition. It is also known to affect reepithelization during wound healing [37-41]. Vitamin A supplementation (10,000–15,000 IU/day) has been shown to reverse delayed wound healing in patients taking steroids [37-42]. Vitamin E is an anti-oxidant and is shown to reduce scar thickness [37, 43]. Vitamin D deficiency is associated with impaired healing in chronic leg ulcers. Wnt/β-catenin signaling is suggested to be an important pathway which may induce hypertrophic scar development in burn patients. Vitamin D has inhibitory effects on Wnt/β-catenin signaling pathway and thus may have important therapeutic implications regarding scar formation [37, 44].

Appropriate dietary protein intake is mandatory for wound healing; enzymes, cells, and collagen formation is dependant on a healthy anabolic state of protein metabolism [37-45]. The amino acid glutamine is crucial for the synthesis of amino acids and nucleotides, and essential for epithelial cells and fibroblasts required for wound healing process [37, 45]. 0.8 g/kg/day protein intake in adults and 1 g/kg/day protein intake for elderly are recommended; which can also be increased to 1.25–1.5 g/kg/day for chronic wounds [37-39, 46].

Patients with scars are also reported to have reduced serum zinc levels. Similarly copper levels are recommended to be evaluated and properly restored [37, 47]. Omega-6 and omega-3 alter pro-inflammatory cytokine production and nutritional deficiency of Omega-3 was found to be correlated with keloid formation [37, 48].

CONCLUSION

Systemic medical therapy of hypertrophic scars and keloids include off-label usage of conservative cytostatic medical treatments like colchicine, doxorubicin, methotrexate, penicillamine, pentoxifylline, sirolimus, tamoxifen, tranilast, and IFNs. These treatment modalities have only been reported in case reports or small case series and are not widely used at the present time. Patients must also be supplied with adequate dietary protein, essential minerals and vitamins considering their potential beneficial effects on wound healing and scarring.

REFERENCES

[1] Berman, Brian, and Andrea Maderal, Brian Raphael. 2017. "Keloids and Hypertrophic Scars: Pathophysiology, Classification, and Treatment." *Dermatologic Surgery* 43:3-18. doi: 10.1097/DSS.0000000000000819.

[2] Lee, Ho J., and Yong J. Jang. 2018. "Recent Understandings of Biology, Prophylaxis and Treatment Strategies for Hypertrophic Scars and Keloids." *International Journal of Molecular Sciences* 19: 711. doi: 10.3390/ijms19030711.

[3] UpToDate. Goldstein, Beth G., and Adam O. Goldstein. 2018. "*Keloids and hypertrophic scars*" Accessed 3 March. https://www.uptodate.com/contents/keloids-and-hypertrophic-scars.html.

[4] Nemeth, Alexandra J. 1993. "Keloids and hypertrophic scars." *The Journal of Dermatologic Surgery and Oncology* 19:738-46.

[5] Mahdavian Delavary, Babak, and Willem M. van der Veer, José A. Ferreira, Frank B. Niessen. 2012. "Formation of hypertrophic scars: evolution and susceptibility." *Journal of Plastic Surgery and Hand Surgery* 46:95-101. doi: 10.3109/2000656X.2012.669184.

[6] Berman, Brian, and Martha H. Viera, Sadegh Amini, Ran Huo, Isaac S. Jones. 2008. "Prevention and management of hypertrophic scars and keloids after burns in children." *Journal of Craniofacial Surgery* 19:989-1006. doi: 10.1097/SCS.0b013e318175f3a7.

[7] Malaviya, Anand N. 2016. "Low-Dose Methotrexate (LD-MTX) in Rheumatology Practice - A Most Widely Misunderstood Drug." *Current Rheumatology Reviews* 12:168- 176. doi: 10.2174/1573397112666160824151801.

[8] Onwukwe, Mba F. 1980. "Treating keloids by surgery and methotrexate." *Archieves of Dermatology* 116:158. doi: 10.1001/archderm.1980.01640260034004.

[9] Muzaffar, Arshad R., and Francisco Rafols, James Masson, Marybeth Ezaki, Peter R. Carter. 2004. "Keloid formation after syndactyly reconstruction: associated

conditions, prevalence, and preliminary report of a treatment method." The *Journal of Hand Surgery* 29:201-8. Doi. 10.1016/j.jhsa.2003.10.017.

[10] Berman, B., and M.R. Duncan. 1990. "Pentoxifylline inhibits the proliferation of human fibroblasts derived from keloid, scleroderma and morphoea skin and their production of collagen, glycosaminoglycans and fibronectin." The *British Journal of Dermatology* 123:339-46. Doi: 10.1111/j.1365-2133.1990.tb06294.x.

[11] Isaac, Cesar, and Mônica B. Mathor, Giovani Bariani, André O. Paggiaro, Marisa R. Herson, Claudia Goldenstein-Schainberg, Solange Carrasco, Walcy R. Teodoro, Natalino H. Yoshinari, Marcus C. Ferreira. 2009. "Pentoxifylline modifies three-dimensional collagen lattice model contraction and expression of collagen types I and III by human fibroblasts derived from post-burn hypertrophic scars and from normal skin." *Burns* 35:701-6. doi: 10.1016/j.burns.2008.11.017.

[12] Wong, T. W., and J. Y. Lee, H. M. Sheu, S. C. Chao. 1999. "Relief of pain and itch associated with keloids on treatment with oxpentifylline." The *British Journal of Dermatology* 140:771-2.

[13] Lefaix, Jean-Louis, and Sylvie Delanian, Marie-Catherine Vozenin, Jean-Jacques Leplat, Yves Tricaud, Michéle Martin. 1999. "Striking regression of subcutaneous fibrosis induced by high doses of gamma rays using a combination of pentoxifylline and alpha-tocopherol: an experimental study." *International Journal of Radiation Oncology Biology Physics* 43:839-47.

[14] Peacock, EE Jr. 1981. "Pharmacologic control of surface scarring in human beings." *Annals of Surgery* 193:592-97.

[15] Vanhaecke Jr, C., and G. Hickman, B. Cavelier-Balloy, V. Masson, J.-B. Duron, M. Gorj, P. May, P. Schneider, C. Vilmer, M. Bagot, M. Battistella, A. Petit. 2015. "Plantar keloids: diagnostic and therapeutic issues in six patients." *Journal of the European Academy of Dermatology and Venereology* 29: 1421-6. doi: 10.1111/jdv.12625.

[16] Mayou, B. J. 1981. "D-Penicillamine in the treatment of keloids." The *British Journal of Dermatology* 105:87-9.

[17] Moynahan, E. J. 1974. "Penicillamine in the treatment of morphoea and keloid in children." *Postgraduate Medical Journal* 50:39-41.

[18] Occleston, Nick L., and Sharon O'Kane, Nick Goldspink, Mark W. J. Ferguson. 2008. "New therapeutics for the prevention and reduction of scarring." *Drug Discovery Today* 13:973-81. doi: 10.1016/j.drudis.2008.08.009 .

[19] Yamada, Haruyoshi, and Shingo Tajima, Takeji Nishikawa, Saood Murad, Sheldon R. Pinnell. 1994. "Tranilast, a selective inhibitor of collagen synthesis in human skin fibroblasts." The *Journal of Biochemistry* 116: 892–7.

[20] Isaji, Masayuki, and Misao Nakajoh, Jun Naito. 1987. "Selective inhibition of collagen accumulation by N-3,4-dimethoxycinnamoyl anthranilic acid (N-50) in

granulation tissue." *Biochemical Pharmacology* 36:469–74. Doi: 10.1016/0006-2952(87)90353-4.

[21] Tredget, Edward E., and Liju Yang, Megan Delehanty, Heather Shankowsky, Paul G. Scott. 2006. "Polarized Th2 cytokine production in patients with hypertrophic scar following thermal injury." *Journal of Interferon & Cytokine Research* 26:179-89. Doi: 10.1089/jir.2006.26.179.

[22] Nedelec, Bernadette, and Heather Shankowsky, Paul G. Scott, Aziz Ghahary, Edward E. Tredget. 2001. "Myofibroblasts and apoptosis in human hypertrophic scars: the effect of interferon-alpha2b." *Surgery* 130:798-808.

[23] Wang, Jianfei, and Haiyan Jiao, Tara L. Stewart, Heather A. Shankowsky, Paul G. Scott, Edward E. Tredget. 2007. "Improvement in postburn hypertrophic scar after treatment with IFN-alpha2b is associated with decreased fibrocytes." *Journal of Interferon & Cytokine Research* 27:921-30.

[24] Wang, Jianfei, and Hong Chen, Heather A. Shankowsky, Paul G. Scott, Edward E. Tredget. 2008. "Improved scar in postburn patients following interferon-alpha2b treatment is associated with decreased angiogenesis mediated by vascular endothelial cell growth factor." *Journal of Interferon & Cytokine Research* 28:423-34. doi: 10.1089/jir.2007.0104.

[25] Ong, C. T., and Y. T. Khoo, A. Mukhopadhyay, D. V. Do, I. J. Lim, O. Aalami, T. T. Phan. 2007. "mTOR as a potential therapeutic target for treatment of keloids and excessive scars." *Experimental Dermatology* 16:394–404. Doi: 10.1111/j.1600-0625.2007.00550.x.

[26] Zhu, J., and J. Wu, E. Frizell, S. L. Liu, R. Bashey, R. Rubin, P. Norton, M. A. Zern. 1999. "Rapamycin inhibits hepatic stellate cell proliferation in vitro and limits fibrogenesis in an in vivo model of liver fibrosis." *Gastroenterology* 117:1198-204.

[27] Wong, Victor W., and Fanglei You, Michael Januszyk, Geoffrey C. Gurtner, Anna A. Kuank. 2014. "Transcriptional profiling of rapamycin-treated fibroblasts from hypertrophic and keloid scars." *Annals of Plastic Surgery* 72:711-9. doi: 10.1097/SAP.0b013e31826956f6.

[28] Park, J., and H. Ha, H. J. Ahn, S. W. Kang, Y. S. Kim, J. Y. Seo, M. S. Kim. 2005. "Sirolimus inhibits platelet derived growth factor-induced collagen synthesis in rat vascular smooth muscle cells." *Transplantation Proceedings* 37:3459–62. Doi: 10.1016/j.transproceed.2005.09.066.

[29] Syed, Farhatullah, and Hitesh J. Sanganee, Ashwani Bahl, Ardeshir Bayat. 2013. "Potent dual inhibitors of TORC1 and TORC2 complexes (KU-0063794 and KU-0068650) demonstrate in vitro and ex vivo anti-keloid scar activity which was found more effective than sirolimus." The *Journal of Investigative Dermatology* 133:1340–50. doi: 10.1038/jid.2012.48.

[30] Kinzbrunner, B., and S. Ritter, J. Domingo, C. J. Rosenthal. 1983. "Remission of rapidly growing desmoid tumors after tamoxifen therapy." *Cancer* 52:2201–4.

[31] Clark, C. P., and D. Vanderpool, J. T. Preskitt. 1991. "The response of retroperitoneal fibrosis to tamoxifen." *Surgery* 109:502–6.

[32] Mancoll, J. S., and J. Zhao, R. L. McCauley, L. G. Phillips. 1996."The inhibitory effect of tamoxifen on keloid fibroblasts." *Surgical Forum* 47:718–20.

[33] Hu, D., and M. A. Hughes, G. W. Cherry. 1998."Topical tamoxifen—a potential therapeutic regime in treating excessive dermal scarring?" *British Journal of Plastic Surgery* 51:462–9.

[34] Mikulec, Anthony A., and Matthew M. Hanasono, Joanne Lum, James M. Kadleck, Magdalena Kita, R. James Koch. 2001. "Effect of tamoxifen on transforming growth factor beta1 production by keloid and fetal fibroblasts." *Archieves of Facial Plastic Surgery* 3:111–4.

[35] Muszynska, A., and J. Palka, S. Wolczynski. 1998. "Doxorubicin-induced inhibition of prolidase activity in human skin fibroblasts and its implication to impaired collagen biosynthesis." *Polish Journal of Pharmacology* 50:151–7.

[36] Sasaki, T., and K. C. Holeyfield, J. Uitto. 1987. "Doxorubicin-induced inhibition of prolyl hydroxylation during collagen biosynthesis in human skin fibroblast cultures. Relevance to imparied wound healing." The *Journal of Clinical Investigation* 80:1735–41.

[37] Amini-Nik, Saeid, and Yusef Yousuf, Marc G. Jeschke. 2018. "Scar management in burn injuries using drug delivery and molecular signaling: Current treatments and future directions." *Advanced Drug Delivery Reviews* 123:135-54. doi: 10.1016/j.addr.2017.07.017.

[38] Stechmiller, Joyce K. 2010. "Understanding the role of nutrition and wound healing" *Nutrition in Clinical Practice* 25: 61–8. doi: 10.1177/0884533609358997.

[39] Stechmiller, Joyce K., and L. Cowan, K. Logan. 2009. "Nutrition support for wound healing" *Support Line* 31:2–8.

[40] Ross, V. 2002. "Micronutrient recommendations for wound healing" *Support Line* 24:3–9.

[41] Langemo, Diane, and Julie Anderson, Darlene Hanson, Susan Hunter, Patricia Thompson, Mary E. Posthauer. 2006. "Nutritional considerations in wound care." *Advances in Skin & Wound Care* 19: 297–303.

[42] Archbold, H. C., and Y. X. Yang, L. Chen, K. M. Cadigan. 2012. "How do they do Wnt they do?: regulation of transcription by the Wnt/beta-catenin pathway" *Acta Physiologica (Oxf)* 204: 74–109. Doi: 10.1111/j.1748-1716.2011.02293.x.

[43] Kavalukas, Sandra L., and Adrian Barbul. 2011. "Nutrition and wound healing: an update" *Plastic and Reconstructive Surgery* 127:38S–43S. doi: 10.1097/PRS.0b013e318201256c.

[44] Pendás-Franco, Natalia, and Óscar Aguilera, Fabio Pereira, José M. González-Sancho, Alberto Muñoz. 2008. "Vitamin D andWnt/beta-catenin pathway in colon

cancer: role and regulation of DICKKOPF genes." *Anticancer Research* 28; 2613–23.

[45] Arnold, Meghan, and Adrian Barbul. 2006. "Nutrition and wound healing" *Plastic and Reconstructive Surgery* 117:42S–58S. doi: 10.1097/01.prs.0000225432.17501.6c.

[46] Campos, Antonio C. L., and Anne K. Groth, Alessandra B. Branco. 2008. "Assessment and nutritional aspects of wound healing." *Current Opinion in Clinical Nutrition and Metabolic* Care 11:281–8. doi: 10.1097/MCO.0b013e3282fbd35a.

[47] Bang, R. L., and H. Dashti. 1995."Keloid and hypertrophic scars: trace element alteration" *Nutrition* 11: 527–31.

[48] McDaniel, Jodi C., and Martha Belury, Karen Ahijevych, Wendy Blakely. 2008. "Omega-3 fatty acids effect on wound healing." *Wound Repair and Regeneration* 16:337–45. doi: 10.1111/j.1524-475X.2008.00388.x.

In: Cutaneous Scars: Biology, Clinics and Management ISBN: 978-1-53615-657-7
Editors: Berna Aksoy, Hasan Mete Aksoy et al. © 2019 Nova Science Publishers, Inc.

Chapter 22

SCAR REVISION SURGERY

Atilla A. Eyuboglu[1], Andac Aykan[2,*] and Muhitdin Eski[3]
[1]Department of Plastic, Reconstructive and Aestetic Surgery,
Memorial Bahcelievler Hospital, Istanbul, Turkey
[2]Department of Plastic, Reconstructive and Aestetic Surgery,
Faculty of Medicine, Yeditepe University, Istanbul, Turkey
[3]Plastic, Reconstructive and Aestetic Surgery, Private Clinic, Ankara, Turkey

ABSTRACT

Hypertrophic scars and keloids are two forms of abnormal cutaneous scarring tissue with unclear pathogenesis. Scar management may require both surgical and non-surgical techniques for a proper scar healing. Scar tissue may behave like a stigmata and cause social and psychological problems in affected patients. In cosmetic manner, scar revision surgery provides conversion of the existing unsighty scar into a better-looking scar with an acceptable appearance. In terms of functionality, scar revision surgery is applied to increase the mobility and correct the limitations in range of motion. Despite the fact that our knowledge about this pathology has increased greatly, we still can not treat pathologic scars completely.

Keywords: flap, geometric broken-line closure, remodeling, relaxed skin tension lines, surgery, Z-plasty, W-plasty, V-Y advancement

[*]Corresponding Author's Email: andac.aykan@yeditepe.edu.tr.

1. Introduction

Hypertrophic scars and keloids are two forms of abnormal cutaneous scarring with unclear pathogenesis [1]. The situations that disrupt the skin integrity and cause inflammatory process, as seen in various types of trauma can result in abnormal scarring. Whatever the reason causing scar is, hypertrophic scar and keloid affect the surgical success functionally and they may cause cosmetic concerns. In cases like these, prevention or reduction of the abnormal scar formation is the first objective of today's treatment protocols.

Less invasive treatment modalities presented in up-to-date literature are cryotherapy, pressure therapy, intralesional corticosteroid injection, topical silicone application, laser treatments and radiation therapy (RT) [2]. Especially for extensive disfiguring scars, *surgery* is another important modality to create a more acceptable scar image.

2. Assessment of Scar and Patient

It is important to make assessment and management of not only the scar tissue but also the patient's complaints and expectations. This is required both for determining the ideal surgical approach and for fulfilling the patient's expectations. It is important to reveal the basic complaints of patient for scar revision *surgery*. The ideal scar assessment tool should demonstrate clinical applicability, validity and inter-observer reliability [3]. There are many grading systems for burn scar index. The most frequently used measure is Vancouver Scar Scale (VSS) [4], and other assessment scales are the Patient and Observer Scar Assesment Scale (POSAS), Visual Analog Scale (VAS) and Stony Brook Scar Evaluation Scale (SBSES) [5]. As there are many modalities for scar assessment, scars are generally assessed according to their erythema, pliability, thickness and pigmentation. Physical examination should include scar tissue's relationship to surrounding tissues as it may be associated with tethering or contracture formation which can cause movement disabilities. After completing the scar assessment, one should examine the patient carefully for additional co-morbidities like diabetes, obesity, nutritional deficiencies and tissue healing problems. Cause of the scar tissue is also an important factor: History of trauma, *surgery,* tattoo, infection, exposure to chemical agents or radiation, tobacco use, self mutilation and even the history of ritual scarring or cicatrization which may be a part of cultural tradition should be questioned [6]. Scar tissue disrupts the body image and also results in psychological effects; patients with significant scarring should be referred to a psychiatrist for a completely successful scar treatment. Treatment of patients with unrealistic expectations will be unsuccessful even if everything is done perfectly.

3. INDICATIONS

Scar revision *surgery* is basically applied for cosmetic and functional improvement. In addition, symptoms that affect everyday life such as discomfort and tightness are an indication for scar revision *surgery*.

Scar tissue may behave like a stigmata and cause social and psychological problems in affected patients. In a cosmetic sense, scar revision surgery provides conversion of the existing scar into a better-looking scar with acceptable appearance.

Scar tissue can restrict movement on joint surfaces and other body parts. Joint contracture which is especially seen in burn patients, is the most common example of functional loss. In terms of functionality, scar revision *surgery* is applied for increasing mobility and correcting the limitations in range of motion.

4. TIMING AND PLANNING

Timing of scar revision is determined according to the condition of the scar tissue and patient's concordance. Both factors can be manipulated by an experienced physician. Understanding of the underlying biology helps physician to determine the requirement and timing of *surgery*.

Immature scars can bleed easily because of neovascularization and surrounding tissues may be edematous restricting the reconstruction following excision. Scar tissue will be ready for revision when it reaches maximum mobility and becomes soft and these often require 12 to 18 months due to collagen remodeling which is associated with 70 - 80% recovery of tensile strength considering uninjured skin [7]. Physican should delay the revision *surgery* if there is any doubt about scar maturity. If so patient should be treated with nonoperative treatment methods like silicone sheets or massage creams to maintain the patient's trust. Motivating the patient is another important factor for successful treatment; patient should be educated and informed about what will happen in future examinations. Sharing of the responsibility is crucial.

Planning is also important for success. Most of the scar revisions are done for lesions which commonly occur in non-vital areas and in the form of a single lesion [8]. Complex reconstructions may be mandatory if multiple areas are involved or scar tissue affects vital organs (especially in the head and neck region). Surgeon must decide if the operation should be performed in multiple stages. Sometimes tissue expansion methods or serial excisions are required for minimizing the scarring [9].

5. Scar Revision Surgery

5.1. Principles of Tissue Revision

Scar revision should be managed by the same principles summarised for scar prevention. Main goal of successful scar treatment should include an atraumatic technique, skin eversion, wound repair without tension, perfect apposition of wound edges and the use of natural skin tension lines [10]. Anatomic landmark restoration like eyelid position, vermillion border or alar base restoration should take priority to minimize scar tissue [11]. Structural and dynamic properties of body parts should be considered. Scar revision on facial tension lines may become apparent as patient changes his/her expression therefore *surgery* should be done according to aesthetic units and subunits [12]. Re-orientation of the scar tissue is also important to distribute the skin tension to avoid contractures. Tight scar tissue can lead to movement limitations and hence cause disabilities. Scar tissue rearrangements can also be done for aesthetic purposes since scar tissue in the form of a straight line will be more apparent.

5.2. Scar Revision Techniques

Scar management may require both surgical and non-surgical techniques for a proper scar healing. Non-surgical techniques are camouflage, topical therapy, cryotherapy, intralesional therapeutic injections, soft tissue fillers, non-ablative lasers, ablative laser resurfacing and other treatment methods like radiation therapy, pressure dressings and positive electrical stimulation therapies [2, 13].

5.2.1. Non-Surgical Techniques

A combination of non-surgical techniques can be used for a finer result. Make-up and accessories can help to camouflage the scar; it may be a good option for patients with unrealistic expectations. Different variations and formulations of topical agents like hydrocortisone, retinoic acid, alpha-hydroxy acid, hydroquinone, kojic acid and mitomycin C have been reported to be effective [13, 14]. Use of topical silicone gel or silicone sheets is also useful for correcting texture and contour of the scar. Cryotherapy is used in combination with other methods. It was reported to be useful in an uncontrolled study of 135 patients and 80% reduction in scar volume was obtained [15]. Intralesional injection agents can be used in the treatment plan. Corticosteroids reduce scar formation by inhibiting inflammatory mediators and by enhancing degradation of collagen [16], and intralesional 5-Fluorouracil (5-FU) acts by inhibiting fibroblast proliferation and expression of TGF- $\beta 1$ and has been shown to be effective [17, 18].

5.2.2. Surgical Scar Revision

Surgical scar revision requires a careful planning and use of techniques according to tissue properties. Surgeon should keep some points in mind to achieve favourable results, and these are; careful incision planning, atraumatic tissue handling, undermining of surrounding tissues, layered wound repair, everting wound edges, adequate haemostasis and using appropriate suture materials [19].

Scar tissues can be revised by total excision and primary closure but various *flap* techniques should be considered for wide scars. Elliptical excision is the most convenient technique for a mature scar which is present on *Relaxed Skin Tension Lines (RSTL)*s [13]. The ratio of length to width should be 3:1 and ends should have an angle of 30 degrees or less to prevent 'dog ear' formation. Even though the 'dog ear' disappears or fades with time, surgeon should avoid it. Scar excision should be done extramarginally to bring healthy normal skin edges together. If the scar tissue needs more than one operation, serial excisions can be done from midline and interior of the scar tissue to avoid additional scar formation on healthy skin.

Different variations of *flap* techniques are used in scar revision. *Z-plasty* is the most commonly used technique for scar revision. *Z-plasty* is a transposition of two triangular *flap*s that are usually equal in size and angle (Figure 1). *Z-plasty flaps* function to lengthen the scar tissue and are used to break up a straight line to make a scar less noticeable. *Z-plasty* also moves tissues from one area to another and can be used to obliterate or create a web or cleft. Planning and performing *Z-plasty* is carried out according to geometric principles. Limberg did the first mathematical analysis in 1929 [20]. He revealed the theoretical gains in length achievable with changes in the angle of the lateral limbs of the *flap*. An angle of 30° lengthens the scar by 25%, an angle of 45° by 50%, an angle of 60° by 75%, an angle of 75° by 100%, and an angle of 90° by 120% (Table 1) [21]. An angle narrower than 60° makes it easier to transpose the *flap*s but results in less scar lengthening. As angle of the triangles increases, the force required for transposition of the flaps increases, therefore scar tension increases simultaneously.

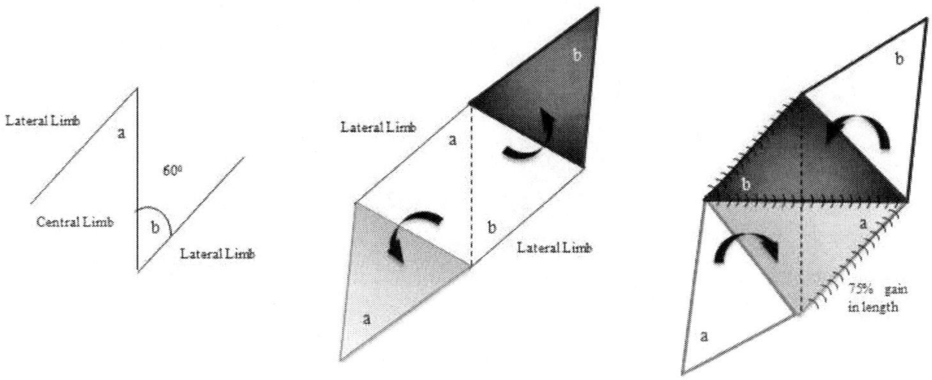

Figure 1. Technique of Simple Z-plasty.

Table 1. Z-plasty gains in length

Angle of Z-plasty (lateral limb) (°)	Theoretical gain in length (central limb) (%)
30	25
45	50
60	75
75	100
90	120

Most of the scar tissues can be corrected with single *Z-plasty* but multiple *Z-plasties* are preferred in large and inelastic scars which will be associated with creation of significant tension at the transverse diagonal after single *Z-plasty*. Multiple *Z-plasties* distribute the tension across various transverse diagonals [22]. It gives similar zigzag lines as the *W-plasty* but there is gain of length in *Z-plasty* (Figure 2). *Z-plasty* can be modified according to the anatomical needs. Double opposing *Z-plasties*, which is a mirror image of the planned Z-plasty, are transposed with interposition of the *flap*s and they are advantageous in areas with limited skin capacity like medial canthal area [23].

Unequal triangles also known as skew *Z-plasty* are useful in areas that lack elasticity and they can be formed by changing the angle of the 'Z' limbs. Half Z-plasty can be used in inelastic areas with an elastic surrounding tissue. An incision is made on inelastic side and a triangular flap from the elastic side is transposed to fill the scar defect.

Limberg's four flap is helpful in releasing scar contractures. Flaps with the angles of 90° are kept at both ends of the 'Z'. Each flap is divided into smaller flaps with 45° angles and transposed (Figure 3).

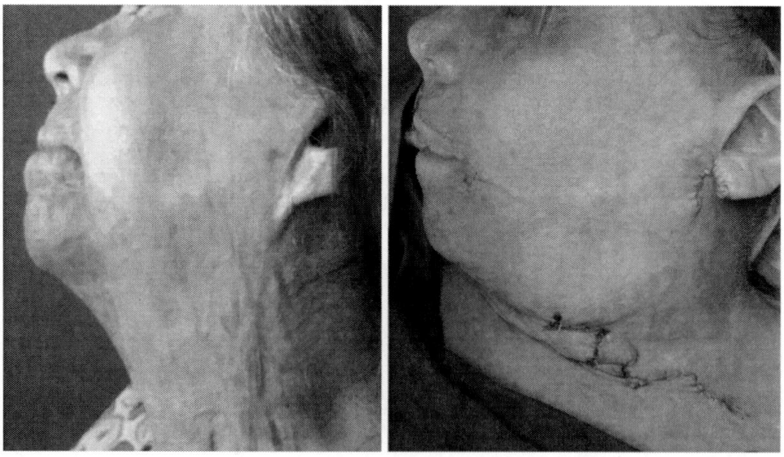

Figure 2. Scar revision patient with single Z-plasties on oral commissure and left ear and multiple Z-plasties on neck region.

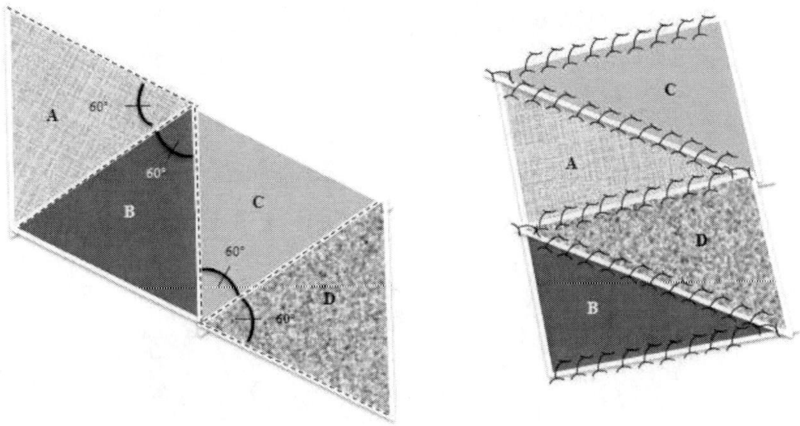

Figure 3. Technique of Limberg's four-flap.

S-plasty is used for areas that are associated with oval defects like ostomy scar tissues. Jumping man procedure is another method that combines *Z-plasty* with *V-Y advancement* methods.

A straight scar with significant length can be distracting and visible. *W-plasty* provides irregular broken line, which conceals the scar tissue. Consecutive triangles are made on one side of the scar with mirror images on the other side (Figure 4). While planning, the apex of the triangles should be placed 5-6 mm apart from each other and 3-5 mm away from the scar. The limbs of the triangles should be 3-5 mm long. If the length is smaller than 3mm it will not break the scar and if it is planned more than 5mm in length it will make the scar more visible. Some scars may require repair of the underlying dermis to decrease the size and for making the scar less prominent (Figure 5). *W-plasty* indications are linear scars measuring longer than 2 cm [13] and being wider than 35° to the *RSTLs*. Closure over curved surfaces, closure of pretrichial areas after browlift or closure after forehead flap and short scars present on cheeks are the other main indications of *W-plasty* [24].

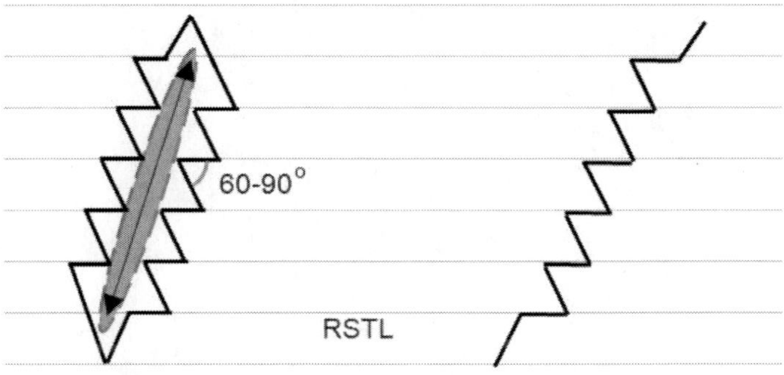

Figure 4. Technique of W-plasty.

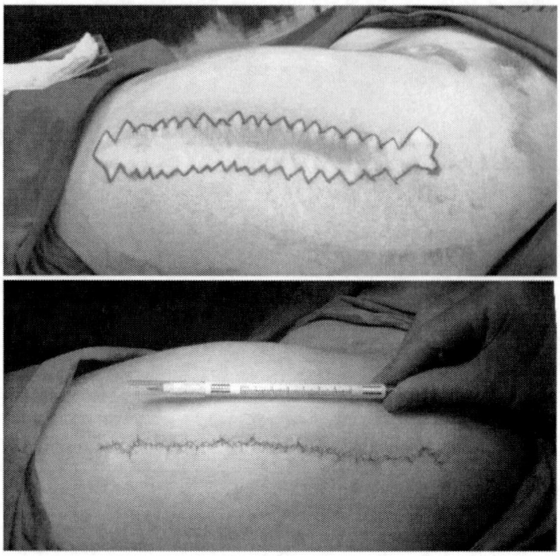

Figure 5. Example of W-plasty performed on a long scar tissue with dermal deficiency and atrophy. Undermining and re-approximation were done to reduce tension on wound edges.

Geometric broken-line closure (GBLC) is a good option for long and irregular scar tissue (Figure 6). *GBLC* is less predictable than *W-plasty* due to its random shape. When performing the surgery, perimeter of the scar should be marked with a distance of 3-6 mm from the border of the scar. Series of irregular geometric designs like squares, triangles, semicircles and rectangles can be drawn with a mirror image on the opposite side of the scar (Figure 7). The angle at the ends of *GBLC* should be less than 30 degrees to avoid dog ear formation and for perfect approximation.

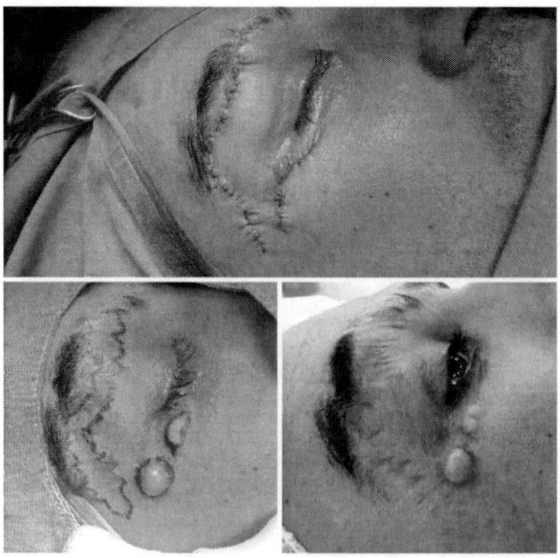

Figure 6. Geometric broken-line closure is a good option for long and irregular scar tissue which will provide good camouflage.

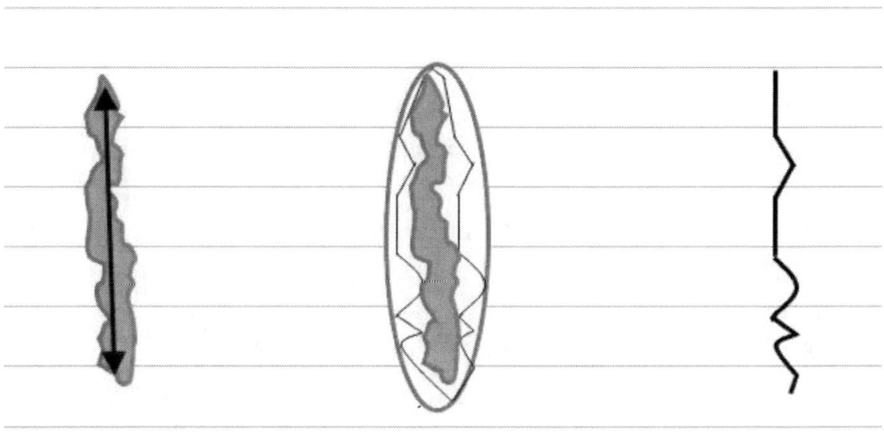

Figure 7. Technique of geometric broken line closure.

Some scars may require reconstruction with advancement flaps. Most commonly used advancement flap is *V-Y advancement* followed by Y-V flap, which is carried out by using similar principles. V-shaped incision is made along the contracted scar along the length of the scar. After wide undermining, flap is pulled in the direction of the base of that flap and the defect is closed side-to-side forming a 'Y' shape when completed (Figure 8).

Various *flaps* or combination of them can be used according to the need of the scar tissue. Large scars may require tissue expansion or skin graft application according to the resulting defect. Scar revision *surgery* can be combined with autologous fat injection which has been shown to be effective in improving the scars and the quality of the overlying tissues via adipose derived stem cells [25].

Scar revision has a tendency of scar widening and hypertrophy so surgeon should be careful when choosing the appropriate suture material. Usage of Steri-Strips© or other wound approximation materials are highly recommended. Careful hemostasis and dead space obliteration are important for preventing hematoma formation which may cause wound infection and wound dehissence.

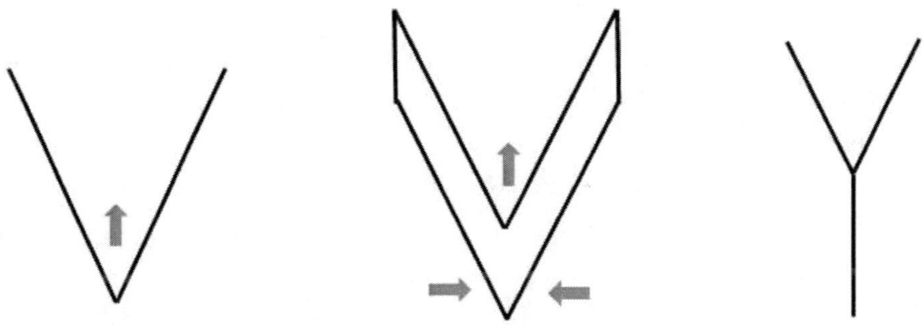

Figure 8. Technique of V-Y advancement.

5.3. Postoperative Care

Scar revision *surgery* requires a close follow up period especially during the first 2 weeks of wound healing [26]. Revision site should be cleaned after 48 hours, which is the optimum time. Cleaning decreases debris of blood clots and eliminates potential zones of infection. Wound should be kept with minimum tension until the sutures are removed. Usage of silicone for scar prevention is important to prevent keloid formation. Patients with scar tissues longer than 5 cm can be treated with Insil© (soft silicone perforated tape) and this will be easier for the patient. Silicone sheets can be used for this purpose but it may require plaster fixation. Some scar revisions may need customized wound dressings for spreading the tension evenly over the wound margins.

Usage of sunscreen is important for preventing hyperpigmentation and early mobilization is effective for preventing scar contracture. Some additional treatments like steroid injections or radiation therapy can be done in accordance with the preference of the surgeon for the prevention of recurrence of keloids.

Conclusion

Scar management may require both surgical and non-surgical techniques for a proper scar healing. Scar revision surgery provides avenues to convert the existing scar into a better-looking scar with an acceptable appearance cosmetically. Scar revision surgery is also applied for increasing the mobility and correcting the range of motion limitations in terms of functionality. Some additional treatments like customized wound dressings, sunscreen, steroid injections or radiation therapy can be performed according to the preference of the surgeon.

References

[1] Atiyeh, Bishara S., and Michel Costagliola, Shady N. Hayek. 2005. "Keloid or Hypertrophic Scar. the controversy: review of the literature." *Annals of Plastic Surgery* 54:676-80.

[2] Reish, Richard G., and Elof Eriksson. 2008. "Scars: a review of emerging and currently available therapies." *Plastic and Reconstructive Surgery* 122:1068-78. doi: 10.1097/PRS.0b013e318185d38f.

[3] Hu, M. S., and E. R. Zeilens, M. T. Longaker, H. P. Lorenz. 2018. "Scar prevention, treatment and revision." In Nelligan Plastic Surgery, edited by Gurtner, G. C., and P. C. Neligan, D. Z. Lui, 196- 213. USA: Elsevier.

[4] Sullivan, T., and J. Smith, J. Kermode, E. McIver, D. J. Courtemanche. 1990. "Rating the burn scar." *The Journal of Burn Care & Rehabilitation* 11:256-60.

[5] Vercelli, Stefano, and Giorgio Ferriero, Francesco Sartorio, Valeria Stissi, Franco Franchignoni. 2009. "How to assess postsurgical scars: a review of outcome measures." Disability and Rehabilitation 31:2055-63. doi: 10.3109/096382 80902874196.

[6] Fisher, A. 1984. Africa Adorned. 304. New York: Harry N. Abrams, Inc.

[7] Scheweinfurth, John M., and Fred Fedok. 2001. "Avoiding pitfalls and unfavorable outcomes in scar revision." Facial Plastic Surgery 17:273-8. Doi: 10.1055/s-2001-18822.

[8] Broughton, George, and Jeffrey E. Janis, Christopher E. Attinger. 2006. "The basic science of wound healing." Plastic and Reconstructive Surgery 117:12-34. Doi: 10.1097/01.prs.0000225430.42531.c2

[9] Lim, Angeline F., and Jennifer Weintraub, Ernest N. Kaplan, Michael Januszyk, Christy Cowley, Peggy McLaughlin, Bill Beasley, Geoffrey C. Gurtner, Michael T. Longaker. 2013. "The embrace device significantly decreases scarring following scar revision surgery in a randomized controlled trial." *Plastic and Reconstructive Surgery* 133:398-405. doi: 10.1097/01.prs.0000436526.64046.d0.

[10] Borges, A. F. 1984. "Relaxed skin tension lines (RSTL) versus other skin lines." *Plastic and Reconstructive Surgery* 73:144-50.

[11] Gillies, H. D., and D. R. Millard. 1957. *The Principles and Art of Plastic Surgery*. Boston: Little, Brown, and Company.

[12] Burget, G. C., and F. J. Menick. 1985. "The subunit principle in nasal reconstruction." *Plastic and Reconstructive Surgery* 76:239-47.

[13] Moran, M. L. 2001. "Scar revision." *Otolaryngology Clinics of North America* 34:767-80.

[14] Sanni, A., and S. Ikponmwosa, D. Golio, K. Therani. 2010. "The use of mitomycin C and keloid scar recurrence." *Plastic and Reconstructive Surgery* 156:682-6.

[15] Rusciani, L., and A. Paradisi, C. Alfano, S. Chiummariello, A. Rusciani. 2006. "Cryotherapy in treatment of keloids." *Journal of Drugs in Dermatology* 5:591-5.

[16] Darzi, M. A., and N. A. Chowdri, S. K. Kaul, M. Khan. 1992. "Evaluation of various methods of treating keloids and hypertrophic scars: A 10-year follow-up study." *British Journal of Plastic Surgery* 45:374-9.

[17] Blumenkranz, M. S., and A. Ophir, A. J. Claflin, A. Hajek. 1982. "Fluorouracil for the treatment of massive periretinal proliferation." *American Journal of Ophtalmology* 94:458-67.

[18] Wendling, Jeanne, and Aime Marchand, Alain Mauviel, Franck Verrecchia. 2003. "5-Fluorouracil blocks transforming growth factor-beta-induced alpha 2 type I collagen gene (COL1A2) expression in human fibroblasts via c-Jun NH2- terminal

kinase/activator protein-1 activation." *Molecular Pharmacology* 64:707-13. Doi: 10.1124/mol.64.3.707.

[19] Watson, Deborah, and Marsha S. Reuther. 2012. "Scar revision techniques-pearls and pitfalls." Facial Plastic Surgery 28:487-91. doi: 10.1055/s-0032-1325642.

[20] Limberg, A. A. 1929. "*Skin plastic with shifting triangle flaps*." In Collection of Scientific works, 862. Leningrad: Traumatological Institute.

[21] Rohrich, R. J., and R. I. Zbar. 1999. "A simplified algorithm for the use of Z-plasty." *Plastic and Reconstructive Surgery* 103:1513-7.

[22] Har-Shai, Yaron, and Micha Amar, Edmond Sabo. 2003. "Intralesional cryotheraphy for enhancing the involution of hypertrophic scars and keloids." Plastic and Reconstructive Surgery 111:1841-52. Doi: 10.1097/01. PRS.0000056868.42679.05.

[23] Hove, Christopher R., and Edwin F. Williams, Bret J. Rodges. 2001. "Z-plasty: A concise review." Facial Plastic Surgery 17:289-94. Doi: 10.1055/s-2001-18828.

[24] Rodgers, Bret J., and Edwin F. Williams, Christopher R. Hove. 2001. "W-plasty and geometric broken line closure." Facial Plastic Surgery 17:239-44. Doi: 10.1055/s-2001-18829

[25] Klinger, M., and M. Marazzi, D. Vigo, M. Torre. 2008. "Fat injection for cases of severe burn outcomes: A new perspective of scar remodeling and reduction." Aesthetic Plastic Surgery 32:465-9. doi: 10.1007/s00266-008-9122-1.

[26] Eyuboglu, Atilla A., and Cagri A. Uysal, Gonca Ozgun, Erhan Coskun, Nilgun Markal Ertas, Mehmet Haberal. 2018. "*The effect of adipose derived stromal vascular fraction on stasis zone in an experimental burn model*." Burns 44: 386-96. doi: 10.1016/j.burns.2017.08.016.

In: Cutaneous Scars: Biology, Clinics and Management ISBN: 978-1-53615-657-7
Editors: Berna Aksoy, Hasan Mete Aksoy et al. © 2019 Nova Science Publishers, Inc.

Chapter 23

SURGICAL TREATMENT OF PROLIFERATIVE SCARS

H. Mete Aksoy*
Department of Plastic, Reconstructive and Aesthetic Surgery,
Faculty of Medicine, Bahcesehir University, Istanbul, Turkey

ABSTRACT

Keloids and hypertrophic scars are challenging disorders to treat and there is so much disagreement on the proper treatment of these proliferative scars. Proliferative scars that do not respond to management via non-surgical methods and that are functionally or aesthetically disabling can be considered for surgical intervention. Surgical treatment of keloids should always be combined with some form of adjuvant therapy as surgical excision alone has been associated with a high recurrence rate. In this chapter, details of surgical management of hypertrophic scars and keloids were covered.

Keywords: 5-fluorouracil, allotransplantation, botulinum toxin, colchicine, corticosteroids, fat transfer, hydrogels, hypertrophic scars, imiquimod, Integra, interferon, keloids, mitomycin C, pressure therapy, radiotherapy, silicone, surgery, tamoxifen, taping, VAC, verapamil

1. INTRODUCTION

Keloids and *hypertrophic scars* are one of the most challenging disorders faced by the surgeon. There is so much disagreement on the proper treatment of these lesions [1].

*Corresponding Author's Email: hasanmeteaksoy@gmail.com.

Wounds can be subjected to tension as a result of motion, body location, or loss of tissue and tension on healing wound is associated with increased risk of scar hypertrophy and spreading [2]. Delayed epithelialization of any wound beyond 10-14 days is also known to increase the incidence of hypertrophic scarring significantly [3]. But *keloids* may be associated with genetic predisposition and they can develop even after minor traumatic injuries [4].

Surgical treatment of proliferative scars requires a careful personalized approach. It is also important that laser and light-based therapies may eliminate the need for scar excision and reconstructive *surgery* in some cases [5].

Surgical excision was one of the earliest forms of treatment of *keloids* and *hypertrophic scars*. In a review study, the cure rate for *surgery* alone ranged from 7-55% in proliferative scars. The major limitation of *surgery* as a sole therapy for proliferative scars is that the recurrence rate is very high. Although the scar mass may be removed, the *surgery* itself causes skin injury in keloid prone patients. To reduce the risk of excessive scar formation, it is imperative to minimize skin tension following wound closure in the operating room. Moreover, careful and meticulous handling of tissues and precise wound edge approximation can help limit pathologic wound healing [6].

Surgical treatment can result in the recurrence of *keloids* and *hypertrophic scars* and recurrent lesions are then often much bigger than the original ones. So, unless the proliferative scar to be treated is a minor hypertrophic scar, the decision to surgically remove an excessive scar should be made very carefully. To reduce the risk of recurrence of these scars, it is also advisable to use special surgical techniques like z-plasties and local flaps in addition to meticulous execution of the surgical procedure [7].

Using fine and atraumatic surgical instruments and intra-cutaneous suture techniques with monofilament suture materials with eversion of wound edges following accurate coaptation of wound layers is of paramount importance for the prophylaxis of scar formation [8]. Intraoperative techniques described as the 5 A's - asepsis, absence of tension, accurate approximation, avoidance of raw surface, and atraumatic tissue handling should be obeyed to when closing wounds [9].

Clinical and experimental findings support the notion that mechanical forces acting on the skin strongly influence the cellular behavior that causes scarring. These observations emphasized the importance of reducing skin tension when *keloids* or hypertrophic are surgically excised to prevent recurrence following *surgery*. Subcutaneous/fascial tensile reduction sutures apply minimal tension on the dermis and are more effective in reducing the risk of recurrence of proliferative scars following surgical treatment than the three-layered sutures used by surgeons for wound closure [10].

Zig-zag sutures like z-plasties are useful for releasing linear scar contractures and tensions. A major advantage of using z-plasty techniques is that segmented scars mature faster than long linear scars. If a proliferative scar crosses over a joint, performing z-plasty significantly reduces the risk of developing pathological scars following operation [7].

2. General Prophylactic Approaches to Minimize the Risk of Postoperative Excessive Scarring

Achieving aesthetic wound closure is based on knowledge of wound healing mechanisms and skin anatomy, as well as appreciation of suture material and wound closure technique. Choosing the proper suture materials and wound closure method ensures optimal healing following *surgery*. Surgical wound closure should directly oppose the tissue layers and this proper coaptation of wound edges serves to minimize new tissue formation within the wound. Atraumatic handling of tissues with fine surgical instruments combined with avoidance of tight-wound closures and excessive tension on wound margins by carefully undermining and loosening the surrounding tissue contribute to a better result [11]. But undermining should not be encouraged in patients with a genetic predisposition for keloid formation [5]. Appropriate surgical wound closure obliterates dead space by approximating the subcutaneous tissues, minimizes scar formation by providing careful epidermal alignment and prevents depressed scars by precise eversion of skin edges. If dead space in a wound following closure is limited with properly opposed wound edges, then new fibrous tissue has limited room for growth. Subcutaneous sutures with, for example, PDS II (polydioxanone) monofilament synthetic absorbable sutures, which provide extended wound support (for up to 6 months) should be employed and they can be combined with absorbable sutures or Steri-stip™ (3M, St Paul, MN, USA) for optimal epidermal wound closure [11].

However, there are other methods which can be used for optimal epidermal wound closure. In a clinical study inframammary skin incisions were sutured with two different synthetic absorbable suture materials; a monofilament suture (monocryl) and a multifilament suture (vicryl-rapide). In this breast reduction scar model development of hypertrophic scar tissue in wounds sutured with monocryl and vicryl-rapide was compared and it was found that the use of monocryl resulted in less conspicuous scars with a reduced tissue reaction and a lower incidence of hypertrophic development. The lower incidence of hypertrophic scarring seen in this breast reduction scar model in wounds sutured with monocryl in comparison with vicryl-rapide is most likely related to the decreased extent of tissue reaction based on the structure of the suture material itself and by the prolonged support, it gives to the coapted wound edges [12]. The use of 2-octyl cyanoacrylate surgical adhesive was similar in terms of scar aspect, closing strength and complication rate when compared to the use of nylon suture in an animal model. The adhesive was found to be at least as safe as the nylon sutures in this study.

Use of the adhesive for skin closure decreases surgical time [13]. There were lower infection and revision rates and a similar hypertrophic scar rate when octyl-2-cyanoacrylate tissue adhesive (Dermabond®) was used instead of Steri-Strips™ in the final stage of unilateral cleft lip repair in a clinical study [14]. So surgical adhesives may also be used for final skin closure without increasing the risk of excessive scarring and time of surgical procedure will be shortened by using this method.

A new modification of the buried vertical mattress suturing technique was developed and this technique was associated with minimal postoperative complications including wound infection, bleeding, dehiscence, and hypertrophic scarring. So this method may be used to decrease scarring following wound closure. The modified buried vertical mattress suturing method uses 4-0 vicryl, 5-0 vicryl, or PDS 4-0 or PDS 5-0 (Ethicon Surgical, Somerville, NJ) suture material and this technique is best performed on body areas where there are uniform tension and thicker skin, like the trunk and proximal extremities. The modified buried vertical mattress suture technique resulted in less hypertrophic scar/keloid formation (2% vs 16%) as well as less wound scar widening (6% vs 24%) compared with conventional bi-layered suturing techniques [15]. This method may be used to decrease scarring following wound closure especially in body areas with thick skin.

3. Mechanism of Action of Surgical Therapy

There are three important mechanisms of action of surgical treatment of proliferative scars:

1- Increased wound tension is a central factor in the development of *hypertrophic scars.* Successful tension-free scar tract removal can be achieved with scar revision s*urgery* employing Z-plasty or W-plasty or similar methods. This can also be achieved by using skin grafts or local skin flaps or other more complex reconstructive techniques like tissue expansion. All these surgical methods lengthen the scar and decrease tension on the healing wound and resulting new scar thus interrupting the vicious circle between tension on the newly formed scar and resulting thickening of this new scar as a result of permanently stimulated collagen production.

2- *Hypertrophic scars* and *keloids* developing as a consequence of delayed wound healing like the healing of deep dermal burns or healing after wound infection or wound dehiscence are transformed by *surgery* into wounds with a shorter healing time by using scar excision and tension-free wound closure (e.g., primary closure, skin grafts or skin flaps).

3- By surgically removing scar tissue a situation corresponding to a fresh healing wound still without excessive fibrosis is achieved, so recurrence of excessive scarring can be prevented by adjuvant therapies like corticosteroid injections and *radiotherapy* [4].

4. Unwanted Effects of Surgical Treatment of Proliferative Scars

The occurrence of wound infections, partial or complete necrosis of skin flaps and partial or total graft loss are associated with delayed wound healing which can result in the development of a possibly even larger scar than the treated scar. If surgical after-treatment does not relieve the increased tension on the scar, which is the most important pathogenic factor for proliferative scar development, a recurrence may occur following surgical treatment [4].

5. Subcutaneous/Fascial Tensile Reduction Sutures

Clinical and experimental research findings support the well-established notion that mechanical forces on the skin strongly influence the cellular behavior that leads to scarring. These observations led researchers to focus on the importance of reducing skin tension when *keloids/hypertrophic scars* are surgically removed to prevent their recurrence. Tension-free closure can just be used to obtain a better scar after wound closure. Clinical studies revealed that subcutaneous/fascial tensile reduction sutures, which provide achievement of minimal tension on the dermis, are more effective in reducing proliferative scar recurrence than three-layered sutures used by surgeons. Ogawa and colleagues use subcutaneous fascial tensile reduction suture technique in their predisposed patient population, where the tension of closure is placed on the layer of deep fascia and superficial fascia. The group uses 2-0 PDS II or 3-0 PDS II sutures for subcutaneous/fascial tensile reduction sutures, and 4-0 or 5-0 PDS II for dermal sutures [10].

The usefulness of subcutaneous/fascial tensile reduction sutures is related to the fact that *keloids* and *hypertrophic scars* originate from the dermis. Dermal buried sutures do not effectively decrease tension on the dermis: to achieve tension reduction, much deeper structures must be assessed, namely, the superficial and deep fascia, and they must be sutured to divert tension from dermal layer of the skin. This type of suturing elevates the wound edges and places minimal tension on the dermis. Wound edges naturally attach to each other by the support of these deeply placed sutures. Only then should dermal and superficial sutures be used to obtain tension free dermal closure. It is very important to realize the fact that dermal sutures on their own cannot reduce the tension placed on the dermis upon wound closure, this concept is very important for the prevention of formation of pathological scars after *surgery* [7].

6. Intralesional or Extralesional Excision

Recurrence of the hypertrophic changes after scar revision *surgery* is not uncommon. It has been claimed that intra-marginal excision method diminishes the chances of recurrent hypertrophic scarring. In a clinical study experience with intra-marginal and extra-marginal excision of *hypertrophic scars* was reviewed. In this study, 50 *hypertrophic scars* were excised in 23 burn patients. Thirty-one (62%) of the excisions were intra-marginal and 19 (38%) excisions were extra-marginal. The results were compared and it was observed that the intra-marginal excisions yielded better results than the extra-marginal excisions [16]. So it may be concluded that intra-marginal excision is superior to extra-marginal excision when treating burn-related *hypertrophic scars.*

Some clinicians recommend that lateral parts of *keloids* should not be excised, but should be joined together and left in situ. However, others objected to this proposal and they consider that the cells located in these lateral parts of the keloid are more active in terms of collagen production [17].

In the case of surgical treatment of mature *keloids*, it is recommended to perform an intra-marginal fusiform excision [5]. Mature *keloids* may contain less active keloid fibroblasts. So intra-scar excision may be performed in mature *keloids.*

In a retrospective study of 75 keloid patients who were treated by using *surgery* and adjuvant therapy, the histopathologic margins of excision materials were studied. Positive margins or incomplete excision correlated with recurrence ($P < 0.001$). Better results were noted with complete excision. All patients received variable adjuvant treatment, which is not accounted for [18]. So for *keloids* in general intra-marginal excision does not seem to be advantageous over extra-marginal excision.

Intra-marginal excision can be useful especially for huge *keloids*, which cannot be closed primarily. However, in the case of *keloids* confined to auricles alone, complete surgical excision with some degree of free surgical margin seems to be reasonable considering the high recurrence rate of *keloids.* This is consistent with the general belief that keloid recurrences generally occur in the surgical margin caused by insufficient lesion excision [19]. Thus large *keloids* can be treated with partial excision to prevent tension on wound closure but small *keloids* should be excised completely.

In another study, the majority of participants chose to operate on *keloids.* The operation was performed by 79 out of 116 (68.1%) participants and operation was not performed by 37 out of 116 (31.9%) participants. Around one-third of participants performed either intra-lesional (20%) or extra-lesional scar excisions (22%); 15% performed both types of excisions and 12% performed unspecified other types of *surgery* [20]. So there is not any common consensus on which type of excision to be used while treating *keloids* among physicians.

In a clinical study performed on 75 patient with intra-marginal excision against extra-marginal excision a significantly lower recurrence rate was observed in completely excised *keloids* in comparison to those that were not completely removed at the edge or the wound base. However, a modification of the intra-marginal excision technique was reported. The skin covering the keloid was lifted as a pedicled flap and then the underlying scar tissue was excised. The previously formed skin flap was used for the closure of keloid excision defect. It was reported that no recurrence was seen in the observation period after keloid removal and that all wounds healed without complications and they were not treated in an adjuvant manner. However, recurrences were observed in four of nine cases (all without adjuvant concomitant therapy) in another study [4].

In conclusion, no final judgment can be made if intra-marginal or extra-marginal excision is to be favored while treating proliferative scars [4].

7. Surgical Treatment of Hypertrophic Scars

Hypertrophic scars become obvious within weeks after healing of cutaneous injury [21]. They rapidly increase in size for 3 to 6 months. Then, after a static phase, they begin to regress [21, 22].

Hypertrophic scars frequently exhibit marked spontaneous regression and mature after about one year [22, 23]. They can show flattening, softening and re-pigmentation along with decreasing contractures even without any physical manipulation [22]. So caution should be exercised when considering surgical treatment of *hypertrophic scars* and expectation of spontaneous regression as a result of scar maturation may render corrective *surgery* for these scars potentially unnecessary [22, 23]. It can be concluded that *surgery* is usually not necessary [22]. However, surgical treatment is indicated for those cases of *hypertrophic scars* that are associated with the formation of scar contractures (especially around joints) with loss of function [3, 21]. Most clinicians recommend surgical treatment of *hypertrophic scars* as first-line treatment when disabling scar contractures are present [5]. *Hypertrophic scars* can impair movement of body parts when they cross joints or they may exert abnormal forces on surrounding tissues creating tension and deformation. Thus, certain hypertrophic burn scars may lead to enough impairment of function (limitation of movement and deformation) to require surgical intervention in a short period of time [24]. So, early *surgery* is always indicated in the case of scar contractures with functional impairment. Surgical release of scar contractures improves the function of affected joints and this release of tension also accelerates the maturation of surrounding *hypertrophic scars* [21]. The most common joints affected by scar contractures following burn injury are the shoulder, elbow, and the knee [24]. *Surgery* may be indicated to release a disabling early stage immature scar in a stable patient with a hypertrophic scar that causes a severe contracture. Because the presence of this contracture impedes proper rehabilitation of the patient in the early periods following burn injury [5]. *Hypertrophic scars* with excessive tension on the wound margins causing joint contractures should be treated surgically in a timely manner to relieve or reduce strain on the scar by using surgical methods like Z-plasty, W-plasty, skin grafts or flaps. This treatment approach becomes particularly important when scar contractures cause significant functional limitations [4, 23].

Surgery may also be performed as a first-line therapy for *hypertrophic scars* caused by delayed wound healing [23]. So, surgical treatment of small, cosmetically distressing *hypertrophic scars* developing as a consequence of disturbed wound healing (prolonged healing and delayed epithelialization) may be recommended [4].

Surgical therapy of *hypertrophic scars* without associated tension (absence of soft tissue deformation and contractures) and without significant cosmetic disfigurement with a scar age of less than one year is generally not recommended [4]. So, experts on this subject recommend scar revision after 12 months of conservative treatment without improvement in the absence of decreased joint mobility from contracture [25]. If the patient has a permanent (>1 year) hypertrophic scar, surgical scar revision may then be considered [17]. In one study *surgery* was the most frequently (85 out of 116/73.3%) used treatment modality among participants (treating clinicians) when there was a history of at least 18 months of hypertrophic scarring [20]. So, after all conservative scar treatment options have failed, scar revision *surgery* can be considered to lengthen, move, or disperse established *hypertrophic scars* [8]. Long-standing or permanent widespread *hypertrophic scars* may also be treated by using surgical therapy [17].

Thus, a hypertrophic scar that does not respond to management via non-surgical methods and that is functionally or aesthetically disabling can be considered for surgical intervention. If primary closure of the defect after excision is not possible or excessive tension is required to close defect then use of local, adjacent, or distant tissue should be considered. Local, regional or distant (free) flaps can be used for tension-free closure of the wound. Difficult reconstructive problems can also be addressed by using tissue expansion, skin grafts, or dermal substitutes [26].

Small and linear *hypertrophic scars* can be treated by surgical treatment directly or nonsurgical multimodal therapy can be used. Ultimately, *hypertrophic scars* unresponsive to nonsurgical treatment modalities can be revised through excision. Aesthetic correction of linear *hypertrophic scars* is usually done by performing a simple resection of the scar and primary closure of the defect with a type of tension-releasing technique such as undermining with approximation of the wound edges, subcutaneous/subfascial sutures, or adding a Z-plasty [17]. So, excision and direct closure can be considered for small *hypertrophic scars* and this procedure is often combined with repositioning of the scar parallel to the lines of minimum skin tension [26]. The use of surgical *taping* or *silicone* gels are strongly advised after wound closure [17]. In the surgical treatment of linear *hypertrophic scars,* a type of tension-releasing technique including Z-plasty, W-plasty, broken line technique or small wave incision technique should be applied to prevent the recurrence of *hypertrophic scars* [21, 27]. If the orientation of the previous incision placed the resulting scar in the line of tension, performing a Z-plasty or W-plasty can transpose the tension vector across the newly created incision [9]. The principle of Z-plasty is based on tissue lengthening and the Z-plasty additionally redirects the scar axes. The principle of V-Y-plasty is also based on tissue lengthening but the V-Y-plasty produces linear lengthening of the scar. Both the broken-line and W-plasty techniques break up straight lines into smaller segments and produce an irregular or zigzag-shaped final scar [8]. These techniques are all discussed in detail in the next chapter. Planimetric elongations are needed for scar corrections on plane skin surfaces [28]. Scar revisions are usually carried out on plane surfaces. So, the planimetric Z-plasty technique can be used to decrease elevations/depressions following scar revision performed on plane skin surfaces [29]. The small wave-incision method can also be used for revision of linear *hypertrophic scars* [30].

In the case of hypertrophic scar-related joint contractures caused by excessive tension on the wound margins, corrective procedures such as Z-plasty or various local flaps can be used [23]. Contracture release after burn injury in areas such as the neck and axilla are best performed with flaps rather than with skin grafts because flaps are usually associated with minimal secondary contraction. Thus, flap reconstruction of defects following contracture release produce excellent functional and aesthetic results [17].

Long standing or permanent widespread *hypertrophic scars* may also be treated surgically. The same techniques used to treat permanent linear *hypertrophic scars* are sometimes used for widespread *hypertrophic scars.* For larger *hypertrophic scars,* serial excision and skin stretching may be used and this procedure involves the advancement of adjacent skin by sufficient undermining after resection of the central part of the hypertrophic scar (Figure 1). Subcutaneous/subfascial sutures are used to relieve the tension from the overlying skin as this procedure involves stretching the skin. Post-burn *hypertrophic scars* can cause severe functional impairment and devastating disfigurement, especially in young patients. Post-burn reconstructive *surgery* is often mandatory to solve problems that are refractory to conservative measures. The armamentarium of post-burn reconstruction comprises free (split thickness and full thickness) skin transplants, cultured keratinocyte grafting, dermal substitute grafting, the use of tissue expanders, and various flap procedures including free flap transfers [5, 31]. All these procedures aim at restoring function and improving aesthetic appearance [31]. These surgical reconstruction procedures should ideally be performed in specialized centers that deal with the treatment of burn complications [17].

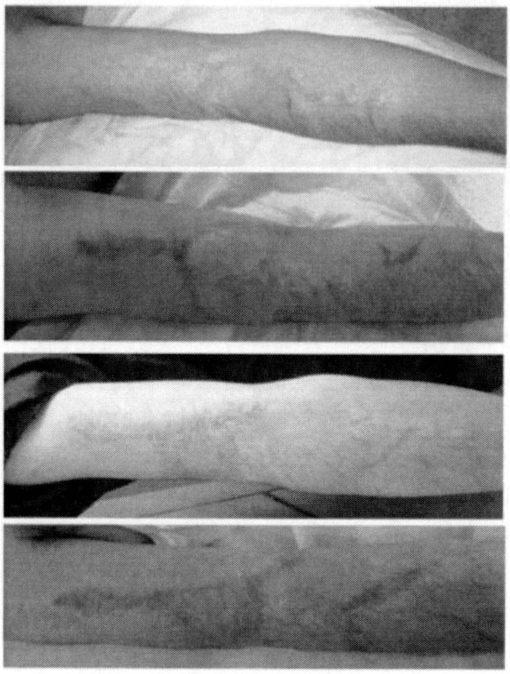

Figure 1. Serial excision and skin stretching for partially regressed hypertrophic burn scars located on the arm (from up to down: before and after 1st session, before and after 3rd session operations).

Surgical skin replacement or resurfacing of unaesthetic widespread *hypertrophic scars* can be performed by using autologous skin grafts. Dermal substitutes like *Integra®* may also be used for skin resurfacing in patients with extensive skin trauma such as those with severe burns. Tissue expansion is a very helpful technique for surgical scar treatment, especially for the treatment of *hypertrophic scars* involving the scalp (Figure 2) [17].

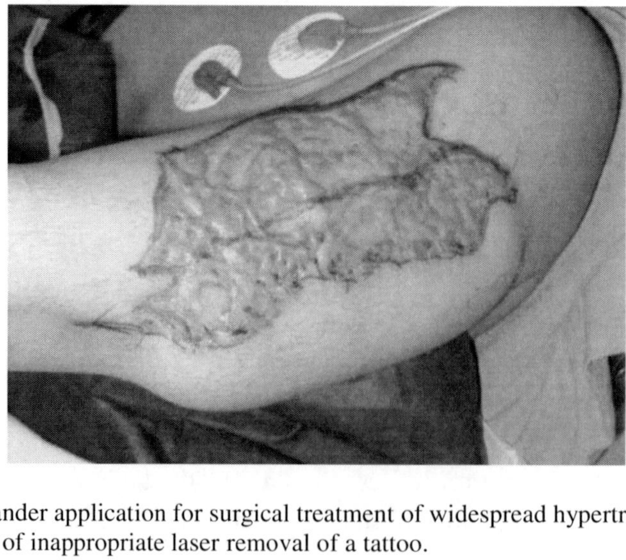

Figure 2. Tissue expander application for surgical treatment of widespread hypertrophic scars that developed as a result of inappropriate laser removal of a tattoo.

With regard to suture materials, it was found that absorbable and nonabsorbable sutures did not differ significantly with regard to recurrence rates in facial hypertrophic scar treatment. However, a similar randomized controlled trial performed on *hypertrophic scars* developing after midline sternotomy incision showed that the use of nonabsorbable sutures diminished the risk of *hypertrophic scars.* So the choice of suture materials depends on the site of usage, with nonabsorbable sutures being more advantageous for high skin tension sites like the anterior chest wall [21].

The combination of *surgery* with adjuvant therapies such as *corticosteroid* injections to avoid recurrence may be used in hypertrophic scar treatment. Intractable recurrent *hypertrophic scars* should be treated according to the keloid treatment algorithm. Thus, the combination of *surgery* and adjuvant therapy should be the treatment of choice for such *hypertrophic scars* [21].

8. Keloid Surgery

A strong tendency for relapse and the presence of genetic predisposition for the development of *keloids* make these lesions the most challenging with regard to scar treatment [8].

Conservative therapeutic options have been currently recommended as the first line treatment for *keloids.* In most cases, surgical therapy of *keloids* is not advised because *surgery* frequently creates an even larger wound than original wound and in light of the pronounced tendency for recurrence, the initial clinical situation may actually be made worse [23]. But surgical intervention remains an indispensable option in the treatment of *keloids*. Primary surgical therapy can be recommended for small based larger *keloids* [4]. So, surgical excision may be used for the removal of narrow base *keloids* but adjuvant measures should be implemented to avoid local recurrence [23]. For all other *keloids,* surgical therapy is recommended only after the failure of conservative therapeutic options [4]. Patients who have failed conservative keloid therapy may complain of a severe impairment of quality of life due to remittent infections or persistent uncomfortable feelings like itchiness or pain. Surgical therapy can be considered after first-line conservative approaches have failed and especially for *keloids* that are therapy-resistant to intralesional corticosteroid injections [8]. If *keloids* do not respond to 12 months of conservative treatment, then surgical excision should be considered [17]. This seems to be a general consensus. But *surgery* can also be used to reduce the size of the lesion or for debulking larger lesions [8, 23]. Surgical treatment of *keloids* has been usually recommended to be used in mature scars to be more effective [5]. Surgical treatment of *keloids* should be avoided in children because of a high risk of recurrence [25].

Surgical therapy can be used to treat *keloids* in two ways: the first one is radically resecting *keloids* and the second one is reducing keloid mass [21]. *Keloids* have been removed by use of a variety of surgical methods ranging from simple core excision with primary closure to complete wide excisions and closure with skin grafts or flaps [9, 32]. If the width of keloid precludes primary wound closure after excision then skin graft or even free flaps must be used to close excision defects without tension. Keloid excisions should be performed with extreme caution and excision should not go beyond the border of the lesion. Keloid excision should be atraumatic *surgery* entirely [8]. For the operative treatment of mature keloid scars, some authors recommend to perform an intra-marginal fusiform excision and this means that lateral parts of *keloids* are not excited and joined together [4, 17]. However, others come against this proposal and they consider that cells located in these lateral parts of the keloid are more active in terms of collagen production and these cells may cause regrowth of keloid after excision [17]. In a study on 75 patients with intra- vs. extra-marginal excision, a significantly lower recurrence rate was seen in completely excised *keloids* in comparison with those not completely removed. So this study favors complete excision of *keloids.* However, a modification of the intra-marginal excision method was reported. The skin above the keloid is lifted as a flap and the underlying scar tissue is excised. The previously formed skin flap is used for closing the defect [4]. There was no recurrence following treatment with this method in that study [4, 33]. However, recurrence was observed in four cases out of nine cases treated with this technique in another study [4]. This excision method was especially successful in resecting *keloids* located in the auricle including earlobe region. In another study, core excision method with skin flaps raised from the surface of the keloid for defect closure and total excision method were compared with regard to recurrence and results showed no statistically significant difference between these two methods of keloid excision. These patients with auricular *keloids* also received postoperative *radiotherapy* and applied self-managed scar stabilization with surgical tape. The overall recurrence rate was 4.8% in this study [34]. No final judgment can be made if intra-marginal or extra-marginal excision is to be favored after reviewing the results of the studies on this subject [4].

As a general rule, closure of the wound following keloid excision should be performed by using sutures with minimal tension and everted wound borders. Z-plasties, W-plasties, and advancement local flaps may indeed be indicated to decrease tension on the closed wound. Sutures are recommended to be applied on several tissue planes to eliminate tension on the healing skin to prevent keloid recurrence. Resorbable sutures are placed into the fascia or subcutaneous tissue (in the form of tensile reduction sutures applied on the deep and superficial fascia) with few or no dermal sutures to prevent foreign body reaction in the dermal layer of the skin. Simple non-absorbable monofilament sutures are usually used for final skin closure. Undermining should not be encouraged during wound closure following keloid excision [5].

Tangential shaving has been described for raised keloidal scars with optimal outcomes [5]. There are also studies on shaving and skin grafting *keloids* with satisfactory results [35].

Radical or complete resection of *keloids* is recommended to be combined with adjuvant therapy because keloid excision alone is associated with a very high rate of recurrence ranging from 45 to 100 percent [4, 17, 21]. Surgical excision alone may even result in enlargement of the keloid [17]. Trauma associated with surgical excision frequently initiates a vicious circle of additional scarring. So resulting scar may be even more marked and more disfiguring than the treated scar [8].

The most important aspect of keloid *surgery* is to reduce wound tension after closure. Tension on healing wound has been widely considered as a dominant factor for keloid development. Small sized *keloids* can be removed surgically and a tension reduction suture can be applied. Postoperative adjuvant therapies such as *radiotherapy* are performed to reduce recurrence risk. A medium-size or large-sized keloid constitutes a considerable challenge for surgeons and transferring tissues from neighboring or distant areas are the options of choice in these circumstances with a risk of keloid development in the donor areas [32].

The skin graft technique is a simple method and has been commonly used instead of direct closure of keloid resection defects [32]. *Keloids* were treated with total excision in combination with the reconstruction of the resulting defect with a full thickness skin graft and intradermal injections of *corticosteroids* at the periphery of both the donor and recipient sites. Ten patients with auricular *keloids* were treated by using this method and during an 11-month follow-up period, no recurrence was observed. So it was concluded that full thickness skin grafts can be used to treat auricular *keloids* without recurrence [36]. However, the skin graft technique has disadvantages in keloid therapy. The early non-vascularized state of the skin graft precluded the immediate use of radiation therapy which is necessary to guarantee the effectiveness of the keloid treatment and this is especially important for *keloids* developing in extracranial locations. Pre-treatment *radiotherapy* was utilized in skin graft *surgery* to circumvent the immediate irradiation issue. With a long-term follow-up, some patients complained of unsightly appearance and poor quality of the irradiated grafted area. Therefore, the flap-based reconstructive approach is recommended to improve the clinical outcomes when *keloids* are treated surgically [32].

Local flaps are useful for treating scar contractures. Local flaps expand naturally after *surgery* and they are not prone to post-surgical contractures. By contrast, skin grafts do not expand and skin grafting tends to generate secondary contractures that result in pathological scars around the grafted skin. Thus, a flap *surgery* is better for keloid treatment. Keloid defect reconstruction with flaps was discouraged in the past because it was thought that *keloids* could develop in the donor site. Such donor site keloid development can be prevented by multimodal therapy such as tension-reduction sutures and radiation therapy. Thus, flap *surgery* is a highly suitable approach especially for severe *keloids* [7].

Surgical treatment of *keloids* has been usually recommended to be combined with complementary conservative therapy strategies like *radiotherapy*, *interferon,* or corticosteroids to avoid recurrence [5]. This approach reduces the risk of keloid recurrence from more than 50% to 8% [5, 9]. However, the risk of keloid recurrence after *surgery* still remains high, even with adjuvant therapies like *radiotherapy* [9, 25]. Recurrence rate is much lower in craniofacial locations and combination therapy yield very good results in the treatment of earlobe *keloids* with 4% recurrence rate after treatment [9, 25, 37]. Interestingly, surgical removal of auricular *keloids* in combination with adjuvant therapy often shows positive long-term results [23]. Postoperative adjuvant treatments are strongly recommended in the surgical therapy of *keloids* and these include *radiotherapy,* intralesional corticosteroids, *silicone*-based therapies, local pressure dressings, *imiquimod* and 5-FU [4, 8, 25]. The combination of surgical keloid therapy with an after-therapy is recommended in principle. The reason for this approach is that due to an underlying genetic predisposition, a recurrence must be expected following surgical removal of *keloids.* But no final judgment can be made on which adjuvant therapy achieves the best results [4].

The treatment options available for cases with huge *keloids* are very limited. However, it has been found that it is possible to treat huge *keloids* successfully by using skin flaps (e.g., perforator flaps and propeller flaps) to release tension on the wound after closure and adjuvant postoperative *radiotherapy* [10].

Non-surgical conservative therapies alone do not seem to be effective for treating large and multiple *keloids.* Careful discussions and goal setting with patients are very important steps in the management of large and multiple *keloids.* Patients with such *keloids* usually have major problems like infections as a result of inclusion cysts and pain. Thus, mass reduction *surgery* and symptomatic multimodal therapy options should be considered on a case-by-case basis [21].

With regard to mass reduction approach, it should be used only to remove infected regions and to reduce enough of the keloid(s) to effect symptomatic improvement. Use of adjuvant therapies after mass reduction *surgery* is not recommended because this may lead to excessive exposure of patients to radiation or the occurrence of the side effects of corticosteroids [21].

A combination therapy approach to the management of *keloids* named 'immuno-surgery' was reported in a clinical study. This immuno-surgery combination therapy included surgical extirpation, reconstruction using artificial dermal replacement by using *Integra®* and split-thickness skin grafting, vacuum-assisted closure *(VAC),* and adjunctive treatment with steroids and *imiquimod.* This combination therapy is based on first; immunologic behavior of *keloids* and methods used to modulate this response; second, recent advances in surgical wound reconstruction by using artificial dermal replacements decreasing the problems associated with scar contracture after grafting; and third; the application of effective wound management techniques such as the *VAC* to promote granulation tissue and immobilize the graft bed. Excellent cosmetic and functional results were reported on the use of *Integra*® dermal grafts to close wounds and the problem of donor site morbidity seen with full thickness skin grafts were not present with this therapeutic approach. *Integra*® was chosen for the post excision reconstruction of keloid patient in this study. The *Integra*® graft was applied to the wound bed following resection of the keloid. *VAC* system (KCI, Inc.) was then placed over *Integra*® graft and maintained at a continuous sub-atmospheric pressure of 125 mmHg. *VAC* was also placed over split-thickness skin grafts used after successful *Integra*® graft take. Results of this study indicate that the management of large recurrent *keloids* is quite difficult and requires a combination of multiple therapeutic modalities. This study concluded that the combination of the use of immunomodulatory agents with surgical therapy performed by using the latest available technology in dermal replacement and *VAC* could yield better control of disfiguring debilitating problem caused by large *keloids.* [38].

Keloid therapy is challenging especially when the defect cannot be closed primarily following resection, necessitating tissue transplantation. A new treatment modality called the sandwich therapy was introduced and used for the treatment of presternal *keloids.* The sandwich therapy consists of pre-*radiotherapy,* superficial circumflex iliac artery perforator (SCIP) flap transplantation, and post-radiotherapy. This procedure also included donor site *radiotherapy* to prevent keloid formation in the donor site area. In this study, 12 patients with presternal *keloids* were treated with this method. All transplanted flaps survived and there was not any complication related to this method. With a mean follow up period of 12 months, only one case with incisional hypertrophic scar development was reported in this study. Main discomfort complaints like pain and itching disappeared in all patients postoperatively. A low-tension or tension-free closure of keloid excision defects was possible with the use of SCIP flap transplantation and peri-operative *radiotherapy* was thought to further lower the risk of keloid recurrence [32].

9. Adjuvant Therapies Used to Reduce Recurrence Following Surgical Treatment of Proliferative Scars

Surgical excision of *keloids* should always be considered in combination with some form of adjuvant therapy because surgical excision alone has been associated with a high recurrence rate of 50-100% and surgical excision may even result in enlargement of the keloid [17].

Thus, surgical treatment of *keloids* has been usually recommended to be used as a part of a combination treatment protocol which contains complementary non-surgical therapies, like *radiotherapy,* or corticosteroid injections, to avoid recurrence. This approach can decrease the risk of recurrence from 50% to as low as 8% [5]. Ear *keloids* seem to respond to combination therapy better than *keloids* located in the other parts of the body.

These adjuvant therapies used following *surgery* are less important in the treatment of *hypertrophic scars*. However, it must not be forgotten that some *hypertrophic scars* are aggressive and may behave like *keloids*. So therapy resistant *hypertrophic scars* should be treated like *keloids* and adjuvant therapy is advised following surgical removal of these scars.

9.1. Radiotherapy

Radiation therapy is another, less common, and less conservative approach for reducing postsurgical recurrence [25, 39]. The combination of proliferative scar resection and immediate postoperative use of *radiotherapy* was proposed many years ago [17]. Corticosteroid injections may be as effective as radiation therapy to prevent recurrence in the surgical treatment of *keloids* limiting the use of radiation therapy for preventing recurrence [4]. Since *keloids* affect relatively young individuals use of *radiotherapy* is a discouraging form of adjuvant therapy. Radiation therapy is generally accepted to be effective as an adjunctive treatment to surgical excisions [9]. Radiation therapy damages proliferating fibroblasts [39]. Both electron beam irradiation and brachytherapy with iridium 192 can be used following surgical removal of *keloids* to reduce recurrence rates [17]. Radiation therapy is usually performed 1 to 3 days after excision of *keloids,* with a total dose of 10 to 15 Gy. The addition of *radiotherapy* to surgical excision reduces recurrence rates of *keloids* to 1% to 35% [39].

In a clinical study, 80 patients who had keloid *surgery* and postoperative radiation were reported. The recurrence rate was reported to be 0% at four weeks, 9% at one year and 16% at 5 years in this study. It was concluded that postoperative radiation was a useful adjunct [18].

The combination of surgical excision with subsequent postoperative *radiotherapy* resulted in freedom from recurrence in 84% after five years with only slight differences between the individual anatomical locations [4].

Appropriate surgical approaches combined with postoperative adjuvant therapies such as *radiotherapy*, and applied self-managed scar stabilization with surgical tape were applied to treat patients with auricular *keloids*. The postoperative *radiotherapy* modalities were 15 Gy administered in three fractions over three days and 10 Gy administered in two fractions over 2 days. The overall recurrence rate was 4.0 percent in 145 patients with 174 auricular *keloids*. Postoperative *radiotherapy* with 10 Gy administered in two fractions over two days was used successfully to treat earlobe *keloids* [37]. So, *radiotherapy* with small doses can be employed to decrease postoperative recurrence of auricular *keloids* successfully.

In a clinical study, 32 *keloids* treated with a combination of *surgery* in the form of extra-marginal excision and postoperative radiation was studied prospectively. A high recurrence rate of 72% at a mean duration of 18 months was found, and this finding contrasts with the previous studies. So, according to the results of this study, it was concluded that postoperative radiation was not useful [4, 18].

Many objections against adjuvant use of *radiotherapy* have been raised and they concern the potential side effects of postoperative *radiotherapy,* especially the potential risk of induction of certain types of malignancy [17]. Although adjunctive radiation therapy seems to reduce recurrence rate following *surgery,* non-discriminate use of radiation is discouraged due to increased risk of cancer with all forms of ionizing radiation [9]. In spite of the fact that radiation therapy carries the risk of carcinogenesis and wound healing problems, those risks seem to be rare [39]. On the basis of an extensive review of the literature on this subject, it has been concluded that the risk of malignancy attributable to keloid radiation therapy is minimal [17]. Reports of cancer cases following irradiation on *keloids* are fortunately rare [9].

9.2. Corticosteroids

Intralesional injection of *corticosteroids* is a mainstay in the treatment and prophylaxis of *hypertrophic scars* and *keloids* [6]. Triamcinolone acetonide inhibits fibroblast growth and promotes collagen degeneration [6, 40]. Triamcinolone acetonide injection into a wound site following keloid excision reduces pro-alpha-1 collagen transcript expression [40].

Important advantages of corticosteroid injections are that it is cost effective and does not require special equipment [40].

Adverse effects of intralesional use of *corticosteroids* include hypopigmentation, dermal atrophy, telangiectasia pain with injection and rarely wound dehiscence (Figure 3) [6, 40]. These complications may occur in approximately half of the patients treated with corticosteroid injections but they frequently resolve without intervention [40].

In one study intralesional injection of *corticosteroids* has been reported to lead to symptomatic improvement in 72% of patients and complete flattening in 64% of lesions [6].

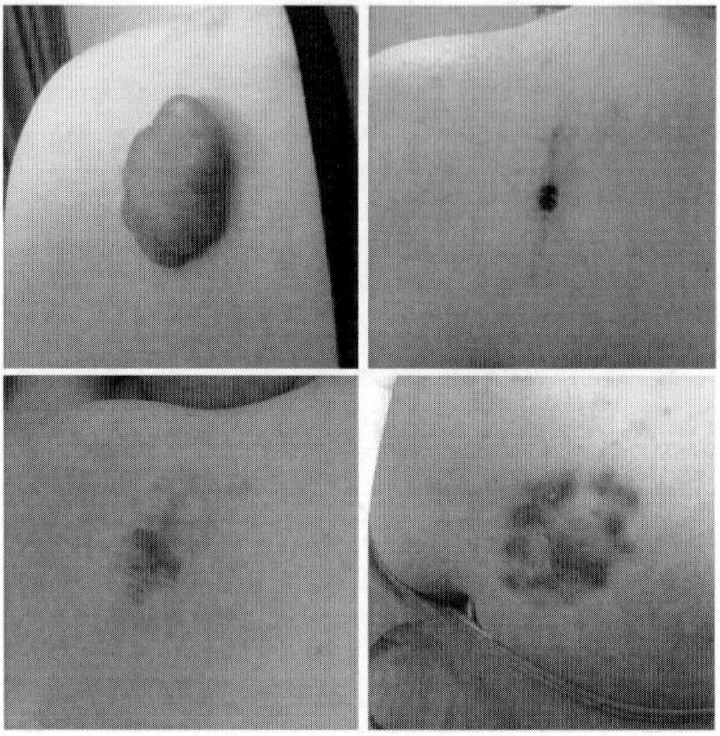

Figure 3. Dermal atrophy, telangiectasia and minor wound dehiscence following surgical treatment of keloid and intraoperative (and then weekly for 2 weeks) application of intralesional corticosteroid injections into wound margins (from top to down and left to right: before, 21st day, 70th day and 8 months after surgery).

Steroids have been tried in different ways for treating *keloids* and *hypertrophic scars.* They have generally been used either alone or in combination with *surgery* with varying results.

There are reports of successful prevention of recurrence by using corticosteroid injections after keloid excision, but the treatment regimens in these studies are highly variable.

The effectiveness of *surgery* combined with intra-operative and serial post-operative local injections of steroids was evaluated in a clinical study. Each proliferative scar lesion was treated by using surgical excision with intra-operative local injection of triamcinolone acetonide, followed by repeat injection of triamcinolone acetonide at weekly intervals for 2-5 weeks depending on the symptomatic relief, and then monthly injections for another 3-6 months. Complete symptomatic relief was obtained in all patients within 5 weeks of *surgery* in this study. No recurrence was noted in 91.9% of patients with *keloids,* and 95.24% of patients with *hypertrophic scars* at a mean follow up of 30.5 months in this study. Local or systemic complications related to corticosteroid use were insignificant in this study [1].

The combination of keloid excision and postoperative intralesional corticosteroid injection (40 mg triamcinolone monthly over at least three months) resulted in no recurrence in twelve patients with earlobe *keloids* with a follow-up period ranging between three and 16 months in a clinical study. So it can be concluded that corticosteroid injections are as effective as radiation therapy to prevent recurrence following the surgical treatment of earlobe *keloids.* However, keloid recurrence was observed in 23% of the patients after using a similar regimen [4].

In another clinical study, the first corticosteroid injection took place after removal of the sutures and then once every 2 weeks after the first injection until it had been done five times. In addition, all post-surgical wounds were treated with self-administered steroid ointment application twice daily for 6 months following suture removal. Postoperative follow-up ranged from 24 to 57 months (median 32 months, mean 32.5 months). Recurrence was observed in three of the 21 keloid cases (14.3%) and one of the six hypertrophic scar cases (16.7%) in this study. Adjuvant corticosteroid therapy in the form of both intradermal injections and topical application were used to prevent recurrence after surgical keloid or hypertrophic scar excision and low recurrence rates were achieved [40]

9.3. 5-Fluorouracil

5-Fluorouracil (5-FU) is an antimetabolite drug that inhibits proliferation of fibroblasts. This agent inhibits fibroblast proliferation by blocking DNA synthesis and transcription via competitive inhibition of thymidylate synthesis. There is strong evidence that 5-FU may be useful in treating *hypertrophic scars* and *keloids* in combination with other treatment modalities including surgical excision or as a sole therapeutic agent. Multiple clinical studies where 5-FU was used as monotherapy have been reported and these studies showed that greater than three-quarters of treated patients experienced a reduction in scar size of at least 50% [6]. It was found that intralesional injection of 5-FU resulted in long-term reduction in scar size. Combination of intralesional triamcinolone, 5-FU, and PDL was evaluated in the treatment of *hypertrophic scars*. It was found that triamcinolone (10mg/mL) injected weekly for 8 weeks significantly improved scar pliability and thickness but the addition of intralesional 5-FU weekly for 8 weeks provided additional benefit in scar height and pliability. A further benefit in scar pliability and thickness was obtained by the addition of 3 PDL treatments [39]. However, 5-FU injections may result in wound ulceration (due to tissue sloughing), hyperpigmentation, and pain, so this form of therapy is generally reserved for the treatment of aggressive *keloids* [6, 39]. Postsurgical adjuvant treatments are recommended following resection of aggressive proliferative scars like *keloids* and they include 5-FU. The evidence for the success of post-excision use of 5-FU is strong [25]. In a clinical study, a total of 94 patients with 102 *keloids* were treated. In this study, 52 *keloids* were treated with intralesional injection of the combination of 5-FU and triamcinolone without excision. In the same study, 24 *keloids* were treated with the combination of 5-FU and triamcinolone with surgical excision and 26 *keloids* were treated with triamcinolone with surgical excision. For patients undergoing excision, drug injections were performed intraoperatively and repeated at 2,4, and 6 weeks postoperatively. Patients who were not operated received drug injections at an average of 4-week intervals. A mixture of 75% 5-FU and 25% triamcinolone was used; 0.1mL of solution per centimeter of the lesion was injected. When steroid adverse effects were observed the corticosteroid concentration was decreased from 40 mg/mL to 10 mg/mL. Follow-up period varied between 6 months to 6 years in this study. Patients treated with combination 5-FU and triamcinolone with surgical excision had a 92% average reduction in lesion size compared with 73% in those patients who were not injected with 5-FU. Patients treated with combination 5-FU and triamcinolone without excision had an average 81% reduction in lesion size. These comparison values were statistically significant in this study displaying the positive effect of the addition of 5-FU to treatment [41].

9.4. Interferon

Interferon therapy, especially *interferon* alfa 2b, has potential therapeutic benefit in the treatment of proliferative scars and this is based on the idea that *interferon* decreases the synthesis of collagen types I and III. In one clinical study, when *interferon* injections used as monotherapy, 75% of patients treated with *interferon* demonstrated a reduction in keloid size. In another study, a recurrence rate of 58% with excision alone was reported and the recurrence rate was 18.7% when *interferon* was added postoperatively. Adverse effects are common with *interferon* treatment and limit the use of this form of proliferative scar treatment. Flu-like symptoms and pain of injection are the most commonly encountered side effects. Although *interferon* therapy is expensive, it still is a viable option in the management of proliferative scars, *keloids* in particular [6].

9.5. Botulinum Toxin A

Botulinum toxin type A (BTA) has classically been used in the rejuvenation of the upper face. A muscle pull is accepted to be the central stimulus to the formation of scar tissue and this idea has led to the application of BTA in the prevention of unpleasant scarring [8]. So, it is possible to reduce wound tension by limiting tissue movement and this is brought about by the help of BTA induced temporary muscle paralysis [42]. It is thought that injections of BTA adjacent to the primary wound margins after closure can eliminate the constant tensile forces leading to cell proliferation and collagen deposition [8].

The first proof came from the use of BTA in the treatment of forehead lacerations. Injection of 15 units of BTA into the facial musculature right next to the site of injury within 24 hours following wound closure resulted in increased wound healing and superior appearance of scars. A regimen that is slightly modified for injection technique and amount of injected units of BTA can usually be applied to reduce scarring 4 to 7 days prior to elective scar revision *surgery* [8]. BTA has also been used postoperatively to improve the appearance of surgical scars [42].

The use of BTA injections can be considered to decrease scar formation at certain localizations that are exposed to mechanical stress and continuous movement such as upper and lower face regions [8]. So, it may be concluded that BTA injections can be used after revision of facial proliferative scars.

Botulinum toxin type A may also regulate the expression of genes related to fibroblast proliferation [42]. It has been studied in the intralesional treatment of established hypertrophic and keloid scars with mixed findings and its efficacy is debatable [8, 42].

9.6. Silicone Gels and Sheets

The studies on excision and *silicone* gel dressings are contradictory. In a Cochrane Database Review, the authors concluded that only weak evidence existed for an advantage of *silicone* gel films in the prevention of HTS and *keloids* after surgical excision [4]. *Silicone* gel is recommended for several months after surgical excision of auricular *keloids* [8].

A clinical study revealed that no significant difference in efficacy existed between *silicone* gel sheets and topical *silicone* gels. While previous studies advised *silicone* gel sheets as first-line therapies in postoperative scar management, similar effects can be expected with topical *silicone* gel [43]. Moreover, topical *silicone* gels are more convenient to use.

9.7. Pressure Therapy

The combination of excision and *pressure therapy* with magnetic buttons was used in more than 1,400 earlobe *keloids* and this combination resulted in a recurrence-free rate of almost 90% after 18 months of follow up. A similar result has been achieved by using an oyster splinter technique [4]. Local pressure dressings using ear clips are recommended for several months after surgical therapy of earlobe *keloids* [8]. Postoperative use of pressure earrings following the removal of auricular *keloids* has positive clinical effects and may be recommended as a preventive measure [23]. However, *keloids* on other parts of the body are not so responsive to *pressure therapy.*

9.8. Imiquimod 5% Cream

Imiquimod is an immune-response modifier and Toll-like receptor (TLR) agonist. This agent was approved for the treatment of genital warts, basal cell carcinoma and actinic keratoses [5]. *Imiquimod* stimulates the production of *interferon* leading to increased collagen breakdown. Some clinical studies reported low recurrence rates of 0-29% following surgical excision of *keloids* and subsequent topical use of *imiquimod* 5% cream. However, other studies reported that *imiquimod* 5% cream was not effective at preventing keloid recurrence with recurrence rates of 89% [17]. Excision and *imiquimod* use was not effective in *keloids* located on the trunk but *imiquimod* 5% cream use after surgical excision of auricular *keloids* seem to be effective.

9.9. Hydrogels

Hydrogels are scaffolds and structurally similar to the extracellular matrix. Dextran-based hydrogel scaffolds were modified and used to promote neovascularization and enhance dermal regeneration during burn wound healing in a murine model. In a clinical study, injection of a porcine gelatin-dextran hydrogel scaffold into the wound margins has been shown to prevent recurrence of earlobe *keloids* following excision [42].

9.10. Mitomycin C

Another adjunct to surgical excision is *mitomycin C.* This drug is an antimetabolite that has been shown to suppress fibroblast proliferation. *Mitomycin C* was used to decrease scarring in a variety of conditions such as esophageal strictures. Clinical studies found that intraoperative topical application of *mitomycin C* (0.4 mg/mL) to the open wound for 3 to 5 minutes after excision of *keloids*, followed by saline irrigation and appropriate wound closure, reduced keloid recurrence rates [39].

9.11. Colchicine

In a randomized study, a total of 27 *keloids* were treated with *surgery* and adjunctive intralesional triamcinolone, and 28 *keloids* were treated with *surgery* and postoperative oral *colchicine*. The improvement was observed in eight (30%) cases in the first group compared to nine (32%) cases in the second group and this represented no difference statistically. Fifty (91%) of the *keloids* were located on the ear in this clinical study [18]. So *colchicine* is not superior to *corticosteroids* but it may be used considering significant potential side effects of steroids.

9.12. Verapamil and Tamoxifen Citrate

In addition to the aforementioned adjuvant treatment modalities, there are other pharmacologic agents that are currently being investigated. These novel therapeutic agents include *verapamil* hydrochloride and *tamoxifen* citrate. When they are used as an adjunct to surgical excision, these agents show promising results; however, further investigation is necessary to determine long-term success rates of these forms of adjuvant therapies [6].

10. Integra and Burn Scar Treatment

Use of artificial dermis *Integra®* (Ethicon ®, Johnson & Johnson Medical, Norderstedt, Germany), a biosynthetic dermal template, is well established in acute burn *surgery*. So, *Integra®* artificial skin is widely used in the treatment of excessive burn injuries [31]. It is also used in reconstructive *surgery* when large soft tissue defects cannot be covered with local or free flaps [44].

The role of *Integra®* in the surgical treatment of postburn scars in a younger population was evaluated in a clinical study. In this study, 17 patients underwent complete excision of *hypertrophic scars* or *keloids* with subsequent implantation of *Integra®* for defect closure. Split-thickness skin graft (STSG) coverage of the *Integra*-derived neodermis was carried out 3 weeks after the first operation. Complications occurred in three patients including minor problems without long-term consequences in 2 patients (seroma formation), and major problems in one patient (hematoma formation). Scar excision and primary *Integra®* implantation were successful in 16 (94%) patients but one patient needed reimplantation in this study. Mean take rate of *Integra®* was 99.7% for all primarily successful patients. Take rate of STSG used to cover *Integra®* derived dermis ranged from 50% to 100% (mean 94%) in this study. Functional and cosmetic long-term results scored 'excellent' in 53%, 'good' in 36%, and 'fair' in 11% in this study. Comparison of pre- and post-operative findings showed a significant functional improvement in all 17 patients and there was a considerable cosmetic improvement in 15 patients in this study [31].

In another clinical study, a 25-year-old patient with an early childhood burn of the trunk and lower extremity was treated with *Integra®* artificial dermal template in combination with the *VAC* (V.A.C., KCI, Texas, U.S.A.) and split-thickness skin grafting. The combination of the artificial dermal substitute with negative pressure therapy resulted in a complete healing of *Integra®* and the skin graft. During the whole treatment, sterile wound conditions were present and time consuming classic dressing changes were not used. Hospital stay was shortened because the patient was discharged from hospital and treated on an outpatient basis by using an ambulant *VAC* device [44].

11. Autologous Fat Transfer

Structural fat grafting has been a substantial advance in achieving improved wound healing and cosmesis. Wound closure can be enhanced by the injection of processed fat around the wound. Fibrosis and scar height is decreased and scar pliability is increased by the use of this technique. To decrease post-burn abnormal scarring, the fat graft is injected into the burn scar every 8-12 weeks and this procedure could be repeated up to four times. These fat graft injections substantially reduce skin hardness as measured with a durometer and decrease scarring as assessed with the POSAS. Adipose-derived stem cells are believed to underlie the beneficial effects of the injected fat graft, with preliminary work suggesting that ECM production by fibroblasts is changed as a consequence of interactions of these cells with adipose-derived stem cells [26].

The emergence of the fat grafting technique has found some applications in the treatment of scars. In an experimental study, it was found that injection of either lipo-aspirate or adipose-derived stem cells into fresh wounds in swine decreased the incidence of hypertrophic scarring. Fat grafting has also been found to make the quality of scar better in cicatricial ectropion, acne scarring, and irradiated surgical scars. The exact mechanism of action of fat grafting on scar tissue is unclear. Fat grafts were used in the filling of depressed scars. The effect of fat grafting on scar tissue is thought to involve more than just a volumetric filling effect of injected fat. Neo-angiogenesis induced by adipose-derived stem cells contained within the injected fat graft is likely to play a role in scar improvement. It was found that fat grafting into irradiated tissue resulted in reduced fibrosis and collagen thickness. Improvement in scar quality after the release of the scar from the underlying tissues and then by lipofilling have been noted. Improvements in burn scar pliability, thickness, and texture have also been shown after fat grafting [39].

12. Composite Tissue Allotransplantation

Composite tissue *allotransplantation* is a discipline of reconstructive plastic *surgery* that makes use of *allotransplantation* of organs and tissues from an appropriate donor to restore deformed or amputated tissue in the recipient. This therapy can potentially be used to treat deforming abnormal scar tissue following severe burns especially when donor sites are not available or insufficient for reconstruction in the patient. Long-term acceptance of the face or limb allotransplants depends on immune tolerance and this makes regulation of the immune response following composite tissue *allotransplantation* a critical issue. So, the modulation of the immune response is necessary for tissue survival and positive functional outcomes following *allotransplantation*. Use of stem-cell therapy or infusion of bone marrow from the donor to increase long-term tolerance is being investigated by researchers to decrease rejection of transplanted tissues. Despite the fact that burn patients may become highly sensitized following use of skin allografts and large blood transfusions, these patients should be considered candidates for composite *allotransplantation* because they can undergo these complex procedures with high success rates. Clinical experience with more than 14 burn patients who received vascularized composite *allotransplantation* for the treatment of deforming burn scars affecting hands and faces has shown good success rates with only one patient showing active rejection [26]. So this advanced form of therapy can be used to treat certain difficult cases of burn scars located on the hands and faces of these patients.

Conclusion

Surgical treatment of proliferative scars necessitates a careful personalized approach because there are alternative less invasive therapeutic options. Using surgery as a sole therapy for proliferative scars is associated with a high recurrence rate. Recurrent lesions are then often much bigger than the original ones. So, the decision to surgically remove a proliferative scar should be made very carefully and proliferative scars that do not respond to non-surgical treatments and that are functionally or aesthetically disabling should be considered for surgical excision. To reduce the risk of recurrence of these scars, it is important to use special surgical techniques like meticulous atraumatic execution of the surgical procedure, intra-marginal/extra-marginal excisions, subcutaneous/fascial tensile reduction sutures, z-plasties and various types of skin flaps. Even techniques like tissue expansion, grafting with artificial dermal substitutes, autologous fat transfer, and composite tissue allotransplantation have been used in the surgical treatment of these scars. Surgical treatment of keloids should always be combined with some form of adjuvant therapy as surgical excision alone has been associated with a high recurrence rate.

REFERENCES

[1] Chowdri, Nisar A., and Mohammad Masarat, Ajaz Mattoo, Mohammad A. Darzi. 1999. "Keloids and hypertrophic scars: results with intraoperative and serial postoperative corticosteroid injection therapy." *The Australian and New Zealand Journal of Surgery* 69:655-9.

[2] Mutalik, S. 2005. "Treatment of keloids and hypertrophic scars." *Indian Journal of Dermatology, Venereology and Leprology* 71:3-8.

[3] Mustoe, Thomas A., and Rodney D. Cooter, Michael H. Gold, F. D. Richard Hobbs, Albert-Adrien Ramelet, Peter G. Shakespeare, Maurizio Stella, Luc Téot, Fiona M. Wood, Ulrich E. Ziegler; International Advisory Panel on Scar Management. 2002. "International clinical recommendations on scar management." *Plastic and Reconstructive Surgery* 110:560-71.

[4] Nast, Alexander, and Sabine Eming, Joachim Fluhr, Klaus Fritz, Gerd Gauglitz, Silvia Hohenleutner, Renato G. Panizzon, Günther Sebastian, Birte Sporbeck, Josef Koller. 2012. "German S2k guidelines for the therapy of pathological scars (hypertrophic scars and keloids)." *Journal der Deutschen Dermatologischen Gesellschaft* 10:747-62. Doi: 10.1111/j.1610-0387.2012.08012.x.

[5] Arno, Anna I., and Gerd G. Gauglitz, Juan P. Barret, and Marc G. Jeschke. 2014. "Up-to-date approach to manage keloids and hypertrophic scars: A useful guide." *Burns* 40:1255–66. doi:10.1016/j.burns.2014.02.011.

[6] Leventhal, Douglas, and Maxwell Furr, David Reiter. 2006. "Treatment of keloids and hypertrophic scars: a meta-analysis and review of the literature." *Archives of Facial Plastic Surgery* 8:362-8. Doi: 10.1001/archfaci.8.6.362.

[7] Ogawa, Rei, and Satoshi Akaishi, Shigehiko Kuribayashi, Tsuguhiro Miyashita. 2016. "Keloids and Hypertrophic Scars Can Now Be Cured Completely: Recent Progress in Our Understanding of the Pathogenesis of Keloids and Hypertrophic Scars and the Most Promising Current Therapeutic Strategy." *Journal of Nippon Medical School* 83:46-53. doi: 10.1272/jnms.83.46.

[8] Heppt, Markus V., and Helmut Breuninger, Markus Reinholz, Gabriele Feller-Heppt, Thomas Ruzicka, Gerd G. Gauglitz. 2015. "Current Strategies in the Treatment of Scars and Keloids." *Facial Plastic Surgery* 31:386-95. doi: 10.1055/s-0035-1563694.

[9] Son, Daegu, and Aram Harijan. 2014. "Overview of Surgical Scar Prevention and Management." *Journal of Korean Medical Sciences* 29:751-7. Doi: 10.3346/jkms.2014.29.6.751.

[10] Ogawa, Rei, and Satoshi Akaishi, Chenyu Huang, Teruyuki Dohi, Masayo Aoki, Yasutaka Omori, Sachiko Koike, Kyoko Kobe, Masataka Akimoto, Hiko Hyakusoku. 2011. "Clinical Applications of Basic Research that Shows Reducing Skin Tension Could Prevent and Treat Abnormal Scarring: The Importance of Fascial Subcutaneous Tensile Reduction Sutures and Flap Surgery for Keloid and Hypertrophic Scar Reconstruction." *Journal of Nippon Medical School* 78:68-76.

[11] Gauglitz, Gerd G. 2013. "Management of keloids and hypertrophic scars: current and emerging options." *Clinical, Cosmetic and Investigational Dermatology* 6:103-14. doi: 10.2147/CCID.S35252.

[12] Niessen, Frank B., and Paul H. Spauwen, Moshe Kon. 1997. "The role of suture material in hypertrophic scar formation: Monocryl vs. Vicryl-rapide." *Annals of Plastic Surgery* 39:254-60.

[13] Freitas-Júnior, R., and R. R. Paulinelli, R. M. Rahal, M. A. Moreira, E. L. Oliveira, K. F. Aiko, M. S. Approbato. 2008. "The use of 2-octyl cyanoacrylate or nylon suture for skin closure produces similar modifications in scar tissue (an animal model)." *Journal of Plastic, Reconstructive & Aesthetic Surgery* 61:990-2. doi: 10.1016/j.bjps.2007.11.052.

[14] Wilson, Andrew D., and Nigel Mercer. 2008. "Dermabond tissue adhesive versus Steri-Strips in unilateral cleft lip repair: an audit of infection and hypertrophic scar rates." *The Cleft Palate - Craniofacial Journal* 45:614-9. doi: 10.1597/07-072.1.

[15] Sadick, Neil S., and Diana L. D'Amelio, Cynthia Weinstein. 1994. "The modified buried vertical mattress suture. A new technique of buried absorbable wound closure associated with excellent cosmesis for wounds under tension." *The Journal of Dermatologic Surgery and Oncology* 20:735-9.

[16] Engrav, L. H., and J. R. Gottlieb, S. P. Millard, M. D. Walkinshaw, D. M. Heimbach, J. A. Marvin. 1988. "A comparison of intramarginal and extramarginal excision of hypertrophic burn scars." *Plastic and Reconstructive Surgery* 81:40-5.

[17] Monstrey, Stan, and Esther Middelkoop, Jan J. Vranckx, Franco Bassetto, Ulrich E. Ziegler, Sylvie Meaume, Luc Téot. 2014. "Updated scar management practical guidelines: non-invasive and invasive measures." *Journal of Plastic, Reconstructive & Aesthetic Surgery* 67:1017-25. doi: 10.1016/j.bjps.2014.04.011.

[18] Pai, Vasudev B., and Ian Cummings. 2011. "Are there any good treatments for keloid scarring after sternotomy?" *Interactive CardioVascular and Thoracic Surgery* 13:415-8.

[19] Park, Tae H., and Ji H. Park, Choong H. Chang. 2014. "Are Auricular Keloids and Persistent Hypertrophic Scars Resectable? The Role of Intrascar Excision." *Annals of Plastic Surgery* 72:369. Doi: 10.1097/SAP.0b013e31827f5131.

[20] Lumenta, David B., and Eva Siepmann, Lars-Peter Kamolz. 2014. "Internet-based survey on current practice for evaluation, prevention, and treatment of scars,

hypertrophic scars, and keloids." *Wound Repair and Regeneration* 22:483-91. doi: 10.1111/wrr.12185.

[21] Ogawa, Rei. 2010. "The Most Current Algorithms for the Treatment and Prevention of Hypertrophic Scars and Keloids." *Plastic and Reconstructive Surgery* 125:557-68. Doi: 10.1097/PRS.0b013e3181c82dd5.

[22] Rabello, Felipe B., and Cleyton D. Souza, Jayme A. Farina Júnior. 2014. "Update on hypertrophic scar treatment." *Clinics (Sao Paulo)* 69:565-73.

[23] Poetschke, Julian, and Gerd G. Gauglitz. 2016. "Current options for the treatment of pathological scarring." *Journal der Deutschen Dermatologischen Gesellschaft* 14:467-77. doi: 10.1111/ddg.13027.

[24] Hudson, Donald A., and Anthony Renshaw. 2006. "An algorithm for the release of burn contractures of the extremities." *Burns* 32:663-8. Doi: 10.1016/j.burns.2006.02.009.

[25] Del Toro, Drew, and Raj Dedhia, Travis T. Tollefson. 2016. "Advances in scar management: prevention and management of hypertrophic scars and keloids." *Current Opinion Otolaryngology & Head and Neck Surgery* 24:322–9. Doi:10.1097/MOO.0000000000000268.

[26] Finnerty, Celeste C., and Marc G. Jeschke, Ludwik K. Branski, Juan P. Barret, Peter Dziewulski, David N. Herndon. 2016. "Hypertrophic scarring: the greatest unmet challenge after burn injury." *The Lancet* 388:1427–36. doi: 10.1016/S0140-6736(16)31406-4.

[27] Baisch, A., and F. Riedel. 2006. "Hyperplastic scars and keloids: part II: Surgical and non-surgical treatment modalities." *HNO* 54:981-92.

[28] Roggendorf E. 1982. "Planimetric elongation of skin by Z-plasty." *Plastic and Reconstructive Surgery* 69:306-16.

[29] Roggendorf E. 1983. "The planimetric Z-plasty." *Plastic and Reconstructive Surgery* 71:834-42.

[30] Huang, Chenyu, and Shimpei Ono, Hiko Hyakusoku, Rei Ogawa. 2012. "Small-wave incision method for linear hypertrophic scar reconstruction: a parallel-group randomized controlled study." *Aesthetic Plastic Surgery* 36:387-95. doi: 10.1007/s00266-011-9821-x.

[31] Stiefel, Dorothea, and Clemens Schiestl, Martin Meuli. 2010. "Integra Artificial Skin for burn scar revision in adolescents and children." *Burns* 36:114-20. doi: 10.1016/j.burns.2009.02.023.

[32] Zeng, Ang, and Kexin Song, Mingzi Zhang, Quancang Men, Youbin Wang, Lin Zhu, Zhifei Liu. 2017. "The "Sandwich Therapy" A Microsurgical Integrated Approach for Presternal Keloid Treatment." *Annals of Plastic Surgery* 79:280-285. Doi: 10.1097/SAP.0000000000000975.

[33] Yang, Jui-Yung, and Shih-Yi Yang. 2012. "Are Auricular Keloids and Persistent Hypertrophic Scars Resectable? The Role of Intrascar Excision." *Annals of Plastic Surgery* 69:637-42. Doi: 10.1097/SAP.0b013e318274d876.

[34] Ogawa, Rei, and Satoshi Akaishi, Teruyuki Dohi, Shigehiko Kuribayashi, Tsuguhiro Miyashita, Hiko Hyakusoku. 2015. "Analysis of the Surgical Treatments of 63 Keloids on the Cartilaginous Part of the Auricle: Effectiveness of the Core Excision Method." *Plastic and Reconstructive Surgery* 135: 868-75. Doi: 10.1097/PRS.0000000000000962.

[35] Moustafa, Mahmoud F., and Abdel F. Abdel-Fattah. 1976. "A reappraisal of shaving and skin grafting for hypertrophic burn scars." *Plastic and Reconstructive Surgery* 57:463-7.

[36] Brown, Nefertiti A., and F. Raymond Ortega. "The role of full-thickness skin grafting and steroid injection in the treatment of auricular keloids." *Annals of Plastic Surgery* 2010. 64:637-8. doi: 10.1097/SAP.0b013e3181dba8aa.

[37] Ogawa, Rei, and Chenyu Huang, Satoshi Akaishi, Teruyuki Dohi, Atsuko Sugimoto, Shigehiko Kuribayashi, Tsuguhiro Miyashita, Hiko Hyakusoku. 2013. "Analysis of Surgical Treatments for Earlobe Keloids: Analysis of 174 Lesions in 145 Patients." *Plastic and Reconstructive Surgery* 132:818e-825e. Doi: 10.1097/PRS.0b013e3182a4c35e.

[38] Chandawarkar, Rajiv Y., and James Piorkowski, Ibrahim Amjad, Peter J. Deckers. 2007. "Combination therapy of a large, recurrent keloid. *Dermatologic Surgery* 33:229-35. Doi: 10.1111/j.1524-4725.2006.33044.x.

[39] Khansa, Ibrahim, and Bridget Harrison, Jeffrey E. Janis. 2016. "Evidence-Based Scar Management: How to Improve Results with Technique and Technology." *Plastic and Reconstructive Surgery* 138:165S-178S. Doi: 10.1097/PRS. 0000000000002647.

[40] Hayashi, Toshihiko, and Hiroshi Furukawa, Akihiko Oyama, Emi Funayama, Akira Saito, Naoki Murao, Yuhei Yamamoto. 2012. "A new uniform protocol of combined corticosteroid injections and ointment application reduces recurrence rates after surgical keloid/hypertrophic scar excision." *Dermatologic Surgery* 38:893-7. doi: 10.1111/j.1524-4725.2012.02345.x.

[41] Davison, Steven P., and Joseph H. Dayan, Mark W. Clemens, Smitha Sonni, Antai Wang, Amy Crane. 2009. "Efficacy of intralesional 5-fluorouracil and triamcinolone in the treatment of keloids." *Aesthetic Surgery Journal* 29:40-6. doi: 10.1016/j.asj.2008.11.006.

[42] Balaraman, Brundha, and Elizabeth R. Geddes, Paul M. Friedman. 2015. "Best Reconstructive Techniques: Improving the Final Scar." *Dermatologic Surgery* 41:S265–S275. Doi: 10.1097/DSS.0000000000000496.

[43] Kim, Sue-Min, and Jung-Sik Choi, Jung-Ho Lee, Young-Jin Kim, Young-Joon Jun. 2014. "Prevention of Postsurgical Scars: Comparsion of Efficacy and Convenience

between Silicone Gel Sheet and Topical Silicone Gel." *Journal of Korean Medical Science* 29:S249-253. Doi: 10.3346/ jkms.2014.29.S3.S249.

[44] Leffler, M., and R. E. Horch, A. Dragu, A. D. Bach. 2010. "The use of the artificial dermis (Integra) in combination with vacuum assisted closure for reconstruction of an extensive burn scar--a case report." *Journal of Plastic, Reconstructive & Aesthetic Surgery* 63:e32-5. doi: 10.1016/j.bjps.2009.05.022.

In: Cutaneous Scars: Biology, Clinics and Management ISBN: 978-1-53615-657-7
Editors: Berna Aksoy, Hasan Mete Aksoy et al. © 2019 Nova Science Publishers, Inc.

Chapter 24

LASER THERAPY OF CUTANEOUS SCARS

G. Isil Kurmus* and Erol Koc
Department of Dermatology and Cosmetology,
Medical Park Ankara Hospital, Ankara, Turkey

ABSTRACT

Surgery, trauma, burns, acne or other inflammatory conditions of the skin can result in multiple types of scars, including keloid, hypertrophic, and atrophic. Previously, several different treatment strategies were used to reduce scarring and showed varying degrees of success for each scar type. The advancement in laser treatment has helped to reduce scarring of all types. The most commonly used non-ablative laser modality for red, hyperemic, hypertrophic scars and keloids has been the pulsed dye laser (PDL) at a wavelenght of 585 – 595 nm. On the other hand, ablative lasers, with carbon dioxide (CO_2) and erbium:YAG (Er:YAG), were first developed for resurfacing the skin. Both of them are most effective for acne scars. Treatment of pathologic scars benefits physical and emotional health. This chapter will provide information on the types of cutaneous scars and the optimal treatments available using laser therapy.

Keywords: acne scars, atrophic scars, hypertrophic scars, keloids, laser, light-based therapies

1. INTRODUCTION

Cutaneous scars resulting from surgery, trauma, burns, and acne generally disrupt emotional and physical health. These skin conditions affect millions of people among

*Corresponding Author's Email: isilkurmus@gmail.com.

different populations and the level of scarring is determined by the wound healing process. There is a complex interaction between neutrophils, macrophages, fibroblasts, growth factors, cytokines, and components of the extracellular matrix during this process [1]. Pathological scars result from a deviation in the orderly pattern of wound healing. The abnormal scar formations pose both cosmetic and physical implications: pruritus, pain, disfigurement, or functional impairment. Currently, there are multiple strategies that include non-invasive and invasive treatments for scarring. In the last decade, there has been an increase in laser therapy for scar reduction or treatment. In this chapter, types of primary cutaneous scars and the vast number of laser therapies for treatment will be discussed.

2. Types of Primary Cutaneous Scars

Hypertrophic Scars and Keloids

Hypertrophic scars are generally elevated, erythematous, firm and are charactarized by an increased type III collagen expression with a parallel orientation to the epidermis [2]. These scars occur as a result of an overabundance of collagen production, persistent fibrosis and inflammation. The growth of these abnormal scars is based on the original wound and their growth is bordered by the size of the scar margins. By definition, they represent a diffuse redness caused by capillary vessel proliferation and chronic inflammation. These scars usually develop after a month following initial injury and reduce in size over time. These scars are classified into two different types as linear hypertrophic and widespread *hypertrophic scars.* They can cause pruritus or dysesthesia [1-3].

Keloids are sharply elevated, irregularly shaped, reddish-purple, papules or nodular scars and are associated with ethnic/genetic determinants. They most frequently occur in higher Fitzpatrick skin phototypes. *Keloids* expand or invade beyond the original wound boundary and often grow in large volumes because of excess collagen type I deposition in the dermis [2, 4]. Unlike the *hypertrophic scars*, they can manifest themselves months after the initial injury or arise spontaneously without any history of trauma [1]. *Keloids* are classified into two different types: minor and major. Minor *keloids* can appear up to 1 year after initial trauma and do not regress with time. They are elevated, pruritic scars extending towards normal tissue. Major *keloids* are big and raised (0.5 cm) abnormal scars that cause pain. These scars may enlarge over many years [3].

Both scarring types typically have a functional, aesthetic, and psychosocial impact. The most important and difficult objective in scar formation is prevention. Both scars are difficult to treat and recurrences are common following conventional treatments such as surgical excision, topical imiquimod, compression, cryotherapy, radiation, silicon sheeting, intralesional or topical corticosteroids, other intralesional therapies including 5-fluorouracil (5-FU), bleomycin, interferon, and *laser* or *light-based therapies. Laser* and *light-based therapies* have been divided into three categories: ablative and non-ablative lasers and non-coherent light sources [4, 5].

Atrophic and Acne Scars

Atrophic scars are skin depressions caused by an absence of dermal collagen/elastin following inflammatory skin diseases such as cystic acne or varicella [1,3,6]. They can also develop following surgeries or skin traumas. The prolonged inflammation leads to collagen destruction with dermal atrophy. They are initially erythematous and later become hypopigmented and fibrotic [6].

Acne vulgaris commonly effects the majority of adolescents and young adults. The development of *acne scars* causes issues with self esteem, social interactions, and patient's psychology. However, *acne scars* pose important treatment challenges for clinicians. *Atrophic acne scars* are classified according to the 3-dimensional scar architecture into three general types as icepick, rolling, and boxcar scars [6, 7]. Icepick scars are narrow, v-shaped epithelial tracts with borders that extend deep into the dermis and sometimes into the subcutaneous tissue. Wider than icepick scars, boxcar scars have edges that descend vertically and are classified as shallow and deep. Lastly, rolling scars are also wide and undulating and develop due to dermal tethering to subcutaneous tissue [7].

Over the years, attempts have been made to improve acne scarring with several treatment strategies including subcision, punch grafting, and punch excision, as well as tissue augmentation with autologous fat transfer, dermal filler injection, dermabrasion, and chemical peels [6]. In addition to these treatments, ablative, non-ablative, and fractional laser therapies have continuously evolved to reduce/prevent scarring. *Laser* treatment options for *atrophic acne scars* have focused on the stimulation of fibroblasts to replace destroyed components including collagen and elastin [6, 7].

3. Laser Therapy of Hypertrophic Scars and Keloids

Laser therapy is one of the most beneficial treatment options for *hypertrophic scars* and *keloids*. Dermatological *laser* treatment has been used to create photothermal effects, which are generated by heat production and direct energy transfer to specific target chromophores in the skin, while minimizing damage to surrounding tissue. This is accomplished through thermal relaxation, which refers to the time necessary for cooling of a given light-absorption in the skin [3]. Many different *lasers* have been used for the treatment of *hypertrophic scars* and *keloids* including CO_2 and Er:YAG ablative *lasers,* fractional ablative and non-ablative lasers, and non-ablative lasers like PDL *lasers.* Presently, PDL (585-595 nm) has been most widely used for the treatment of *hypertrophic scars* and *keloids*, respectively [3, 4].

The first *lasers* used for treating *hypertrophic scars* and *keloids* were continuous wave argon, CO_2, and neodymium:yttrium-aluminum-garnet 1064 (Nd:YAG) *lasers.* The Nd:YAG *laser* reduces/blocks the production of collagen through direct photobiologic effects and generates an infarction of the tissue. However, early results were inconsistent and scar recurrence as well as other side effects including pain, atrophy, and dyspigmentation were common with a response rate between 36% and 47% [3]. Similarly, scars that were removed by using a continuous-wave CO_2 *laser* reappeared within 1 year and often between 6 and 12 months following treatment [8, 9].

Later, the 585 nm PDL was shown to be effective in treating vascular lesions including port-wine stains and telangiectasias. Based on this, Alster and Williams (1994) reported the first study showing PDL treatment of *hypertrophic scars* and *keloids* located on median sternotomy scars. Results from this study demonstrated a 57-83% clinical/textural improvement following one to two PDL treatments [3]. *Keloids* and very thick or proliferative *hypertrophic scars* may require additional *laser* treatments or the simultaneous use of intralesional corticosteroid or 5-fluorouracil injections to enhance clinical results.

To date, no consensus on mechanism of action has been described how PDL delineates its clinical effects. Epidermal melanin absorption may be a concern in patients with darker skin. The PDL is based on the concept of selective photothermolysis [9-11].

PDL therapy is routinely done as an outpatient service with no need for anesthesia. If local anesthesia is needed, then a cream or gel with lidocaine can be given 30 minutes prior the procedure. It should be noted that the skin must be clean and flammable reagents must be avoided during the preparation. Wet gauze can be used to protect hairy regions from the laser and prevent unnecessary thermal injury. In addition, eyewear must be worn to protect against retinal damage [1].

Fluences are selected based on the patient's skin phototype, scar type, and history of treatments to target area. In general the *laser* parameters for *hypertrophic scars* and *keloids* consist of non-overlapping laser pulses ranging from 6.0 to 7.5 J/cm^2 (5 or 7-mm spot) or 4.5 – 5.5 J/cm^2 (10-mm spot), which should be applied over the entire surface of the scar [12, 13]. Pulse durations that range from 0.45 to 1.5 milliseconds are recommended [14] and low energy densities should be initiated for follow up visits if postoperative oozing, crusting, or vesiculation are observed [1]. Energy densities should be decreased by at least 0.5 J/cm^2 in patients with darker skin phototypes and for scars in more sensitive or thin skin body sites such as the chest or neck [12, 14]. Intralesional corticosteroids or 5-fluorouracil can provide benefit when scar proliferation continues [15, 16]. Intralesional corticosteroid (20mg/mL triamcinolone) injections are better tolerated immediately after PDL treatment when the scar becomes edematous due to the *laser* treatment [1]. The 585 nm PDL has been shown to be effective, not only in the treatment, but also in the prevention of *hypertrophic scars* [17].

PDL treatment can have some side effects including edema, cutaneous purpura, and transient hyperpigmentation/hypopigmentation, which typically resolves within a period between 48 hours to more than several weeks [1].

A topical ointment and bandage for healing can be used to protect the skin following the *laser* procedure. The lasered region can be daily wiped with a mild soap and water. Sun exposure should be avoided to prevent pigment variation. If hyperpigmentation occurs treatment should be discontinued to allow for normal resolution of the pigment. During this time, topical bleaching creams including hydroquinone, azelaic acid, tretinoin, or kojic acid can aid in acceleration of pigment resolution. Treatments are typically performed at 6-8 week intervals to allow for sufficient healing time [1].

The use of other non-ablative *lasers,* such as Nd:YAG laser, can cosmetically improve these scars. Nd:YAG may offer advantages over PDL in the treatment of thicker or proliferative *hypertrophic scars* and *keloids* since it has a deeper skin penetration capability compared to PDL [4]. Koike et al. treated *hypertrophic scars* and *keloids* with 1064 nm Nd:YAG *laser* 3-4 times weekly for 52 weeks, using *laser* pulses ranging from 65 to 75 J/cm^2 (5 mm spot) and significant improvement was observed after one year [18].

Cho and colleagues lowered the fluence of the 1064 nm q-switched Nd:YAG *laser* and used it for 5-6 passes at 1-2 weekly intervals and found a significant improvement in pigmentation, vascularity, and scar pliability and height at 3 months post procedure [19].

The most routinely used fractional ablative *lasers* are the Er: YAG and CO_2 *lasers* (Figure 1). In 1984, Henderson and colleauges first demonstrated the use of continuous wave argon and CO_2 *lasers* for *keloids* [20]. Nicoletti et al. demonstrated that the high energy CO_2 *laser* can reduce keloid scars but recurrence was an issue and may be due to the incomplete removal of fibroblasts. [21]. CO_2 *laser* therapy combined with other therapies including intralesional corticosteroid, interferon alfa 2b injections, or occlusive agents may help reduce recurrences [4].

4. Laser Therapy of Atrophic and Acne Scars

Atrophic scarring, which is caused by cystic acne, varicella, trauma, or surgery, is a very difficult problem to treat. *Acne scars* can create disfiguring facial indentations. To date, *acne scar* treatments make a spectrum from dermal fillers, chemical peels, microdermabrasion, subcision, punch excision to *laser* resurfacing and the recommended treatment strategy must consider the patient's skin and scar type [22].

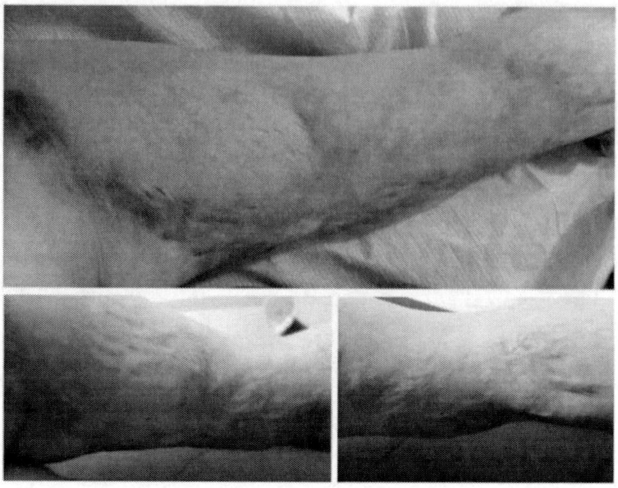

Figure 1. Atrophic and hypertrophic burn scars before (top) and following 4 sessions (bottom) of combined fractional CO_2 laser and fractional microneedle radiofrequency.

The ablative CO2 and Er:YAG resurfacing *lasers* are short-pulsed, high-powered lasers and they offer reproducible tissue vaporization via selective ablation of water-containing tissues. Pulsed Er:YAG *lasers* at a 2,940 nm wavelength are more selective for water than their CO_2 counterparts at 10,600 nm and hence this laser minimizes thermal damage [22, 23]. The photothermal effect of these ablative *lasers* on the skin lead to shrinkage of collagen, neocollagenesis and collagen remodelling [24]. Collagen remodelling and scar improvement may proceed till 12-18 months following the procedure [8, 25].

The CO_2 *laser* is typically used at 250 to 350 mj fluence and 60 watts for a single pass removal of the epidermis, whereas the short-pulsed Er:YAG *laser* requires 2-3 passes using a 5 mm spot size at 5-15 j/cm^2. Long-pulsed Er:YAG systems can be operated at higher fluences (22.5 j/cm^2) to achieve comparable results with a single pass [1, 3, 8]. The Er:YAG *laser* has an average depth and zone of thermal necrosis of 2-5 μm per J/cm^2 and 10-15 μm, respectively [26-27]. Pintpoint bleeding appears after several passes with dermal penetration and limited coagulative necrosis. The vaporized skin appears erythematous and edematous immediately after *laser* treatment with generalized worsening of the skin's apperance within 24-48 hours. Re-epithelialization generally occurs 4-7 days after Er:YAG *laser* and 7-10 days after CO_2 *laser* resurfacing. Therefore, the first 7 days is crucial and strict observation is paramount to obtain optimal outcomes. Short-term complications including transient erythema, pruritus, milia formation, and acneiform pustules can occur. Transient hyperpigmentation which appears 3 to 4 weeks after treatment is often seen in darker skin types. Although hyperpigmentation is relatively common, hypopigmentation is rarely observed [28]. The fractional CO_2 *laser* is most effective for the treatment of mild or moderate *acne scars* (Figure 2) and the Er:YAG *laser* is better tolerated and has less down-time. It should be noted that different scar types may respond differently to *laser* resurfacing. Elevated scars and shallow boxcar scars improve the most with *laser* resurfacing.

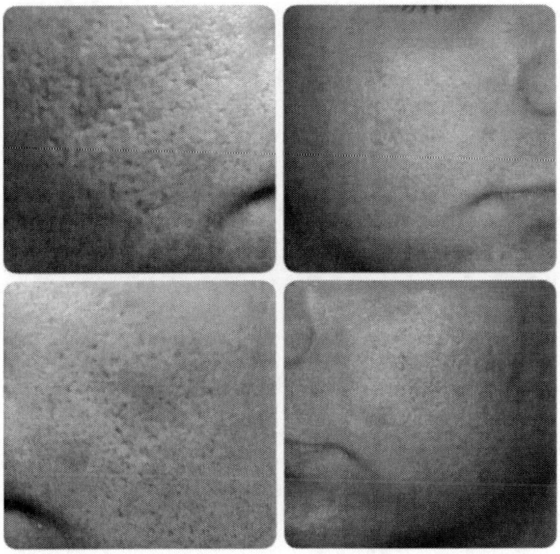

Figure 2. Pre- (left hand side) and post- (right hand side) treatment photographs of atrophic acne scars with 6 sessions of fractional CO_2 laser.

The combination *laser* approach of CO_2/Er:YAG can deliver the Er:YAG ablation wavelength and a deeper-penetrating sub-ablative thermal pulse of CO_2, simultaneously. Studies have shown that the combined approach minimized postoperative crusting, swelling, and itching compared the conventional CO_2 *laser* resurfacing [29, 30]. Others have shown similar results with similar added postoperative benefits [31, 32].

Recently, non-ablative *laser* therapy has been used for scarring and aging skin reduction. Non-ablative therapy reduces posttreatment care, giving patients the ability to resume normal daily activities. Non-ablative *lasers* cause thermal injury to the papillary/reticular dermis, while preserving the epidermis. The non-ablative *lasers* commonly used for acne scars are mid-infrared *lasers* that include 1064 q-switched Nd:YAG, 1320 nm Nd:YAG, 1450 nm diode, and 1540 nm erbium:glass *lasers* [25]. Most widely used nonablative *lasers* are the Nd:YAG and the 1450 nm diode *laser* for the treatment of facial *atrophic scars*. Interestinlgy, however, clinical improvement using non-ablative *lasers* is less than the ablative *lasers*. On the other hand, the adverse effects of non-ablative *lasers* are typically mild. Blistering, crusting, scarring, and post-inflammatory hyperpigmentation are rarely seen and present most commonly in darker skin types [3].

In a comparative study, the 1450 nm diode *laser* was better for the treatment of atrophic facial scarring (mild to moderate) compared to the 1320 nm Nd:YAG *laser*. However, scar improvement was determined to be between 25% and 50% at a 6 month follow up for both *lasers* [33]. It was noted in this study as well as in other reports that scarring type rather than scarring extent may be the best predictor of response rate to *laser* therapy [34, 35].

Bernstein and colleagues found a mild to moderate improvement of *acne scars* following three sessions of a pulse/frequency-doubled Nd:YAG (532 nm) *laser* treatment [36].

Conclusion

In summary, laser therapy is effective for the reduction/prevention of all types of scars. Currently, there are no treatments available for full scar resolution. For this reason, both the patient skin type and scar level must be evaluated before a decision on optimal treatment is made. Even thought laser therapy is recommended for scarring, more studies are still necessary to determine the efficacy, safety, and recurrence rates for all laser treatment modalities.

References

[1] Alster, Tina, and Larissa Zaulyanov. 2007. "Laser scar revision: a review." *Dermatologic Surgery* 33:131-40. DOI: 10.1111/j.1524-4725.2006.33030.x.

[2] Brewin, M. P., and T. S. Lister. 2014. "Prevention or treatment of hypertrophic burn scarring: a review of when and how to treat with the pulsed dye laser." *Burns* 40:797-804. doi: 10.1016/j.burns.2013.12.017.

[3] Khatri, Khalil A., and Danielle L. Mahoney, Melisa J. McCartney. 2011. "Laser scar revision: A review." *Journal of Cosmetic and Laser Therapy* 13:54-62. doi: 10.3109/14764172.2011.564625.

[4] Forbat, E., and F. R. Ali, F. Al-Niaimi. 2017. "Treatment of keloid scars using light-, laser- and energy-based devices: a contemporary review of the literature." *Lasers in Medical Science* 32:2145-54. doi: 10.1007/s10103-017-2332-5.

[5] Mamalis, A. D., and H. Lev-Tov, D. H. Nguyen, J. R. Jagdeo. 2014. "Laser and light-based treatment of Keloids-a review." *Journal of the European Academy of Dermatology and Venereology* 28:689-99. doi: 10.1111/jdv.12253.

[6] Sobanko, Joseph F., and Tina S. Alster. 2012. "Management of acne scarring, part I: a comparative review of laser surgical approaches." *American Journal of Clinical Dermatology* 13:319-30. doi: 10.2165/11598910-000000000-00000.

[7] Cohen, Brandon E., and Jeremy A. Brauer, Roy G. Geronemus. 2016. "Acne scarring: A review of available therapeutic lasers." *Lasers in Surgery and Medicine* 48:95-115. doi: 10.1002/lsm.22410.

[8] Nouri, K., and T. S. Alster, C. J. Ballard, V. Vejjabhinanta. 2008. 'Laser revision 2. of scars.' *eMedicine Dermatology* Accessed 2009 December 22. http://emedicine.medscape. com/article/1120673-overview.

[9] Nouri, Keyvan, and Kelley Vidulich, Maria P. Rivas. 2006. "Lasers for scars: a review." *Journal of Cosmetic Dermatology* 5:14-22. doi: 10.1111/j.1473-2165.2006.00217.x.

[10] Alster, T. S. 1994. "Improvement of erythematous and hypertrophic scars by 585-nm flashlamp-pumped pulsed dye laser." *Annals of Plastic Surgery* 32:186-90.

[11] Oliaei, Sepehr, and John S. Nelson, Richard Fitzpatrick, Brian J. Wong. 2012. "Laser treatment of scars." *Facial Plastic Surgery* 28:518-24. doi: 10.1055/s-0032-1325646.

[12] Alster, T. S. 2000. *Laser treatment of scars and striae*. 89–107. Philadelphia: Lippincott Raven.

[13] Kauver, A. N. B, and G. J. Hruza. 2005. *Principles and practices in cutaneous laser surgery*. 12-29. Boca Raton, FL: Taylor and Francis Group.

[14] Macedo, Otavio, and Tina S. Alster. 2000. "Laser treatment of darker skin tones: a practical approach." *Dermatologic Therapy* 13:114–26.

[15] Alster, Tina S. 2002. "Laser scar revision: comparison of pulsed dye laser with and without intralesional corticosteroids." *Dermatologic Surgery* 29:25–9.

[16] Manuskiatti, Woraphong, and Richard E. Fitzpatrick. 2002. "Treatment response of keloidal and hypertrophic sternotomy scars: comparison among intralesional corticosteroid, 5-fluorouracil, and 585-nm flashlamppumped pulsed-dye laser treatments." *Archives of Dermatology* 138:1149–55.

[17] Bouzari, Navid, and Stephan C. Davis, Keyvan Nouri. 2007. "Laser treatment of keloids and hypertrophic scars." *International Journal of Dermatology* 46:80-8. doi: 10.1111/j.1365-4632.2007.03104.x.

[18] Koike, Sachiko, and Satoshi Akaishi, Yuki Nagashima, Teruyuki Dohi, Hiko Hyakusoku, Rei Ogawa. 2014. "Nd:YAG laser treatment for keloids and hypertrophic scars: an analysis of 102 cases." *Plastic and Reconstructive Surgery. Global Open* 2: 272. doi: 10.1097/GOX.0000000000000231.

[19] Cho, S. B., and J. H. Lee, S. H. Lee, S. J. Lee, D. Bang, S. H. Oh. 2010. "Efficacy and safety of 1064-nm Q-switched Nd:YAG laser with low fluence for keloids and hypertrophic scars." *Journal of the European Academy of Dermatology and Venereology* 24:1070-74. doi: 10.1111/j.1468-3083.2010.03593.x.

[20] Henderson, D. L., and T. A. Cromwell, L. G. Mes. 1984. "Argon and carbon dioxide laser treatment of hypertrophic and keloid scars." *Lasers in Surgery and Medicine* 3:271-7.

[21] Nicoletti, Gianfranco, and Francesco De Francesco, Carmine M. Mele, Chiara Cataldo, Roberto Grella, Sergio Brongo, Marina Accardo, Guiseppe A. Ferraro, Francesco D'Andrea. 2013. "Clinical and histologic effects from CO_2 laser

treatment of keloids." *Lasers in Medical Science* 28:957-64. doi: 10.1007/s10103-012-1178-0.

[22] Carniol, Paul J., and Lauren Meshkov, Lisa D. Grunebaum. 2011. "Laser treatment of facial scars." *Current Opinion in Otolaryngology & Head and Neck Surgery* 19:283-8. doi: 10.1097/MOO.0b013e32834896b9.

[23] Alster, Tina S., and Amy B. Lewis, Alan Rosenbach. 1998 "Laser scar revision: comparison of CO_2 laser vaporization with and without simultaneous pulsed dye laser treatment." *Dermatologic Surgery* 24:1299-302.

[24] Fitzpatrick, Richard E., and Elizabeth F. Rostan, Nancy Marchell. 2000. "Collagen tightening induced by carbon dioxide laser versus erbium:YAG laser." *Lasers in Surgery and Medicine* 27:395-403. Doi: 10.1002/1096-9101(2000)27:5<395::AID-LSM1000>3.0.CO;2-4.

[25] Alexiades- Armenekas, Macrene R., and Jeffrey S. Dover, Kenneth A. Arndt. 2008. "The spectrum of laser skin resurfacing: nonablative, fractional, and ablative laser resurfacing." *Journal of the American Academy of Dermatology* 58:719-37. doi: 10.1016/j.jaad.2008.01.003.

[26] Alster, Tina S. 1999. "Clinical and histologic evaluation of six erbium:YAG lasers for cutaneous resurfacing." *Lasers in Surgery and Medicine* 24:87-92.

[27] Majaron, Boris, and Shyam M. Srinivas, Huai-en L. Huang, J. Stuart Nelson. 2000. "Deep coagulation of dermal collagen with repetitive Er:YAG laser irradiation." *Lasers in Surgery and Medicine* 26:115.

[28] Nanni, Christopher A., and Tina S. Alster. 1998. "Complications of carbon dioxide laser resurfacing." *Dermatologic Surgery* 24:315-20.

[29] Fitzpatrick, Richard E. 1999. "Treatment of inflamed hypertrophic scars using intralesional 5-FU." *Dermatologic Surgery* 25:224-31.

[30] Alster, T. S., and T. B. West. 1997. "Treatment of scars: A review." *Annals of Plastic Surgery* 39:418-32.

[31] Goldman, Mitchel, and Nancy Marchell, Richard Fitzpatrick. 2000 "Laser resurfacing of the face with a combined CO_2/Er:YAG." *Dermatologic Surgery* 26:102-4.

[32] Trelles, M. A., and L. Garcia-Solana, R. G. Calderhead. 1999. "Skin resurfacing improved with a new dual wavelength Er:YAG/CO_2 laser system:comparative study." *Journal of Clinical Laser Medicine & Surgery* 17:99-104. Doi: 10.1089/clm.1999.17.99.

[33] Tanzi, Elizabeth L., and Tina S. Alster. 2004. "Comparison of a 1450-nm diode laser and a 1320-nm Nd:YAG laser in the treatment of atrophic facial scars: A prospective clinical and histologic study." *Dermatologic Surgery* 30:152-7.

[34] Lee, Dong H., and Yu S. Choi, Seong U. Min, Mi Y. Yoon, Dae H. Suh. 2008. "Comparison of a 585-nm pulsed dye laser and a 1064 nm Nd:YAG laser treatment

of acne scars: A randomized split-face clinical study." *Journal of the American Academy of Dermatology* 60:801-7. doi: 10.1016/j.jaad.2008.11.883.

[35] Kim, Sangeun, and Kyeong H. Cho. 2009. "Clinical trial of dual treatment with an ablative fractional laser and a nonablative laser for the treatment of acne scars in Asian patients." *Dermatologic Surgery* 35:1089-1098. doi: 10.1111/j.1524-4725.2009.01193.x.

[36] Bernstein, Eric F., and Mauren Ferreira, Dan Anderson. 2001 "A pilot investigation to subjectively measure treatment effect and side effect profile of nonablative skin remodelling using a 532 nm, 2 ms pulse-duration laser." *Journal of Cosmetic and Laser Therapy* 3:137-41. doi: 10.1080/147641701753414942.

In: Cutaneous Scars: Biology, Clinics and Management ISBN: 978-1-53615-657-7
Editors: Berna Aksoy, Hasan Mete Aksoy et al. © 2019 Nova Science Publishers, Inc.

Chapter 25

OTHER TREATMENTS

N. Burcu Ozturk[*]
Specialist of Dermatology, Private Practice, Kocaeli, Turkey

ABSTRACT

Cutaneous scarring of the skin may occur as a result of various reasons. Scars may be erythematous, hyperpigmented, hypopigmented, hypertrophic, keloidal, atrophic or dystrophic. There are many types of scar treatments currently available, each appropriate for particular type of these scars. In this chapter, chemical peeling, microneedling, filler applications and radiation, as well as other treatment methods recommended for scar treatment will be discussed.

Keywords: filler, microneedling, peeling, percutaneous collagen induction, plasma, radiation, radiofrequency

1. INTRODUCTION

Cutaneous scarring of the skin may occur as a result of various reasons such as following trauma or various diseases. A scar is the end result of wound healing process that ensures dermal integrity. Scarring is formed after the restructuring process by the collagen fibrils in the dermis and occurs as a result of trauma or inflammatory processes [1]. Scars may be erythematous, hyperpigmented, hypopigmented, hypertrophic, keloidal, atrophic or dystrophic [2, 3]. There are many types of scar treatments currently available. These include topical, intralesional and systemic medical treatments, surgical methods,

[*]Corresponding Author's Email: nadideburcuozturk@gmail.com.

laser systems, chemical *peeling*, *microneedling*, *filler* applications, and *radiation* treatments. Goodman graded scar types and suggested a suitable treatment plan including those treatments mentioned above and tried to determine the most appropriate one for the patient. He further stated that this grading system could be used not only for post-acne scarring but also for all types of scars developing as a result of diseases or trauma [2]. In this chapter, chemical *peeling*, *microneedling*, *filler* applications and *radiation*, as well as other treatment methods recommended for scar treatment will be discussed.

2. Chemical Peeling

Chemical *peeling* is the process of production of controlled chemical injury to the skin followed by regeneration of the skin through the use of various chemical agents [4]. Its aim is to induce a loss of keratinocytes and dermal structures at the epidermal and dermal level, depending on the potency of the agent being used [5].

Chemical *peeling* is classified as very superficial, superficial, medium or deep, according to the penetration depth of the agent being used. Very superficial peel is the exfoliation of the stratum corneum and its effect does not reach the stratum granulosum layer whereas, superficial peel is the destruction of the full thickness of epidermis including the basal cell layer located below the stratum granulosum. Medium peel is the destruction of epidermis and papillary dermis, and deep peel is the destruction of epidermis, papillary dermis, and reticular dermis [6]. These effect levels can vary according to the concentration of the chemical agent used, the number of applications, the use of other chemical agents, and the pH status [7].

In the chemical *peeling* process, contraindications are present being both absolute and relative ones. Absolute contraindications include pregnancy, breastfeeding, the use of isotretinoin in the previous six months, active herpes simplex infections/cold sores, Fitzpatrick skin-type V-VI for superficial *peeling* and IV-VI for medium and deep *peeling*, and the presence of kidney failure in the phenol *peeling*. The periods when relative contraindications are seen include: a period of 4-6 weeks after a cold sore infection is healed, a period of 1-2 weeks following the injection of botulinum toxin, a 2-week period before or after a collagen injection, a 6-week period after the occurrence of edema following facial surgery, an 8-week period after laser treatment, and three weeks following waxing and the use of epilators. Relative contraindications also include: a noncompliant patient, regular exposure to sun, excessive cigarette consumption, inactive but recurrent herpes infections, oral estrogen use, a history of hypertrophic scarring, connective tissue disorders, and advanced AIDS [8].

Herpes virus reactivation may be seen in patients with a history of recurrent herpes virus infections in the regions where *peeling* will be applied. Therefore, *peeling* should be performed with an acyclovir prophylaxis. In the prophylaxis, acyclovir of 400 mg three times a day or valacyclovir of 500 mg two times a day should be started one day prior to the procedure and should be continued for five days after the procedure [9]. With deep *peeling*, the prophylaxis should be continued for 15 days and for 10 days for medium *peeling* [10].

Preparing the skin with topical skin care products prior to the application of chemical *peeling* increases the effectiveness of the *peeling*, accelerates recovery after treatment and reduces the risk of complications [11]. It is recommended to start topical treatment up to six weeks prior to the procedure, in order to increase the epithelization rate, stabilize melanocyte activity, and reduce local inflammation. For this purpose, topical tretinoin, hydroquinone (HQ) and topical steroids are generally used in combination [12]. The use of retinoids before the application reduces the thickness of the stratum corneum, helps make the application area flatter for the *peeling* application and ensures an increase in penetration. It is recommended that topical retinoids are discontinued one or two weeks prior to the *peeling* application. In this way, epidermal healing is completed before the *peeling* and skin integrity is ensured during *peeling* [11].

Peeling agents generally consist of alpha hydroxy acids (AHA), beta hydroxy acids (BHA), trichloroacetic acid (TCA), tretinoin, and various phenolic compounds (HQ, resorcinol, and carbolic acid) [7].

Additionally, chemical *peeling* agents can be classified according to their penetration depths within the skin. Very superficial peels are 20 - 50% glycolic acid and 20 - 30% salicylic acid. Superficial peels are Jessner's solution, 10 - 30% TCA and 70% glycolic acid. Medium peels include different concentrations of TCA and various combined *peeling* agents. In deep *peeling*, Baker-Gordon phenol solution is used [13].

2.1. Glycolic Acid

Glycolic acid is the most commonly used alpha hydroxy acid. It is used in daily skin care with concentrations of 5 - 15%. It is used for chemical *peeling* at 30 - 70% concentrations. It is a non-toxic, systemically safe and easily tolerable *peeling* agent. As with all AHA *peeling* agents, they must be neutralized to cease their effects on the skin. This agent can be best neutralized with an alkaline solution such as sodium bicarbonate. It is not beneficial to wash the face with water, as it may not remove the agent completely [6].

2.2. Salicylic Acid

This is a superficial *peeling* agent that is included in the beta hydroxy acid group. Owing to its oil-soluble properties it can mix with epidermal lipids [14]. It penetrates well into the pilosebaceous units and reduces intercellular lipid [15]. It is the best *peeling* agent for acne scars and its most effective concentration is 30%. Treatment is repeated 3 to 5 times every 3 to 4 weeks. It has very few side effects and these are temporary. Dehydration and erythema may be observed. Resistant post-inflammatory hyperpigmentation and scarring are very rarely seen. When applied at a concentration of 20% to 50% of the body surface area, salicylic acid toxicity (salicylism) may be seen. This is characterized by increased respiratory rate, hearing loss, tinnitus, abdominal cramps, and dizziness [16].

2.3. Jessner's Solution

This consists of three synergistic keratolytic agents, formulated by Dr. Max Jessner. It constitutes a mixture of 14% lactic acid, 14% resorcinol, and 14% salicylic acid in 95% ethanol and is used in superficial *peeling*s [15, 16]. Resorcinol is structurally and chemically similar to phenol and increases the penetration of other agents by breaking down the weak hydrogen bonds of keratin. Jessner's solution is very well-tolerated and rarely leads to allergic contact dermatitis or systemic contact dermatitis [16]. Resorcinol may cause post-inflammatory hyperpigmentation in patients with skin phototype IV-VI [15].

2.4. Trichloroacetic Acid (TCA)

TCA has long been used as a *peeling* agent. Its application leads to cellular necrosis in the epidermis, as well as collagen necrosis in the papillary and reticular dermis [17]. *Peeling* depth depends on the concentration of TCA. If the concentration is between 10-30%, it can be used as a superficial peel; however, at concentrations higher than 30% it can be used as medium depth peel. Generally, the concentration used does not exceed 50%. The depth of penetration is not only related to the concentration but also to the method of application. For this reason, the use of TCA can vary depending on the practitioner. Neutralization is not required [8]. There is no systemic absorption even when used at high concentrations because TCA neutralizes itself. Therefore, toxicity and pain are not serious [15]. Nowadays, it can be used on focal atrophic acne scars with the chemical reconstruction of skin scars (CROSS) technique, in order to induce collagenization at high concentrations. The solution is applied to the base of the scar using a sharp, slender wooden applicator. This technique has been found to increase dermal thickening and collagen production [15]. In a study by Lee et al. containing 65 patients with atrophic acne scarring, 65% TCA was applied to 33 and 100% TCA was applied to 32 of them by CROSS technique. The improvement in the group treated with 100% TCA was found to be significant [18].

2.5. Phenol Peeling

Phenol is a deep chemical *peeling* agent that has been used for the last two decades. It causes full-thickness epidermolysis and dermal elastosis. Fibroblast stimulation can occur and this results in neocollagenesis. When it is systemically absorbed, it can cause fatal arrhythmia, hepatotoxicity, nephrotoxicity, and depression in the respiratory system. The cutaneous side effects include hypo-/hyper-pigmentation, hypertrophic scarring, keloid and prolonged erythema [15]. General anesthesia or deep sedation should be administered as the procedure is painful [8]. Among the various modern phenol peel formulae, the Baker-Gordon formula is the best-known, consisting of 2.05% croton oil (Baker Gordon Phenol Formula: 3 mL Phenol 88%; 2mL distilled water; 8 drops Septisol liquid soap; 3 drops Croton oil). The basic components of the Brown, Hetter, Stone, Litton, and Exoderm formulae are identical but they contain different concentrations. Croton oil increases the penetration of phenol. If the phenol concentration is increased without the addition of croton oil, *peeling* will be ineffective. For this reason, the *peeling* depth is more contingent on the concentration of croton oil rather than the phenol concentration [19].

2.6. Combined Chemical Peeling Methods

Combined *peelings* are used to increase the penetration of low-concentration TCA or other acids. As a result of this, the acidity can be as deep as TCA of 50% and the risk of scarring is reduced [6]. Combined *peelings* are used in medium-depth chemical *peelings*. Brody *peeling*, Monheit *peeling*, Coleman *peeling*, and Moy *peeling* are the most commonly used *peeling* combinations.

2.6.1. Monheit Peeling

The Jessner's + TCA *peeling* combination was developed by Monheit. It is a safe and moderately effective *peeling* method that can be used in superficial acne scars, photoaging, and actinic keratoses. By using this method, a 35% TCA peel will be capable of penetrating deeper into the skin and increasing its efficiency while safety is maintained [20].

2.6.2. Solid Carbon Dioxide and TCA

This combination, developed by Dr. Hal Brody, is used for *peeling* at different levels and various depths. It is used in cases where deeper *peeling* is required, such as for scarring or wrinkles. First, solid carbon dioxide is applied. It is immersed in a solution of acetone and alcohol, which makes it easier to spread over the skin. The *peeling* depth increases as the length of application is prolonged and the amount of applied pressure is increased. When the paresthesia diminishes, which occurs as a result of carbon dioxide, 35% TCA can be applied to the whole face [6].

2.6.3. Glycolic Acid and TCA

Glycolic acid 70% is applied to the skin for two minutes. Trichloroacetic acid 35% is applied afterwards. This combination is thought to result in a smoother and deeper *peeling* than TCA when used alone [21].

2.6.4. Jessner Solution and Glycolic Acid

With this *peeling* technique, which was developed by Dr. Larry Moy, between 1 and 3 coats of Jessner's solution is applied until diffuse erythema occurs over the entire area of skin to be treated. Then 70% glycolic acid is applied to the skin. In this way, the exfoliative effect of the Jessner's solution and the stimulating effect of glycolic acid are combined [6].

3. MICRONEEDLING

Microneedling, also known as *percutaneous collagen induction* (PCI) therapy, is a minimally invasive technology used to treat numerous dermatologic conditions [22]. *Microneedling* is usually applied with devices comprising multiple needles on a cylinder called a dermaroller. The needles are 0.1 – 0.25 mm in diameter and 0.5–3 mm in length. There are also miniature devices, whose needles are 0.12 mm in diameter and 2 mm in length. These are called dermastamp and are used for localized scarring such as those caused by varicella [23]. In addition, there is an electronic pen-shaped device that has adjustable settings to control the speed and depth of needle penetration [24].

The needles on the device create holes and microchannels in the skin without damaging the epidermis. The production of new collagen and elastin is stimulated in the papillary dermis, owing to release of growth factors. Additionally, new capillaries are produced and the neovascularization process begins. Scarring is reduced through neocollagenation and neovascularization. This treatment is therefore called *percutaneous collagen induction* therapy [25]. Regeneration of the tissue will continue for a period lasting from eight weeks to a year [23].

Microneedling can also be used to augment transdermal drug delivery (TDD) through the creation of pores in the stratum corneum [26].

Topical products and *radiofrequency* treatments may be used together with the *microneedling* method. Through combination of the topical products with microneedling, the penetration and efficacy of these products are enhanced. Extra growth factors are produced with the use of platelet-rich plasma (PRP) and human stem cell products and in this way, percutaneous collagen induction will be increased. Fractionated Microneedle *Radiofrequency* (FMRF) devices directly transmit the *radiofrequency* current to the dermis over the microneedles and create thermal damage [24].

Microneedling is a well-tolerated treatment method. Erythema may be seen following the treatment and can last for two to three days. Sun protection is recommended for a week. Cream with a topical antibiotic is recommended after the application. It can be used on all skin types and in areas such as the eye contour area, where laser and peeling methods cannot be applied very easily [25].

In the literature, there are many studies on *microneedling* applications and acne scarring.

Sharad has reported that the combination of *microneedling* and glycolic acid *peeling* is effective in the treatment of acne scars [27]. In another study, 20 patients with acne scarring with Fitzpatrick skin phototypes ranging from 1 to 5 underwent *microneedling* procedures 3 times with 2 weeks intervals. Two different dermatologists evaluated the photographs of the patients according to the Goodman and Baron rating system (GBSG). During the 6-month follow-up period, there was a statistically significant decrease in the patients' scores compared with the control group and no side effects were reported [28]. In a case series, 32 patients with rolling scars underwent two *microneedling* procedures. The scars of the patients were evaluated by using GBSG. At the end of the treatment, a significant decrease was observed in the scar grades [29]. In another case series, 36 patients with Fitzpatrick skin phototypes IV-V who had acne scarring, underwent five *microneedling* applications and an improvement rate of 50 – 75% was observed. Ecchymosis and pain were observed as side effects. Moreover, five patients left the study due to the development of post-inflammatory hyperpigmentation and tram-track scarring [30]. Figure 1 depicts typical effect of microneedling in atrophic acne scarring.

In another study involving 49 patients with acne scarring, *microneedling* and TCA application were performed alternatively at 2 weeks intervals and levels of improvement were evaluated according to the GBSG system. At least one degree of improvement was observed in each one of the patients. Additionally, ice pick scarring have been reported to be more treatment-resistant. In terms of side effects, post-inflammatory hyperpigmentation was observed in three patients after 5 months of topical treatment [31].

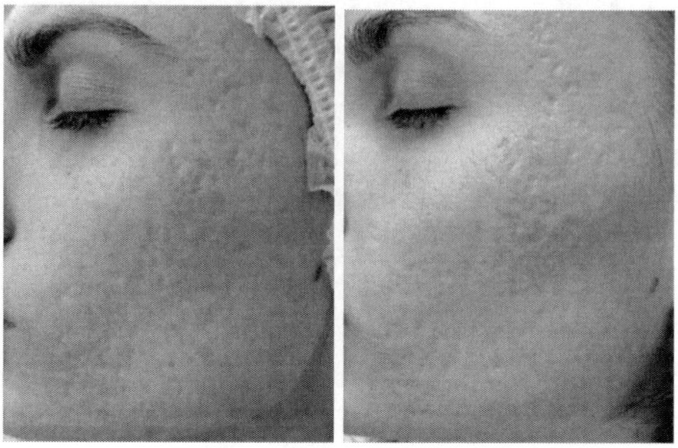

Figure 1. (a) Before and (b) 7 months follow up photographs of 4 monthly sessions of microneedling performed by electronic pen-shaped device for atrophic acne scarring (Courtesy of Berna Aksoy, MD).

In another study, in which 45 patients with acne scarring were randomly selected, PRP, topical TCA 100% and *microneedling* treatment methods were used. No statistically significant difference was observed in the three groups [32].

Microneedle fractional *radiofrequency* (MFR) therapy is also used for acne scarring. This treatment provides dermal remodeling and new collagen formation without damaging the epidermis. The four-session MFR treatment method was performed on 31 patients with Grade 3-4 acne scarring. Considering all patients, 2 degrees of improvement was observed in 80.6% and 1 degree of improvement was observed in 19.4% of them. Transient post-inflammatory hyperpigmentation developed in five patients, and transient tram-track marks developed in two patients [33]. Figure 2 depicts result of 2-session MFR therapy.

Microneedling has been studied as a treatment for a variety of other scars, including burns, striae, and other atrophic scars [34-36].

In a case series, 3-4 sessions of *microneedling* therapy were performed on a patient group with atrophic scarring which was graded from 2 to 4, and scars developed as a result of various reasons (acne, varicella, trauma, post-herpetic). The best response was obtained on rolling and boxcar scars, while a moderate response was obtained on pitted scars and a minimal response was obtained from applications on deep tunnels and complicated scarring. In patients with postherpetic scarring, 2 degrees of improvement was observed; whereas, in patients with posttraumatic and postvaricella scarring, 1 degree of improvement was observed [37].

Conversely, the effects of *microneedling* on hypertrophic scarring and keloids have not been fully examined and therefore further research is required [24].

There is also a study which has reported that collagen and elastin in the extracellular matrix of the reticular dermis were normalized following *microneedling* treatment performed for hypertrophic scarring in patients with burn injury [36].

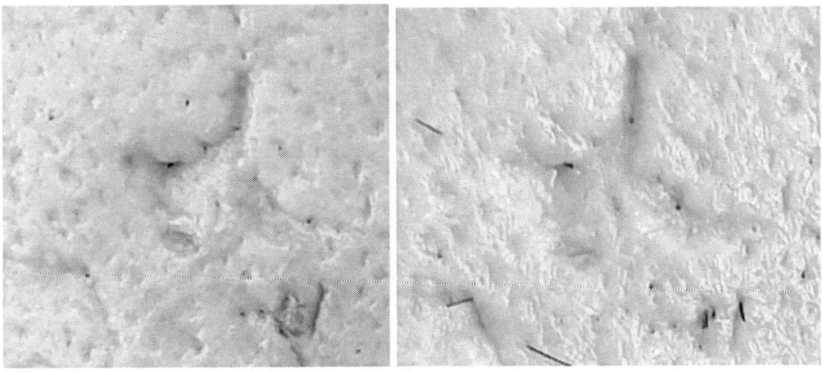

Figure 2. (a) Before and (b) after 2 monthly sessions of MFR therapy used for atrophic acne scars.

Practitioners prefer the *microneedling* method as an alternative method in the treatment of scarring, as it is easy to apply, comparatively safer than the other methods and patients are able to return to their daily lives more quickly following this procedure.

4. Filler Injections

Filling is one of the treatment methods used for scarring. Atrophic or depressive scars are usually seen as flat and soft-edged or deep and narrow like ice pick scars. Most of the stretchable, soft, and rounded atrophic scars can be improved with dermal *filler*s [38].

Filler materials can be classified as temporary, semipermanent, and permanent. The half-lives of temporary and semipermanent fillers vary across a wide range and are biodegradable; however, permanent fillers are not biodegradable [39]. In addition, *filler*s can be classified histopathologically, according to the extracellular matrix response in the area to which they are applied. For example, hyaluronic acid fillers stimulate collagen production. The most potent collagen stimulation is achieved by biostimulator semipermanent and permanent fillers, such as poly L-lactic acid (PLLA) and calcium hydroxylapatite (CaHA) [40]. The effect of temporary fillers lasts for up to 18 months and for this hyaluronic acid may be given as an example. The duration of action of semipermanent fillers such as PLLA and CaHA lasts for up to 2 years. The duration of action of permanent fillers, such as poly-methyl methacrylate (PMMA), silicone, polyacrylamide, and polyalkylimide, lasts longer than 3 years [41].

Filler materials should not be used on pregnant or breastfeeding women, patients with an impaired immune system, individuals with allergies to *filler*s, and in the presence of infection [42].

A good dermal *filler* should be safe, cost-effective, hypoallergenic, easy to dispense, easy to store, injectable over a short period of time and painless. An allergy test should not be necessary. It should not impact on the daily life of the patient and there should be no risk of complications. Additionally, there should be a feeling of naturalness following the application. The results should be long-term or permanent, and predictable but it should be easy to remove the filler if required [43].

To correct depressive scars, dermal *filler*s are injected from the surface to the mid dermis. Usually, two or four fan injections are made, depending on the size of the scar. Injections are applied directly adjacent to the scar and opposite to each other. The use of fine dermal fillers, using a small quantity of *filler*, applying only slight pressure to the piston of the injector, intradermal implantation, and the slow retrograde movement of the needle during injection, can reduce the risk of vascular damage during the application. *Filler* can accumulate on the edges of some scars. In such cases, the injection should be stopped, the filler should be flattened and the injection should be continued from a different side of the scar. In cases where there is a noticeable decrease in the volume of the dermal *filler* product and the scars re-emerge, it is recommended to repeat the *filler* application. For scars that cannot be adequately filled, the results may be improved by applying the subcision method prior to the filling procedure (Figure 3) [38].

Benefits of the *filler* treatment in acne scars can vary according to the type of scarring. The benefit of *filler* treatment on depressed or broad-based scars is rather limited, due to the fibrous properties of pitted and ice-pick type scars [44-46]. Atrophic and/or rolling scars are the acne scars that have the best response to injections [42]. Therefore, soft atrophic scarring, in which dermal tissue loss is apparent, are the main indications for *filler* injections. Dermal *filler* injections that are made under scars enable the surface of the scar to reach the level of the surrounding skin [44].

Silicone has long been used for filling scars. Good results can be obtained, particularly in widespread and stretched scarring developed as a result of various reasons like acne, excoriation, trauma, varicella, infections, and surgery. The silicone is injected into the deep dermis in very small quantities at distances of 2-10 mm, by multiple injections using the microdrop serial injection method [47].

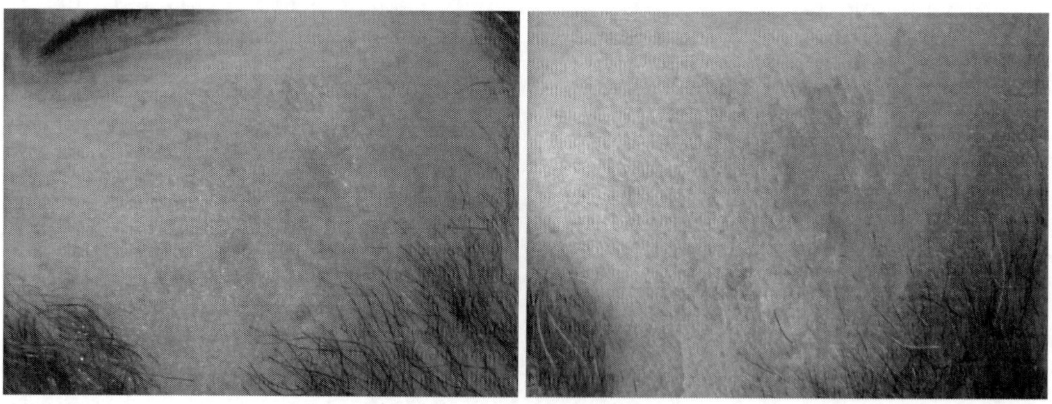

Figure 3. Rolling acne scars (a) before and (b) one month after subsicion and hyaluronic acid filler injection (Courtesy of Berna Aksoy, MD).

PLLA is considered to be a deep tissue regenerator, as it provides soft tissue improvement by stimulating the collagen production by fibroblasts. It is a synthetic polymer that stimulates collagen synthesis through a foreign body reaction with an effect that is similar to absorbable suture materials [48]. In a study by Sadove, two cases with acne-related dermal fat atrophy on their cheeks were successfully treated with PLLA injections. In this type of scarring, the volume increase produced by, PLLA has been reported to be more permanent when compared with other filler materials [45]. Beer et al. investigated the efficacy and safety of PLLA in acne and varicella scars. In this study, PLLA was prepared by diluting a dry powder with 4 mL of sterile water containing 1 mL of lidocaine and 1/100,000 epinephrine. The diluted product was left at room temperature for 2 to 48 hours so that it could become hydrated. The application was made at monthly intervals. The needle was inserted under the scar and the filling material was injected until the scar reached the same level as the surrounding skin. Massaging after each treatment prevented the formation of subcutaneous papules. At the end of the investigation, rolling type scars were reported to be the scars that best responded to the PLLA applications, however, ice pick scars were observed not to respond so well. The study reported that the most suitable scars for PLLA treatment were those that were not deeper than 2-3 mm, and those scars whose depths were not higher than their widths [49].

In scar filling, PMMA is used as a long-acting permanent filler [50-52]. PMMA is an inert synthetic permanent *filler* material that induces fibrous capsule formation in animals [53]. It is commercially available as 80% collagen solution containing 20% PMMA microspheres. In addition, 0.3% lidocaine is added to reduce the pain at the injection site. As PMMA is in a collagen solution, to prevent a possible hypersensitivity reaction, an allergy test is advised, which should be performed 4 weeks prior to the injection. It is very effective for mature mildly-depressed rolling acne scars. Horizontal filling can be made for these scars at a distance of 5-10 mm. With boxcar scars, filling should be performed by moving the needle backwards and forwards after inserting it perpendicularly from the center of the scar. Incipient scars should not be treated as they may not improve and they may even become worse [51, 52].

CaHA is a synthetic, biodegradable, semipermanent, and biostimulatory *filler*. CaHA stimulates collagen production. Soft-tissue augmentation lasts for up to 18 months [54]. Goldberg et al. investigated the efficacy and safety of CaHA in the treatment of acne scars. In their study, CaHA in a gel carrier was injected into the mid-depth dermis with a 27 G injector. This study concluded that it could be an effective and safe alternative treatment for boxcar type scarring; however, no improvement was observed in cases with ice pick scars [55].

Collagen *filler*s are temporary *filler*s of either porcine, bovine or recombinant human origin. It is recommended that two intradermal tests are performed at 2-4 weeks intervals due to the allergic potential of bovine collagen; however, this is not necessary for porcine collagen or recombinant human collagen. Collagen *filler*s should not be used in patients with collagen hypersensitivity or auto-immune disease. Soft-tissue augmentation usually continues for up to six months [56-58].

Hyaluronic acid (HA) is a glycosaminoglycan polysaccharide and a physiologic component of the extracellular matrix. Cross-linked stabilized hyaluronic acid *fillers* (HAFs) are created through many different technological methods. Modern HAFs are produced by bacterial fermentation [59]. There are several case reports using HA in scar treatment. A HAF application was performed on a patient with traumatic atrophic depressed scarring, which has developed in the cheek area approximately 20 years following a traffic accident. In this case, two different filler materials were applied one for the deeper scarring and one for the superficial scarring. An effective improvement was noted after the application and a more symmetrical appearance was obtained between the right and left sides of the face. The effect was observed to continue throughout the 6-month follow-up period. No side effects were reported [60]. In another case report, cross-linked HA was applied in two cases with acne scarring, using the pneumatic injection method. At the end of the treatment, a degree of regression was observed in the degree of the patients' acne scarring. It was reported that no side effects developed [61]. In another case with an atrophic skin area, which developed following steroid injections administered for keloid treatment, was successfully treated with HA injections and no side effects were reported. They have, however, recommended that patients should be informed that the efficacy of this application is temporary [62]. At the control of the patient, which was made 24 months after the HAF treatment, improvement in scar volume and appearance was observed to continue, even though no further HAF injection had been performed in the lesion [63].

5. RADIATION

Radiation therapy can also be used as a treatment method for scarring. It is predominantly used in keloid treatment. In terms of the mechanism of action, *radiation* therapy is primarily effective during the early period of wound healing. Endothelial vascular bulbs are more susceptible to *radiation*. It reduces the proliferation of new fibroblasts [64]. Accordingly, it is recommended that *radiation* therapy is applied as soon as possible following surgical excision in keloid treatment. Radiotherapy is reported to provide better results when it is performed between one to three days after the surgery [65, 66]. In the literature, there is a study comparing the recurrence rates of adjuvant corticosteroids and adjuvant radiotherapy performed following surgical excisions of earlobe keloids. The study observed that there were lower rates of recurrence reported following adjuvant radiotherapy treatment [67]. Another recent study compared the efficacy of intralesional 5-fluorouracil and triamcinolone acetonide treatment and radiotherapy applied to earlobe keloids after surgery. Intralesional 5-fluorouracil and triamcinolone acetonide treatment was found to be statistically more effective [68]. In a review examining the effective treatment methods for earlobe keloids following surgical excision, an evaluation was made for post-operative adjuvant treatment modalities and recurrence rates. To this end point, 25 studies in the literature have been examined. Based on their examination results, among the adjunctive therapies used after surgery triamcinolone therapy and radiation therapy have been reported to provide somewhat better treatment results for ear keloids but without a significant difference between the two treatment methods, although it has been stated that a large-scale and randomized study is required [69]. In another study, an investigation on the efficacy of high-dose, single-fraction radiotherapy treatment was made and this method was applied to patients following surgical excisions of resistant keloids (resistant to surgical excision, steroid injection, and laser treatment) located in different parts of the body. The study concluded that this treatment is an effective and reliable method for preventing recurrence. It was further emphasized that radiotherapy was non-invasive and painless when compared with other treatments, such as steroid injections. Nevertheless, due to the risk of radiation-induced malignancy, it is not recommended to be used in young patients, exception is those cases for whom treatment has been ineffective for many years, or cases who suffer from a complaint of severe pain. Due to this malignancy risk, use of radiotherapy for keloids should be evaluated by both plastic surgeons and dermatologists and only then radiotherapy administration should be decided [70].

6. Plasma

Plasma skin regeneration (PSR) creates a thermal effect on the skin using *plasma* energy and is currently being used as a new resurfacing method. Unlike laser systems, PSR is not chromophore-dependent. It stimulates wound healing without vaporizing the tissue. In histological studies that included patients for whom *plasma* resurfacing treatment was performed, increased collagen production, decreased elastosis, and progressive skin rejuvenation were shown to continue even a year after treatment [71]. When various studies on the use of PSR in acne scarring and traumatic scars are examined, this treatment appears to be effective and considering the small number of complications and the short duration of downtime it can be used as an alternative treatment [72, 73]. Likewise, Goodman GJ, who graded acne scarring, has recommended the use of PSR for the treatment of grade 3 scars [3].

As this is a new treatment method, it appears that further studies should be carried out about its use.

CONCLUSION

Cutaneous scars pose important therapeutic challenges for the practitioner. There are various treatment modalities. Of them, chemical peeling can be performed by different agents, inducing different depths of epidermal and dermal injury and are usefull in different types of atrophic acne scarring. Microneedling is effective in various types of cutaneous scarring. Filler materials may be used principally for the recovery of the lost volume and the correction of cosmetic appearance, especially in rolling and soft atrophic scars. Radiotherapy seems to be an effective and safe treatment method that may be preferred, particularly for resistant keloids. Plasma treatment is a new modality and needs further studies.

REFERENCES

[1] Busam, Klaus J. 2010. Dermathopathology. USA: Elsevier Health Sciences

[2] Goodman, Greg J. 2012. 'Treating Scars: Addressing Surface, Volume, and Movement to Optimize Results: Part 1. Mild Grades of Scarring.' Dermatologic Surgery 38:1302-9. doi: 10.1111/j.1524-4725.2012.02434.x.

[3] Goodman, GJ. 2012. 'Treating Scars: Addressing Surface, Volume, and Movement to Expedite Optimal Results. Part 2: More-Severe Grades of Scarring.' Dermatologic Surgery 38:1310-21. doi: 10.1111/j.1524-4725.2012.02439.x

[4] Roenigk, R. K. 1998. 'Facial chemical peel.' In Textbook of Cosmetic Dermatology, edited by Baran, R., and H. I. Maibach, 585-94. London: Martin Dunitz.

[5] Matarasso, S. L., and R. G. Glougau. 1991. 'Chemical face peels.' Dermatologic Clinics 9:131-49.

[6] Clark, Eileen, and Lawrence Scerri. 2008. 'Superficial and medium- depth chemical peels.' Clinics in Dermatology 26:209-18. doi: 10.1016/j.clindermatol.2007.09.015.

[7] Rullan, Peter, and Amir M. Karam. 2010. 'Chemical peels for darker skin types.' Facial Plastic Surgery Clinics of North America 18:111-31. doi: 10.1016/j.fsc.2009.11.010.

[8] Fischer, T. C., and E. Perosino, F. Poli, M. S. Viera, B. Dreno, Cosmetic Dermatology European Expert Group. 2010. 'Chemical peels in aesthetic dermatology: an update 2009.' Journal of the European Academy of Dermatology and Venereology 24:281-92. doi: 10.1111/j.1468-3083.2009.03409.x.

[9] Hirsch, Ranella, and Meghan Stier. 2009. 'Complications and their management in cosmetic dermatology.' Dermatologic Clinics 27:507-20. doi: 10.1016/ j.det.2009.08.013.

[10] Monheit, Gary D. 2004. 'Chemical peels.' Skin Therapy Letter 9:6-11.

[11] Small, Rebecca, and Dalano Hoang, Jennifer Linder. 2013. A Practical Guide to Chemical Peels, Microdermabrasion, &Topical Products. USA: Lippincott Williams & Wilkins, Wolters Kluwer Health

[12] Been, Mark J., and Devinder S. Mangat. 2014. 'Laser and face peel procedures in non-Caucasians.' Facial Plastic Surgery Clinics of North America 22:447-52. doi: 10.1016/j.fsc.2014.04.012.

[13] Salam, A., and O. E. Dadzie, H. Galadari. 2013. 'Chemical peeling in ethnic skin: an update.' The British Journal of Dermatology 169:82-90. doi: 10.1111/bjd.12535.

[14] Brackett, W. 1997. 'The chemistry of salicylic acid.' Cosmetic Dermatology 10:s5-s6.

[15] Handog, Evangeline B., and Maria S. L. Datuin, Ivan A. Singzon. 2012. 'Chemical peels for acne and acne scars in asians: evidence based review.' *Journal of Cutaneous and Aesthetic Surgery* 5:239-46. doi: 10.4103/0974-2077.104911.

[16] Fabbrocini, Gabriella, and M. C. Annunziata, V. D. Arco, V. D. Vita, G. Lodi, M. C. Mauriello, F. Pastore, G. Monfrecola. 2010. 'Acne scars: pathogenesis, classification and treatment.' *Dermatology Research and Practice* 2010:893080. doi: 10.1155/2010/893080.

[17] Fabbrocini, G., and S. Cacciapuoti, N. Fardella, F. Pastore, G. Monfrecola. 2008. 'CROSS technique: chemical reconstruction of skin scars method.' *Dermatologic Therapy* 21:S29–S32. doi: 10.1111/j.1529-8019.2008.00239.x.

[18] Lee, Jung B., and Woo G. Chung, Ho Kwahck, Kwang H. Lee. 2002. 'Focal treatment of acne scars with trichloroacetic acid: chemical reconstruction of skin scars method.' Dermatologic Surgery 28:1017-21.

[19] Hetter, Gregory. 2000. 'An examination of the phenol-croton oil peel: Part I. Dissecting the formula.' *Plastic and Reconstructive Surgery* 105:239-48.

[20] Monheit, G. D. 1995. 'The Jessner's-trichloroacetic acid peel. An enhanced medium-depth chemical peel.' *Dermatologic Clinics* 13:277-83.

[21] Coleman, W. P., and I. M. Futrell. 1994. 'The glycolic acid–trichloroacetic acid peel.' *The Journal of Dermatologic Surgery and Oncology* 20:76-80.

[22] Fernandes, Desmond. 2005. 'Minimally invasive percutaneous collagen induction.' Oral and Maxillofacial Surgery Clinics of North America 17:51–63. Doi: 10.1016/j.coms.2004.09.004.

[23] Deepali, Bhardwaj. 2012. 'Collagen induction therapy with dermaroller.' *Community Based Medical Journal* 1:35-7.

[24] Ramaut, Lisa, and Henk Hoeksema, Ali Pirayesh, Filip Stillaert, Stan Monstrey. 2018. 'Microneedling: Where do we stand now? A systematic review of the literature.' *Journal of Plastic*, Reconstructive & Aesthetic Surgery 71:1-14. doi: 10.1016/j.bjps.2017.06.006.

[25] Doddaballapur, Satish. 2009. 'Microneedling with dermaroller.' *Journal of Cutaneous and Aesthetic Surgery* 2:110-1. doi: 10.4103/0974-2077.58529.

[26] Vandervoort, J., A. Ludwig. 2008. 'Microneedles for transdermal drug delivery: a minireview.' *Frontiers in Bioscience* 13:1711–5.

[27] Sharad, Jaishree. 2011. 'Combination of microneedling and glycolic acid peels for the treatment of acne scars in dark skin.' *Journal of Cosmetic Dermatology* 10:317-23. doi: 10.1111/j.1473-2165.2011.00583.x.

[28] Alam, Murad, and Sansra Han, Marisa Pongprutthipan, Wareeporn Disphanurat, Rohit Kakar, Michael Nodzenski, Natalie Pace, Natalie Kim, Simon Yoo, Emir Veledar, Emily Poon, Dennis P. West. 2014. 'Efficacy of a needling device for the treatment of acne scars: a randomized clinical trial.' *JAMA Dermatology* 150:844–9. doi: 10.1001/jamadermatol.2013.8687.

[29] Fabbrocini, G., and N. Fardella, A. Monfrecola, I. Proi- etti, D. Innocenzi. 2009. Acne scarring treatment using skin needling. *Clinical and Experimental Dermatology* 34:874-9. doi: 10.1111/j.1365-2230.2009.03291.x.

[30] Dogra, Sunil, and Savita Yadav, Rishu Sarangal. 2014. 'Microneedling for acne scars in Asian skin type: an effective low cost treatment modality.' *Journal of Cosmetic Dermatology* 13:180-7. Doi: 10.1111/jocd.12095

[31] Garg, Shilpa, and Sukriti Baveja. 2014. 'Combination therapy in the management of atrophic acne scars.' *Journal of Cutaneous and Aesthetic Surgery* 7:18-23. doi: 10.4103/0974-2077.129964.

[32] Nofal, Eman, and Afaf Helmy, Ahmad Nofal, Rania Alakad, Mohammad Nasr. 2014. 'Platelet-rich plasma versus CROSS technique with 100% trichloroacetic acid versus combined skin needling and platelet rich plasma in the treatment of atrophic acne scars: a comparative study.' *Dermatologic Surgery* 40:864–73. doi: 10.1111/dsu.0000000000000091.

[33] Chandrashekar, Byalekere S., and Rashmi Sriram, Rajdeep Mysore, Sapnashree Bhaskar, Abhishek Shetty. 2014. 'Evaluation of microneedling fractional radiofrequency device for treatment of acne scars.' *Journal of Cutaneous and Aesthetic Surgery* 7:93–7. doi: 10.4103/0974-2077.138328.

[34] Costa, Izelda M., and Mariana C. Costa. 2014. 'Microneedling for varicella scars in a dark- skinned teenager.' Dermatologic Surgery 40:333-4. doi: 10.1111/dsu.12396.

[35] Aust, Matthias C., and Karsten Knobloch, Peter M. Vogt. 2010. 'Percutaneous collagen induction therapy as a novel therapeutic option for Striae distensae.' Plastic and Reconstructive Surgery 126:219e–220e. doi: 10.1097/PRS. 0b013e3181ea93da.

[36] Aust, Matthias C., and Karsten Knobloch, Kerstin Reimers, Jörn Redeker, Ramin Ipaktchi, Mehmet A. Altintas, Andreas Gohritz, Nina Schwaiger, Peter M. Vogt. 2010. 'Percutaneous collagen induction therapy: an alternative treatment for burn scars.' *Burns* 36:836–43. doi: 10.1016/j.burns.2009.11.014.

[37] Majid, Imran. 2009. 'Microneedling therapy in atrophic facial scars: an objective assessment.' *Journal of Cutaneous and Aesthetic Surgery* 2:26–30. doi: 10.4103/0974-2077.53096.

[38] Small, Rebecca, and Dalano Hoang. 2012. *A Practical Guide to Dermal Filler Procedures*. USA: Lippincott Williams & Wilkins, Wolters Kluwer Health

[39] Ahn, Christine S., and Babar K. Rao. 2014. 'The life cycles and biological end pathways of dermal fillers.' *Journal of Cosmetic Dermatology* 13:212–23. doi: 10.1111/jocd.12100.

[40] Mercer, S. E., and R. Kleinerman, G. Goldenberg, P. O. Emanuel. 2010. 'Histopathologic identification of dermal filler agents.' *Journal of Drugs in Dermatology* 9:1072–8.

[41] Forbat, E., and F. R. Ali, F. Al-Niaimi. 2017. 'The role of fillers in the management of acne scars.' *Clinical and Experimental Dermatology* 42:374–80. doi: 10.1111/ced.13058.

[42] Alam, Murad, and Hayes Gladstone, Edward M. Kramer, Jack P. Murphy Jr, Keyvaan Nouri, Isaac M. Neuhaus, James M. Spencer, Elisabeth Spenceri, Susan Van Dyke, Roger I. Ceilley, Ken K. Lee, Greg Menaker, Gary D. Monheit, David S. Orentreich, Benjamin Raab, Kevin C. Smith, Nowell J. Solish; American Society for Dermatologic Surgery. 2008. 'ASDS guidelines of care: injectable fillers.' *Dermatologic Surgery* 34:S115–S148. doi: 10.1111/j.1524-4725.2008.34253.x.

[43] Ballin, Annelyse C., and Fredric S. Brandt, Alex Cazzaniga. 2015. 'Dermal Fillers: An Update.' *American Journal of Clinical Dermatology* 16:271–83. doi: 10.1007/s40257-015-0135-7.

[44] Khunger, Niti, and IADVL Task Force. 2008. 'Standard guidelines of care for acne surgery.' *Indian Journal of Dermatology, Venereology and Leprology* 74:28-36

[45] Sadove, Richard. 2009. 'Injectable poly-L: -lactic acid: a novel sculpting agent for the treatment of dermal fat atrophy after severe acne.' *Aesthetic Plastic Surgery* 33:113-6. doi: 10.1007/s00266-008-9242-7.

[46] Barnett, Jay G., and Channing R. Barnett. 2005. 'Treatment of acne scars with liquid silicone injections: 30-year perspective.' *Dermatologic Surgery* 31:1542-9.

[47] Duffy, D. M. 2006. 'Liquid Silicone for Soft Tissue Augmentation: Histological, Clinical, and Molecular Perspectives.' In Tissue Augmentation In Clinical Practice edited by Klein, A.W., 141-238. New York, NY: Taylor & Francis Group.

[48] Goldberg, David, and Adriana Guana, Andrea Volk, Elizabeth Daro-Kaftan. 2013. 'Single-arm study for the characterization of human tissue response to injectable poly-L- lactic acid.' *Dermatologic Surgery* 39:915–22. doi: 10.1111/dsu.12164.

[49] Beer, Kenneth. 2007. 'A single-center, open-label study on the use of injectable poly-L-lactic acid for the treatment of moderate to severe scarring from acne or varicella.' *Dermatologic Surgery* 3:S159-S167. Doi: 10.1111/j.1524-4725.2007.33356.x.

[50] Haneke, E. 2004. 'Polymethyl methacrylate microspheres in collagen.' *Seminars in Cutaneous Medicine and Surgery* 23:227-32. Doi: 10.1016/j.sder.2004.08.002.

[51] Lemperle, G. 2006. 'ArteFill augmentation of wrinkles and acne scars.' In Tissue Augmentation In Clinical Practice edited by Klein, A. W., 267-90. New York, NY: Taylor&Francis Group.

[52] Lemperle, Gottfried, and James J. Romano, Mariano Busso. 2003. 'Soft tissue augmentation with artecoll: 10-year history, indications, techniques and complications.' *Dermatologic Surgery* 29:573-87.

[53] Lemperle, G., and H. Ott, U. Charrier, J. Hecker, M. Lemperle. 1991. 'PMMA microspheres for intradermal implantation: Part I. Animal research.' *Annals of Plastic Surgery* 26:57–63.

[54] Jacovella, PF. 2008. 'Use of calcium hydroxylapatite (Radiesse) for facial augmentation.' *Clinical Interventions in Aging* 3:161–74.

[55] Goldberg, David J., Snehal Amin, Mussarrat Hussain. 2006. 'Acne scar correction using calcium hydroxylapatite in a carrier-based gel.' *Journal of Cosmetic and Laser Therapy* 8:134–36. Doi: 10.1080/14764170600891632.

[56] Elson, M. L. 1988. 'Clinical assessment of Zyplast implant: a year of experience for soft tissue contour correction.' *Journal of the American Academy of Dermatology* 18:707–13.

[57] Varnavides CK, Forster RA, Cunliffe WJ. 1987. 'The role of bovine collagen in the treatment of acne scars.' *The British Journal of Dermatology* 116:199–206.

[58] Sage, Robert J., and Matteo C. Lopiccolo, Austin Liu, Basel H. Mahmoud, Emily P. Tierney, David J. Kouba. 2011. 'Subcuticular incision versus naturally sourced porcine collagen filler for acne scars: a randomized split-face comparison.' *Dermatol Surgery* 37:426–431. doi: 10.1111/j.1524-4725.2011.01918.x.

[59] Wollina, Uwe, Alberto Goldman. 2013. 'Dermal fillers: facts and controversies.' *Clinics in Dermatology* 31:731–736. doi: 10.1016/j.clindermatol.2013.05.010.

[60] Hussain, Syed N., and Greg J. Goodman, Eqram Rahman. 2017. 'Treatment of a traumatic atrophic depressed scar with hyaluronic acid fillers: a case report.' Clinical, *Cosmetic and Investigational Dermatology* 10:285–287. doi: 10.2147/CCID.S132626.

[61] Patel, T, and O Tevet. 2015. 'Effective treatment of acne scars using pneumatic injection of hyaluronic acid.' *Journal of Drugs in Dermatology* 14:74–76.

[62] Elliott, Lauren, and Rashid M. Rashid, Maria Colome. 2010. 'Hyaluronic acid filler for steroid atrophy.' *Journal of Cosmetic Dermatology* 9:253–5. doi: 10.1111/j.1473-2165.2010.00508.x.

[63] Richards, Kristen N., Rashid M. Rashid. 2010. 'Twenty-four-month persistence of hyaluronic acid filler for an atrophic scar.' *Journal of Cosmetic Dermatology* 10:311–2. doi: 10.1111/j.1473-2165.2011.00589.x.

[64] Levy, D. S., and M. M. Salter, R. E. Roth. 1976. 'Postoperative irradiation in the prevention of keloids.' AJR. *American Journal of Roentgenology* 127:509–10.

[65] Deigert, F. A., and K. D. Allen. 1973. 'Keloids: Reassessment of irradiation therapy.' *Rocky Mountain Medical Journal* 70:35–37.

[66] Abdus-salam, A. A., and A. A. Orekoya, M. A. Jimoh A. A. Olabumuyi. 2016. 'Radiotherapy treatment of keloids in Ibadan.' *Journal of the West African College of Surgeons* 6:104–16.

[67] Sclafani, A. P., and L. Gordon, M. Chadha, T. Romo. 1996. 'Prevention of earlobe keloid recurrence with post-operative corticosteroid injections versus radiation therapy: A randomized, prospective study and review of the literature.' *Dermatologic Surgery* 22:569–74.

[68] Khalid, Farrukh A., and Usman K. Farooq, Muhammad Saleem, Jibran Rabbani, Muhammad Amin, Kamal U. Khan, Younas Mehrose, Moazzam N. Tarar. 2018. 'The efficacy of excision followed by intralesional 5-fluorouracil and triamcinolone acetonide versus excision followed by radiotherapy in the treatment of ear keloids: A randomized control trial.' Burns 44:1489-95. doi: 10.1016/j.burns.2018.02.017.

[69] Shin, Jin Y., and Jin-Won Lee,Si-Gyun Roh, Nae-Ho Lee, Kyung-Moo Yang. 2016. 'A Comparison of the Effectiveness of Triamcinolone and Radiation Therapy for Ear Keloids after Surgical Excision: A Systematic Review and Meta-Analysis.' Plastic and Reconstructive Surgery 137:1718-25. doi: 10.1097/PRS.0000000000 002165.

[70] Song, Changhoon, and Hong-Gyun Wu, Hak Chang, Il H. Kim, Sung W. Ha. 2014. 'Adjuvant single-fraction radiotherapy is safe and effective for intractable keloids.' *Journal of Radiation Research* 55:912-6. doi: 10.1093/jrr/rru025.

[71] Foster, K. Wade, and Ronald L. Moy, Edgar F. Fincher. 2008. 'Advances in plasma skin regeneration.' *Journal of Cosmetic Dermatology* 7:169–79. doi: 10.1111/ j.1473-2165.2008.00385.x.

[72] Kono, Taro, and William F. Groff, Hiroyuki Sakurai, Takashi Yamaki, Kazukata Soejima, Motohiro Nozaki. 2009. 'Treatment of traumatic scars using plasma skin regeneration (PSR) system.' *Lasers in Surgery and Medicine* 41:128–30. doi: 10.1002/lsm.20723.

[73] Gonzalez, Michele J., and William H. Sturgill, E. Victor Ross, Nathan S. Uebelhoer. 2008. 'Treatment of acne scars using the plasma skin regeneration (PSR) system.' *Lasers in Surgery and Medicine* 40:124–7. doi: 10.1002/lsm.20617.

In: Cutaneous Scars: Biology, Clinics and Management ISBN: 978-1-53615-657-7
Editors: Berna Aksoy, Hasan Mete Aksoy et al. © 2019 Nova Science Publishers, Inc.

Chapter 26

TREATMENT OF ACNE SCARS

Asli Tatliparmak*
Department of Dermatology,
Faculty of Medicine, Bahçeşehir University, Istanbul, Turkey

ABSTRACT

Acne scarring is a common problem that affects significant number of acne patients. Currently there is no standart treatment for acne scars, and often several modalities may be combined to achieve best results.

Keywords: Ablative, acne scar, boxcar scar, carbon dioxide (CO2), chemical, dermabrasion, Er:YAG, filler, fractional, icepick scar, laser, microneedling, non-ablative, peels, rolling scar, subcision, radiofrequency

1. INTRODUCTION

Acne vulgaris is a common skin disease with 80% prevalence in adolescents [1, 2]. Lesions can lead to scars which may have negative effect on quality of life. *Acne scars* affect approximately 14% of individuals who have *acne* [3]. Effective treatment of *acne scars* can minimize the physical disfigurement [4].

Acne scars can be divided into three categories morphologically; atrophic, hypertrophic and keloidal. Most of the *acne scar* patients have atrophic scars (80-90%), rarely they have hypertrophic scars and keloids (commonly on the shoulders and chest).

*Corresponding Author's Email: aslitatliparmak@gmail.com.

Atrophic *acne scars* can be subdivided as *ice pick, rolling* and *boxcar scars. Ice pick scars* are the most common type (60-70%) of atrophic *acne scars*. They are narrow, < 2 mm in diameter, sharply demarcated tracts that can extend into deep dermis or even subcutaneous tissue. Their depth makes them diffucult to treat with skin resurfacing options [2]. *Boxcar scars* are wider at the base and U shaped tracts. They are 15-20% part of atrophic *acne scars. Rolling scars* are wider (4-5 mm) and characterized by the tethering of the dermis and subcutis. They constitute 20-30% of atrophic *acne scars*. [1, 2, 4]. Hypetrophic scars remain within the borders of the original wound and in contrast keloid scars extend beyond the marjin of original wound. The clinical appearence of both atrophic and hypertrophic scars may be erythematous.

Scar classification is important in the choice of treatment. *Ice pick scars* may be resistant to conventional skin resurfacing modalities. *Rolling scars* may need subdermal treatments. *Boxcar scars* are more amenable to skin resurfacing treatments. But in daily routine most of the patients may have different types of scars at the same time. Therefore pre-treatment patient assessment is an essential component of *acne scar* teratment. To minimize the side effects and achive best results; type of scars, history of acne treatment, history of abnormal wound healing (keloid or postinflammatory hyperpigmentation), history of skin disease (disorders which may have Koebner phenomenon like psoriasis and lichen planus) must be identified before the treatment. More attention should be given to the patients with bleeding disorders, immunosuppression and those who had recieved radiation therapy as they may have disturbed wound healing and infection [5, 6]. Before *ablative* treatments such as *ablative laser* or *dermabrasion,* prophylactic antiviral treatment should be given. And finally patients' expectations should be discussed in detail. Before and after photographs should be taken for every patient [6].

The treatment can be categorized as energy based and non-energy based modalities.

2. Energy Based Treatments

Energy based treatments include ablative and non ablative lasers, fractional lasers and radiofrequency.

2.1. Ablative Lasers

Carbon dioxide and erbium:yttrium aluminum garnet *(Er:YAG) lasers* are the most commonly used *ablative lasers* for the treatment of *acne scars* [5]. These ***lasers*** target water in the skin as chromophore and induce collagen remodelling [5].

Traditional 10,600 nm *ablative carbon dioxide laser* emits light in the far infrared spectrum [2]. It vaporizes the tissue at a depth of 20 to 60 μm with a zone of thermal necrosis ranging another 20 to 50 μm [7].

The *Er:YAG laser* has 2490 nm wavelength and causes less side effects than 10,600 nm *carbon dioxide laser*. Water absorbs energy better in 2,490 nm wavelength than 10,600 nm and this reduces surronding tissue damage [5]. *Er:YAG* vaporizes the tissue at a depth of 20 to 25 μm with an additional 5 to 10 μm zone of thermal necrosis [7]. But intraoperative bleeding is more common in treatment with *Er:YAG laser* [8].

Ablative lasers have good clinical results in *acne scar* treatment but also they are associated with procedural discomfort, prolonged recovery and significant risks of dyspigmentation and scarring [2].

2.2. Non-Ablative Lasers

Non-ablative lasers used in the treatment of *acne scars* have become popular recently. These *lasers* target water as cromophore and make thermal induction in dermis which results in collagen remodeling in the treated tissue. They also have variable amounts of absorption by hemoglobin and melanin. These *lasers* deliver the energy to dermis without ablating epidermis thus epidermal damage and post treatment downtime are minimized [2]. Most commonly used *non-ablative lasers* are 1320 and 1064 nm neodymium doped yttrium aluminum garnet (Nd:YAG) and the 1450 nm diode *lasers*. But the clinical results of non *ablative lasers* in the treatment of *acne scars* are limited [5, 9].

2.3. Fractional Lasers

Fractional lasers target water as cromophore. *Fractional* photothermolysis creates micro thermal damage zones (MTZs) in the skin which improve skin healing. MTZs may vary in diameter and depth as a result of *laser* settings. These thermal damage zones which are known as microthermal zones, are columns of cougulated tissue extending into the deep portion of dermis. The untreated tissue around the microthermal zone provides rapid healing and remodelling [2, 5]. The stratum corneum contains little water and hence remains intact after treatment so the recovery time is shorter than *ablative lasers* [2].

Advantages of these *lasers* are short downtime and fewer side effects when compared to *ablative lasers* and more tissue regeneration compared to non-*ablative lasers* [5]. Erythema, edema, crusting, scaling are the side effects that reside in less than two weeks. Postinflammatory hyperpigmentation is one of the major complications of fractional *laser* treatments [10].

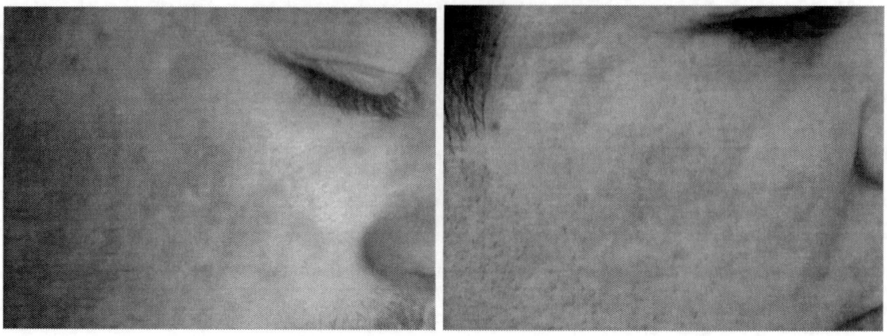

(a) (b)

Figure 1. Rolling acne scars a) before and b) after 5 sessions of combined fractional microneedle RF and fractional carbon dioxide laser treatments (Courtesy of Erol Koc, MD).

2.4. Radiofrequency

These devices deliver the bipolar *radiofrequency* (RF) energy directly into the dermis using needles that stimulate dermal remodelling [9]. *Fractional* RF uses an array of electrodes to create zones of thermal wounds that stimulate remodelling. Microneedle bipolar RF and *fractional* RF treatments have the best results for *acne scars* compared to monopolar RF [2]. *Radiofrequency* (RF) can be applied as monotherapy or combined with *fractional lasers* (Figure 1).

3. Non-Energy Based Treatments

Subcision, dermabrasion, microneedling, dermal *fillers* and *chemical peels* are non-energy based treatment options.

3.1. Subcision

Subcutaneous incisionless surgery *(subcision)* is a technique which is made with a needle being inserted subcutaneously and moved to untether the fibrous bands and stimulate new collagen formation to elevate the *scar* surface. The success rate of the subsicion is reported to be 50-60% in the treatment of *rolling scars* [5]. Releasing the fibrous strands from dermis is essential in this technique. The needle is introduced into the subdermis backward and forward motions followed by horizontally rotating the needle in a fanning manner. These motions loosen the fibrotic adhesions that cause the bound down appearence of *rolling scars* [8]. When the treatment is successful new collagen is produced through physiological healing [2].

There have been a few needle types used in *subcision*; cataract blade, wires, tribeveled hypodermic needle and blunt blade needle. Blunt blade *subcision* is made with a stainless steel blade which is noncutting at the tip. Blunt blade prevents neorovascular injury [11].

Edema, local tenderness or infection, ecchymoses or hematoma formation are the side effects that may be seen after ***subcision*** treatment [12].

3.2. Dermabrasion

Dermabrasion is an old resurfacing technique. In this treatment epidermis is totally removed under local or general anesthesia to stimulate new collagen remodeling and reepithelization [4, 5]. It is best used for well defined *scars* with distinct borders or broad based scars with indistinct borders but not for *ice pick* or deep *boxcar scars* [2]. *Dermabrasion* can be performed with brush or diamond fraze. Brush *dermabrasion* is more diffucult to perform but more effective for *acne scars* compared to use of diamond fraze [6].

Microdermabrasion is a technique made with aluminum oxide crystals that are ejected from a nozzle. It is used in *rolling* or *boxcar scar* subtypes to minimize the borders of the scar [5].

Dermabrasion has risks of postinflammatory hyperpigmentation, infection, scaring and milia formation [2]. Viral infections should be suspected when erythema or ulcerations occur especially after 7-10 days after treatment. Persistant erythema may herald scarring, so preventive treatment should be started by high potency corticosteroids when it is determined [6].

3.3. Microneedling

Skin needling has been used since 1995 for collagen stimulation in *acne scar* treatment [13]. Manual rollers or *microneedling* devices (Figure 2) have 0.5-2.5 mm length needles that penetrate into dermis and create microchannels. These channels induce collagen production and remodelling via wound healing mechanisms. Wound healing has three phases. Phase one is inflammatory phase that starts immediately after needling. Phase two is proliferation phase that growth factors (platelet derived growth factor, fibroblast growth factor, transforming growth factors alpha and beta) are released. Fibroblast activation and collagen production occurs. Keratinocytes then start producing all the constituents for remodeling of the basement membrane. Phase three is skin remodeling phase which continues for months after treatment [13].

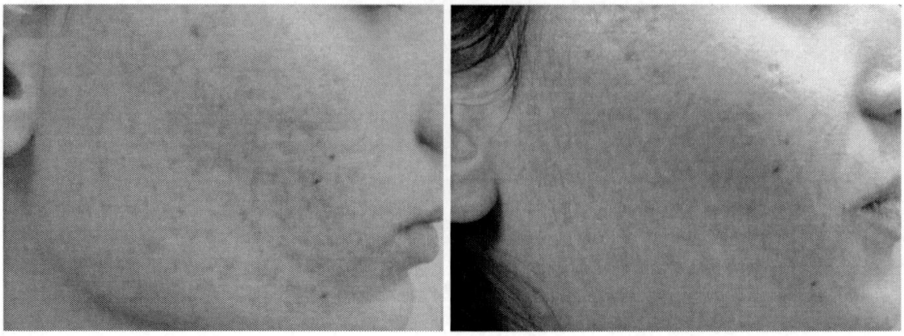

(a) (b)

Figure 2. a) Before and b) 7 months follow up photographs of 4 sessions of monthly microneedling treatments performed by electronic pen-shaped device in boxcar and icepick scarring (Courtesy of Berna Aksoy, MD).

Microneedling can be performed in all types of scars and colors of skin safely [5]. Furthermore *microneedling* provides channels for absorption of topical agents including platelet rich plasma and remodelling agents [2].

The standart dermaroller used for *acne scars* is a drum-shaped roller studded with 192 fine microneedles in eight rows. Microneedles are available in different lengths and the needle diameter is 0.1 mm [14].

3.4. Dermal Fillers

Level V evidence supports the use of *fillers* for atrophic *acne scars;* especially for atrophic *rolling* or *boxcar scars* to augment soft tissue [2]. Microinjection of the filler under the scar provides immediate amendment in atrophic *acne scars* [5]. Types of injection include serial punctures, linear threading, fanning and cross-hatching, deep bolus and superficial micro-droplet injections. Most common adverse effects are pain, erythema, lumps and abscess formation. *Fillers* are categorized as temporary, semi-permanent and permanent [2].

Temporary *fillers* last for a few months. The most commonly used temporary filler agent in atrophic *acne scars* is hyaluronic acid. The injection of hyaluronic acid *fillers* stimulates collagen production and augmentation of soft tissue (Figure 3) [2].

Semi permanent *fillers* last for up to two years. Poly L-lactic acid and calcium hydroxlyapatite are semi-permanent *fillers* used in *acne scars* especially in *rolling scars* [2, 8].

Permanent *filler* choices are silicone and polymethylmethacrylate. They are intended to last for lifelong [2, 8].

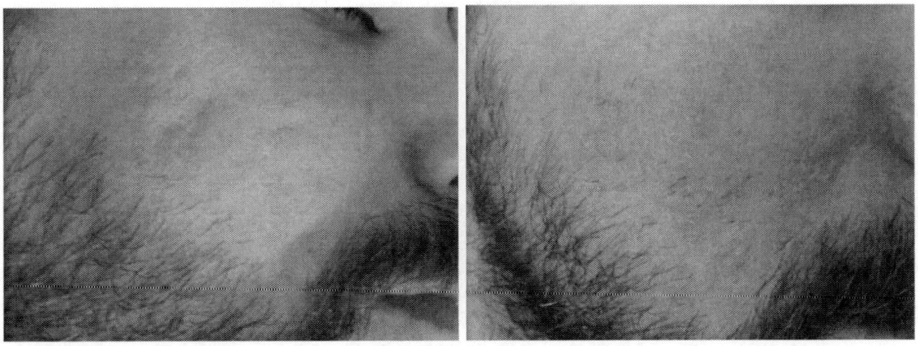

(a) (b)

Figure 3. Rolling acne scars a) before and b) one month after subsicion and hyaluronic acid filler injection (Courtesy of Berna Aksoy, MD).

3.5. Chemical Peels

Chemical peels are used to make a controlled injury on the skin stimulating skin remodelling and regeneration. Salicylic acid, glycolic acid, pyruvic acid, Jessner's solution, trichloroacetic acid, phenol, lactic acid and mandelic acid are the most commonly used peeling agents [3]. Superficial *peels* such as lactic acid, salicylic acid, glycolic acid, Jessner's solution and 10 to 25% trichloroacetic acid only affect epidermis. Medium depth *peels* such as 35 to 50% trichloroacetic acid combined with Jessner's solution affect epidermis and papillary dermis. Deep *peels* such as phenol affect epidermis and mid reticular dermis [2].

Salicylic acid peeling may reduce the postinflammatory hyperpigmentation of *acne scars*. The effective concentration in *acne scars* is 30%. The treatment is perfomed in every 3-4 weeks for a total of 3-5 sessions [3].

Glycolic acid is the most commonly used alpha hydroxy acid as a peeling agent [7]. It increases hyaluronic acid in dermis and induces collagen production by stimulating interleukin 6 secretion. It is effective and safe at the concentrations of 10% -70% in the treatment of superficial *acne scars* [3, 7]. The advantages of glycolic acid are mild erythema, mild desquamation and short healing period. In recent years, combination of *microneedling* and glycolic acid *peels* have been shown to be effective in acne *scars* [15].

Pyruvic acid is an alpha-ketoacid. It has keratolytic effect and stimulates new collagen production. The use of 40 to 70% pyruvic acid has been proposed for the treatment of *acne scars*. The advantages of this *peel* are homogeneous penetration and mild desquamation. Burning sensation, desquamation, irritating vapors for the upper respiratory mucosa may be seen after the treatment [3].

Jessner's solution consists of 14% salicylic acid, 14% resorcinol or citric acid and 14% lactic acid in 95% ethanol [3]. The depth of *peel* (level of peeling) depends on the number of layers applied. Level 1 peeling is made with the application of *peel* 1 to 3 layers of Jessner's solution and it has very superficial effect. Level 2 peeling is made with the application of *peel* in 4 to 10 layers. It has increased erythema, mild to moderate burning which lasts for 15 to 30 minutes and exfoliation lasts 2 to 4 days. Further layers of *peel* makes it a level 3 peeling, where exfoliation lasts 8 to 10 days with prominent erythema. Penetration of the *peel* depends on various factors such as thickness of the stratum corneum, sensitivity of the skin, and preparation of the skin [7].

Trichloroacetic acid (TCA) is the most commonly used peeling agent in *acne scars.* Depth of peeling depends on the concentration; 10% to 20% TCA is used as superficial *peel,* 35% is used as medium depth *peel* [7]. TCA causes protein denaturation which results in frosting. This peeling is not indicated in patients with dark skin types because of the hyperpigmentation risk. A new tecnique called chemical reconstruction of skin scars (CROSS) has been recently described as local application of TCA into individual *acne scars.* In this technique high concentrations of TCA (50% - 100%) is applied with wooden applicators to the scars until frosting happens. CROSS technique is useful for *ice pick* and narrow *boxcar scars.* The treatment shoud be repeated at 4 week intervals and up 2 to 3 sessions. This technique increases the efficiency and reduces the risk of hyperpigmentation even in darker skin types [3, 16].

Phenol is a deep peeling agent which induces neocollagenesis. The use of phenol has decreased in recent years due to side effects. In addition to local side effects, it has the risk of excessive systemic absorption leading to cardiac toxicity [3, 17].

The latest guidelines recommend waiting for 6 months after isotretinoin use to avoid the development of hypertrophic scars and keloids [12]. However, some authors suggested that isotretinoin is not a contraindication for CROSS technique [16,18].

CONCLUSION

Various treatment options have been reported for acne scars in the literature. Each of these procedures has different roles in the treatment. When deciding on treatment, the morphology of the scar, skin type, previous treatments and expectations of the patient should be considered.

REFERENCES

[1] Agarwal, Nidheesh, and Lalit K. Gupta, Ashok K. Khare, C. M. Kuldeep, Asit Mittal. 2015. "Therapeutic response of 70% trichloroacetic acid CROSS in atrophic acne scars." *Dermatologic Surgery* 41:597-604. doi: 10.1097/DSS.00000000 00000355.

[2] Alexiades, Macrene. 2017. "Laser and light-based treatments of acne and acne scarring." *Clinics in Dermatology* 35:183-9. doi: 10.1016/j.clindermatol.2016.10.012.

[3] Barikbin, Behrooz, and Zahra Akbari, Maryam Yousefi, Yahya Dowlati. 2017. "Blunt Blade Subcision: An Evolution in the Treatment of Atrophic Acne Scars." *Dermatologic Surgery* 43:S57-S63. doi: 10.1097/DSS.0000000000000650.

[4] Connolly, Deirdre, and Ha L. Vu, Kavita Mariwalla, Nazanin Saedi. 2017. "Acne Scarring-Pathogenesis, Evaluation, and Treatment Options." *The Journal of Clinical and Aesthetic Dermatology* 10:12-23.

[5] Dogra, Sunil, and Savita Yadav, Rishu Sarangal. 2014. "Microneedling for acne scars in Asian skin type: an effective low cost treatment modality." *Journal of Cosmetic Dermatology* 13:180-7. doi: 10.1111/jocd.12095.

[6] Fabbrocini, G., and N. Fardella, A. Monfrecola, I. Proietti, D. Innocenzi. 2009. "Acne scarring treatment using skin needling." *Clinical and Experimental Dermatology* 34:874-9. doi: 10.1111/j.1365-2230.2009.03291.x.

[7] Frith, M., and C. B. Harmon. 2006. "Acne scarring: current treatment options." *Dermatology Nursing* 18:139-42.

[8] Gozali, Maya V., and Bingrong Zhou. 2015. "Effective treatments of atrophic acne scars." *The Journal of Clinical and Aesthetic Dermatology* 8:33-40.

[9] Hession, Meghan T., and Emmy M. Graber. 2015. "Atrophic acne scarring: a review of treatment options." *The Journal of Clinical and Aesthetic Dermatology* 8:50-8.

[10] Kontochristopoulos, Georgios, and Eftychia Platsidaki. 2017. "Chemical peels in active acne and acne scars." *Clinics in Dermatology* 35:179-82. doi: 10.1016/j.clindermatol.2016.10.011.

[11] Kravvas, Georgios, and Firas Al-Niaimi. 2017. "A systematic review of treatments for acne scarring. Part 1: Non-energy-based techniques." *Scars, Burns & Healing* 3:2059513117695312. doi: 10.1177/2059513117695312.

[12] Landau, Marina. 2007. "Cardiac complications in deep chemical peels." *Dermatologic Surgery* 33:190-3. doi: 10.1111/j.1524-4725.2006.33037.x.

[13] Lee, Jung B., and Woo G. Chung, Ho Kwahck, Kwang H. Lee. 2002. "Focal treatment of acne scars with trichloroacetic acid: chemical reconstruction of skin scars method." *Dermatologic Surgery* 28:1017-21.

[14] Magnani, Lauren R., and Eric S. Schweiger. 2014. "Fractional CO2 lasers for the treatment of atrophic acne scars: a review of the literature." *Journal of Cosmetic and Laser Therapy* 16:48-56. doi: 10.3109/14764172.2013.854639.

[15] McGoldrick, Rory B., and Evgenia Theodorakopoulou, Ernest A. Azzopardi, Maxwell Murison. 2017. "Lasers and ancillary treatments for scar management Part 2: Keloid, hypertrophic, pigmented and acne scars." *Scars, Burns & Healing* 3:2059513116689805. doi: 10.1177/2059513116689805.

[16] Nast, A., and B. Dreno, V. Bettoli, Z. Bukvic Mokos, K. Degitz, C. Dressler, A. Y. Finlay, M. Haedersdal, J. Lambert, A. Layton, H. B. Lomholt, J. L. Lopez-Estebaranz, F. Ochsendorf, C. Oprica, S. Rosumeck, T. Simonart, R. N. Werner, H. Gollnick. 2016. "European evidence-based (S3) guideline for the treatment of acne - update 2016 - short version." *Journal of the European Academy of Dermatology and Venereology* 30:1261-8. doi: 10.1111/jdv.13776.

[17] Pavlidis, Athanasios I., and Andreas D. Katsambas. 2017. "Therapeutic approaches to reducing atrophic acne scarring." *Clinics in Dermatology* 35:190-4. doi: 10.1016/j.clindermatol.2016.10.013.

[18] Sharad, Jaishree. 2011. "Combination of microneedling and glycolic acid peels for the treatment of acne scars in dark skin." *Journal of Cosmetic Dermatology* 10:317-23. doi: 10.1111/j.1473-2165.2011.00583.x.

In: Cutaneous Scars: Biology, Clinics and Management ISBN: 978-1-53615-657-7
Editors: Berna Aksoy, Hasan Mete Aksoy et al. © 2019 Nova Science Publishers, Inc.

Chapter 27

TREATMENT OF STRIAE

G. Isil Kurmus** and Erol Koc
Department of Dermatology and Cosmetology,
Medical Park Ankara Hospital, Ankara, Turkey

ABSTRACT

Striae distensae (SD), with the other commonly known name "stretch marks," are frequent, aesthetically undesirable and therapeutically challenging form of dermal scarring. Striae distensae are hypothesized to represent atrophic dermal scars associated with abnormal collagen and elastic fibers. Therefore, the majority of treatments intend to increase collagen production. In this chapter a vast number of treatment modalities will be discussed briefly, ranging from topicals and chemical peel treatments to more invasive methods such as microdermabrasion, microneedling, subcision and laser therapies.

Keywords: centella asiatica, chemical peels, hyaluronic acid, infrared light, intense pulse light, laser, microdermabrasion, microneedling, platelet rich plasma (PRP), radiofrequency, silicon gel, stretch marks, striae, striae alba, striae distensae, striae rubra, subcision, tretinoin, ultraviolet light

1. INTRODUCTION

Striae distensae (SD) are a common, permanent skin condition, particularly in young healthy women. SD occur twice as often in women than men, with the majority of them arising during pregnancy and puberty [1, 2]. The incidence and prevalence of SD is

*Corresponding Author's Email: isilkurmus@gmail.com.

poorly documented within the literature, ranging from 11% to 88% [3, 4]. Although benign, they can cause significant emotional and psychological distress. Dyspigmentation, ulceration, urticaria, edema, dehiscence, subcutaneous emphysema, and koebnerization of primary lesions within SD are rarely seen complications [5-15]. Internal connective tissue disorders such as mitral valve prolapse and pelvic prolapse may be seen together with SD [16-18]. They have also been described in association with Cushing's Syndrome, Marfan's Syndrome, genodermatoses, following the administration of both short- and long-term oral and topical corticosteroids, growth spurts, and chronic liver disease. SD are also associated with obesity, rapid increase or decrease in weight such as bodybuilders, anorexia nervosa, after slimming diets and postbariatric surgery or prolonged periods of skin stretching such as breast augmentation or tissue expansion surgery [3, 19-24]. Other rarely reported causes of SD include cachetic states, such as tuberculosis and typhoid. SD have been seen rarely in patients positive for the human immunodeficiency virus receiving the protease inhibitor indinavir [24]. Due to their high prevalence and impact on patients' quality of life, there is great need for a consistently effective treatment [25].

Clinically and histopathologically recognizable forms of SD have been mentioned as *striae rubrae* (SR), *striae albae* (SA), and *striae* gravidarum (SG) [1, 3]. Ultimately the diagnosis is a clinical one. The initial erythematous and violaceous-appearing lesions associated with ruptured capillaries are named as SR. They can be raised and symptomatic flesh-toned atrophic linear marks. These progress to wrinkled, hypopigmented, atrophic scar-like dermal depressions referred to as SA, which have been known as a permanent, chronic form of SD. The term SG mentions to the same entity seen in pregnancy, usually developing after the 24th week of gestation [1-4]. High-resolution epiluminescence colorimetric assesment of SD defined four different types including *striae albae* (white color), *striae rubrae* (pink/red color), striae caerulea (dark blue/purplish color), and striae nigrae (dark grey/black color) [24]. SD most commonly occur on the abdomen, breasts, lower back, buttocks, thighs, upper arm and knee [1-3, 24].

The pathophysiology underlying *striae* is poorly understood. Endocrine imbalance, mechanical stretching of the skin, reduced genetic expression of fibronectin, collagen and elastin are aetiological theories that have been proposed [1, 3]. Hormonal alterations involving estrogens, androgens, and glucocorticoid levels and their receptors modulate cellular production of extracellular matrix (ECM) components [1]. High serum levels of steroid hormones have a catabolic effect on the activity of fibroblasts and decrease the deposition of collagen in dermal ECM [24].

The histopathologic findings of *striae* match a scar. Early histopathological changes may be determined on electron microscopy. In the early stages, a deep and superficial perivascular lymphocyctic infiltrate around the venules, mast cell degranulation and macrophage activation resulting in elastolysis of the middermis can be seen. Straight collagen bundles on the upper third of the reticular dermis are stretched and parallel to the dermoepidermal junction (DEJ). In the late phases, atrophy of epidermis can be seen due to flattening of the rete ridges and loss of collagen, elastin, and fibrillin. Uninvolvement of the DEJ and papillary dermis suggest that laminin, collagen IV and VII are unaffected [1-3, 24].

Several treatments for SD have been proposed but a treatment modality that is consistently effective with minimal adverse effects does not exist to date [3]. No single therapy is considered to be pivotal for this skin condition. It has always been reported that effective treatment of SD be applied during the active stage, well before the scarring process is complete [24]. Therapeutic outcomes also depend on both the type of SD and the patients' Fitzpatrick skin phototype. Most adverse effects, particularly with laser therapies, are seen in patients with darker skin types. Lifestyle measures such as exercise and diet restrictions have no effect on SD as indicated by one study [3].

In this chapter, we will discuss all of the treatment modalities of SD to enable clinicians to make an evidence-based decision about the best treatment option for their patients.

2. Treatment of Striae

2.1. Topical Therapies

Tretinoin (retinoic acid) has been shown to improve the clinical appearance of the *striae* during the active stage. It has maximal efficacy in *striae rubrae*, although not much effect is present in *striae albae.* It is believed to increase dermal collagen through modulation of transforming growth factor beta and stimulation of fibroblasts [1-3, 24]. A double-blind randomized vehicle controlled trial reported that daily application of 0.1% *tretinoin* cream for 24 weeks resulted in a statistically significant reduction in the mean length and width (14% and 8%, respectively) of SD. On the other hand, significant increase in collagen or elastin was not found on histopathological assessments [26, 27].

Centella asiatica, which contains asiaticoside, madecosside and thiosulfinates, is a plant used in Asian herbal medicine [25]. It has antagonistic effect against glucocorticoids and stimulates fibroblasts for ECM synthesis. Furthermore, it has been reported that thiosulfinates have antiseptic and fibrinolytic properties and asiaticoside enhances Type 1 collagen production and scar maturation [1]. *Centella asiatica* and boswellic acid combination has also antiinflammatory effects. Application of this combination twice daily for three months decreased *striae* severity in a recent study. However, side effects such as pruritus, erythema and burning were observed [28].

Hyaluronic acid, a humectide, is thought to work through its ability to enhance skin's water retention and wound healing. It also increases collagen production through stimulation of fibroblasts and decreases collagen loss induced by hormonal fluctuations or mechanical stretch [24]. Two randomized, controlled trials have reported a significant improvement in mean overall, appearance, softness, color, and texture of lesions after pregnancy [29, 30].

Silicone gel, and occlusive bandages are believed to have a similar mechanism for treating SD as a form of dermal scarring. Ud-Din et al., reported a double-blind randomized controlled trial evaluating the effect of *silicone gel* versus placebo. Following daily application, significantly increased Type 1 collagen levels and pliability, decreased melanin, vascularity of treated lesions and a reduction of length of rete ridges were observed as histopathological findings at six weeks. Although this study demonstrates positive results, large-scale studies are needed to suggest *silicone gel* for the treatment of SD [31].

Herbal topical oils and topical oil massage are some unconventional therapies and some of the anecdotal reports suggest applying herbal topical oils with massage. The underlying principle for this use is unclear. Taavoni et al., reported a randomized controlled clinical trial evaluating the effect of topical olive oil in the development of SD. No significant differences were reported in the development of SD between olive oil treatment and control groups [32]. A nonrandomized controlled clinical trial evaluating the prophylactic daily use of almond oil at 19th-32nd week gestation has reported significant difference in frequency of SD between groups: almond oil and massage 20%, almond oil alone 38.8%, control 41.2%. Large- scale randomized controlled trials are needed to support the recommendation of herbal oils [33].

2.2. Chemical Peel Treatments

Acid-peel treatments including glycolic acid (GCA) and trichloroacetic acid (TCA) act by inducing an initial inflammatory process and increase in collagen synthesis. No epidemiological study on the application of GCA in pregnancy or no data on the efficacy of GCA to prevent *striae* has been found in the scientific literature. Mazzarello et al., reported that using a total of six peels with 70% GCA over six months resulted in significant decrease in the furrow width and haemoglobin of the SR; the SA group also showed a similiar decrease in furrow width and an increase in melanin levels [34]. Low concentrations [15-20%] of TCA is reported to improve the texture and color of *striae* [35, 36]. However, side effects include postinflammatory hyperpigmentation and erythema. One study comparing 20% GCA/10% ascorbic acid, 2% zinx sulphate, and 0.5% tyrosine versus 20% GCA/tretinoin 0.05% cream found that both regimens improved SD on abdomen or thighs and they both increased epidermal thickness and decreased papillary dermal thickness on histopathology. Elastin content is also reported to be increased with topical 20% GCA and 0.05% tretinoin [37]. In another study a 70%

GCA and 35% TCA has been recommended for improving the texture and appearance of SD. The follow-up period of the reviewed *chemical peels* trials was 6 months or less [38]. It is necessary to conduct trials with longer follow-up periods for evaluating the long-term efficacy of *chemical peels* for treatment of SD.

2.3. Mechanical Techniques

Microneedling or percutaneous collagen induction therapy results in epidermal and dermal thickening through stimulation of Type I and III collagen and elastin production [39, 40]. One case series investigated the efficacy of *microneedling* versus fractional CO_2 *laser* and showed significant improvement and higher patient satisfaction from *microneedling* in comparison with fractional CO_2 laser [41]. Another comparative trial observed *microneedling* achieved better clinical and histological results in comparison with fractional CO_2 *laser.* Aust et al., reported improvement in skin texture, skin tightening, dermal neovascularization and no change in pigmentation by using a single 30 minute *microneedling* procedure [42]. Park et al., also reported that three *microneedling* treatments at 4-week intervals resulted in increased collagen in the dermis and post-treatment normalization of fragmented dermal elastin fibers [43]. However, both of these two studies have no control group and no randomization. A trial compared *microneedling* favorably against *microdermabrasion* combined with sonophresis and demonstrated greater clinical and histological improvement with *microneedling* [44]. It is needed to study an objective assessment method with longer follow-up periods in future studies.

Subcision is a surgical technique which is used to treat depressed scars. A recent case series study observed no significant difference among treatment with *subcision* versus *tretinoin* 0.1% cream versus *subcision* with *tretinoin* 0.1% cream for treating SD. Stria necrosis was seen in three patients after *subcision* treatment in this case series. *Subcision* is not recommended due to its unfavorable results [45].

Microdermabrasion mechanically ablates damaged skin by using physical agents, typically aluminum oxide. *Microdermabrasion* has efficacy in many skin conditions such as acne scars, mottled pigmentation, and fine wrinkles [1]. It also allows adjuvant topical therapies to penetrate the dermis more effectively. It is thought that this injury induces neocollagenesis by epidermal signal transduction pathways that causes remodeling of dermal matrix and deposition of elastin [46, 47]. A randomized trial investigated *microdermabrasion* versus *platelet-rich plasma* (PRP) versus combination therapy of *microdermabrasion* and PRP and this trial has reported that combination treatment has better effects requiring fewer treatment sessions compared with either treatment [48]. A more recent Egyptian study included 20 patients with SD receiving five *microdermabrasion* treatment sessions at weekly intervals on half of the body; SD on the other half of the body served as a control. The authors reported "good to excellent" clinical improvement in SD in 50% of treated subjects. Significantly increased type 1 procollagen α1 mRNA levels were detected in histopathology sections of treated patients by using real-time reverse transcriptase polymerase chain reaction [47]. Combination *microdermabrasion* and *chemical peel* therapies have been reported to improve SD in case series; however, further studies on a larger scale are needed to identify the efficacy of using such techniques for treatment of SD [35].

Galvanopuncture is a needling therapy that applies a continuous microcurrent, inducing an inflammatory reaction with the production of collagen. Bitencourt et al., demonstrated clinical improvements in SA, and erythema was the only side effect. However, randomized controlled studies with histological analysis are needed to assess its efficacy [49].

2.4. Platelet- Rich Plasma Treatment

PRP means concentrated solution of autologous platelets including growth factors and cytokines injected intradermally. The released growth factors by degranulation of platelets' α granules are platelet-derived growth factor (PDGFα, β), transforming growth factor (TGFα, β), vascular endothelial growth factor (VEGF), epidermal growth factor (EGF), fibroblast growth factor (FGF), and insulin-like growth factor (ILGF 1). *PRP* stimulates fibroblast growth and induces the expression of Type I collagen and metalloproteinases (MMP) in fibroblasts. So, *PRP* induces collagen and elastic fiber formation along with ECM remodeling. *PRP* has a crucial role in angiogenesis and epithelialization in wound healing [50]. In scientific literature some case series have combined *PRP* with fractional RF, *microneedling* and *microdermabrasion,* all reporting varying degrees of clinical improvement of *striae* and patient satisfaction (3,24]. Gamil et al., reported a study in the treatment of SD comparing the efficacy of *PRP* versus 0.05% *tretinoin.* Authors demonstrated significant improvement and higher patient satisfaction with *PRP* compared with topical 0.05% *tretinoin* [50]. However, small sample sizes and paucity of data are limits to draw significant conclusions from these studies.

2.5. Light and Radiofrequency Devices

Intense pulse light (IPL) is characterized by a noncoherent, polychromatic light energy with a broadband spectrum (515-1200 nm). Three case series have evaluated the efficacy of IPL treatment of SD. IPL improves epidermal atrophy and dermal elastosis, and induces neo-collagen formation [51]. It is reported that IPL use results in decrease in the number, total length, and width of SD, reduction in the erythema and improvement in skin elasticity. Histologically, an increase in the quality and amount of the collagen was found [52]. IPL has demonstrated greater results in reduction of erythema and discoloration of SD [52-55]. However, additional large-scale randomized controlled trials are needed to assess this therapy.

Infrared light, which is applied to the skin results in heating of the dermis and collagen denaturation with subsequent neocollagenesis [25,56]. Trelles et al., investigated the use of broadband *infrared light* between 800 and 1800 nm to treat ten patients with SA for four treatments at 2 week intervals. No adverse effects were observed. This case series showed improvement of clinical apperance by assessing 3-D photographs [53]. Large sample sized trials and comparison with other therapeutic methods are necessary to further assess this modality.

Ultraviolet (UV) *light* may only provide a temporary increase in pigmentation that reduces the appearance of striae [51,56]. Sadick et al., evaluated the combined use of UVB (296-315 nm) and UVA1 (360-370 nm) light in nine patients with mature SA with 10 treatment sessions . All patients reported some form of repigmentation in their lesions with different percentages. However, the pigmentation was transient and greater than 50% of patients had postinflammatory hyperpigmentation (PIH). No changes were observed on biopsy to indicate an effective collagen remodelling effect of the therapy [57]. More research will be needed for better outcomes using the different treatment regimens with UV light.

Radiofrequency (RF) devices transfer higher-energy fluences to the skin through a coupling method. The transmitted energy is converted to heat upon interacting with the skin's resistance and this results in collagen remodeling. Furthermore, activation of cellular signaling cascades stimulates fibroblast neocollagenesis [1]. It is observed that collagen fibril contraction occurs immediately after RF treatment sessions, which induces new collagen formation [24]. A randomized study reported significant clinical improvement and decrease in *striae* depth from treatment with bipolar RF potentiated with *infrared light* used in combination with fractional bipolar RF [58]. Another randomized study observed combination treatment with fractional microneedle RF and fractional CO_2 *laser* had significantly higher SA improvement compared with fractional microneedle RF alone [59]. Manuskiatti et al., demonstrated a case series with tripolar RF (40-50 W energy, 1 MHz frequency) treatment alone for six, weekly treatments in 17 subjects. It has been reported that 38.2% and 11.8% of subjects had 25% to 50% and 51% to 75% SD improvement respectively, at 6 month follow-up [60]. Monopolar RF and pulsed dye *laser* (PDL) combination therapy showed modest results with reduction in SD width at 12-week follow-up. Histopathology demonstrated increased collagen in upper- and mid-dermal areas and increase in the number of elastic fibers [61]. Other studies have also evaluated subjective improvement of *striae* using microneedle RF combined with an ablative fractional CO_2 *laser* and bipolar RF combined with *PRP* [62-64]. It has been suggested that RF may be considered as a potential treatment option for patients with Fitzpatrick skin types IV and V in these studies.

2.6. Laser Therapies

Laser therapies offer a variety of wavelengths that can target specific chromophores at varying fluences. This poses an advantage by allowing individualized treatments based on SD type and location, as well as patient's skin phototype. Some lasers target selectively oxyhemoglobin in the dilated blood vessels in SR to reduce the appearance. In mature SA, laser therapies work to induce collagen formation and the production of elastin. They have also been used with other treatment modalities to improve efficacy and decrease adverse effects. Several *lasers* with different parameters have been studied for the treatment of SR, SA, or both, with vastly different results [51, 56].

308- nm xenon chloride (XeCl) excimer *laser* emits light energy close to that of narrow-band UVB and is classically used to treat hypopigmented disorders, psoriasis and depigmentation of vitiligo. The excimer *laser* offers increased efficacy over standard phototherapy through its ability to deliver higher fluences with greater precision in less time. It treats *striae* by causing dermal injury and initiating formation of collagen and elastin [51, 56]. Goldberg et al., reported the use of excimer *laser* for the treatment of mature hypopigmented SA in 75 subjects with Fitzpatrick skin types II-IV. All patients achieved a substantial increase in pigmentation after a mean of 8.4 treatment sessions. 31% of patients had increased pigmentation beyond the treated area, or splaying to normal surrounding skin. Mild to moderate erythema was observed in each patient at some time point during sessions; however, there was no correlation between degree of erythema and extent of pigmentation [65]. Similar efficacy data was documented by Alexiades-Armenakas et al., who revealed pigment correction rates of 60-70% in comparison to control after nine sessions at biweekly intervals with excimer *laser*. The authors subtracted 50 mj/cm^2 from each subjects' minimal erythema dose for use during treatment. No adverse effects were seen other than transient erythema, which was authors' desired end point. The treated *striae* demonstrated increased melanin content and hypertrophy of melanocytes; however no improvement in skin atrophy was reported [66]. Ostovari et al., also reported the use of excimer *laser* for an average of 9.1 treatments at weekly intervals using 50 mj/cm^2 less than their minimal erythema dose in ten subjects with SA. It was shown to increase pigmentation, although only one patient had near complete repigmentation. Splaying of pigmentation was a notable adverse effect [67]. The excimer *laser* may therefore be considered for temporary repigmentation of mature SA with an acceptable success rate and a low incidence of adverse effects.

585- nm pulsed dye *laser* (PDL) is an effective treatment option of erythema by targeting hemoglobin selectively in dilated vessels. PDL treatment has also been shown to stimulate reorganization of dermal collagen and elastin in the papillary and reticular dermis of SD. This *laser* is less suitable for Fitzpatrick skin types V-VI due to possibility of PIH or permanent dyspigmentation [51, 56]. McDaniel et al., demonstrated the use of short pulse (0.4 ms pulse widht) 585 nm PDL in 39 female subjects with SA. The authors reported improvement of the texture and significantly decreased shadow ratios of SA after treatment at 6 months follow up. Histopathologically, increased elastin fibers and amount of collagen were seen, even in SA that had minimal clinical improvement. A correlation between posttreatment erythema and resolution of SA has also been reported. The authors revealed that the optimal treatment fluence was 3 j/cm^2 using a 10-mm spot size [68]. Jimenez et al., reported the use of short pulsed 585-nm PDL in 20 patients with SD who received two sessions at 6 week intervals and were analyzed 6 weeks after last session. Only four SR had a pigmentation change after treatment. No improvement was observed in any of the SA; however, histopathological analysis revealed an increase in collagen in both SR and SA [69]. The PDL is significantly more effective for treating SR owing to their increased vascularity [51,56]. Although textural improvements were observed in some recent studies, the primary endpoint for treating SA is normalization of pigmentation, for which PDL is virtually ineffective.

Copper bromide *laser* emits light energy at 577 nm. It is characterized by the maximum absorption peak of hemoglobin and it has greater range of parameter settings. Longo et al., reported the use of copper bromide *laser* to treat SD in 15 female patients. Patients received one to five sessions using a 1.5 mm spot size, 4 j/cm^2 for SD on the breast or 8 j/cm^2 for SD on other parts of the body. In this study, five patients achieved complete resolution of their SD while the remaining patients displayed a 50-90% improvement in depth, width, and color at both 1- and 2-year follow-up [70]. The authors suggest that the copper bromide *laser* is an efficacious, safe, and long term solution to treat SD, although further studies are needed to determine ideal parameters and the number of sessions for better response.

1064 nm neodyium:yttrium-aluminum-garnet *laser* (Nd: YAG) is useful for the treatment of vascular lesions and induces dermal collagen formation. The ability of vascular selectivity and collagen induction has beneficial effects in the treatment of immature SR [51,56]. A recent study used 1064 nm Nd: YAG *laser* in immature SD of 20 subjects. Subjects underwent an average of 3.5 treatment sessions every 3-6 weeks. The authors reported that the best results were observed after three sessions. Complications are rarely seen even in dark skinned patients when the appropriate settings and cooling are employed [71].

1450 nm diode *laser* has demonstrated efficacy in the treatment of rhytides, active acne and atrophic facial scars in recent clinical trials. Only one study revealed the efficacy and safety of diode *laser* in eleven patients with SA nad SR. Patients who have Fitzpatrick skin types IV to VI underwent three treatment sessions, receiving either 4, 8, or 12 J/cm^2 at 6 -week intervals. Dynamic cooling with cryogen spray was also applied. The authors observed no improvement in any lesions at any fluences while they revealed post procedural erythema, two months after the last session. Also, transient hyperpigmentation was seen in 64% of cases [72]. The authors concluded that, for dark skinned patients, treatment of *striae* with the 1450 nm diode *laser* is not effective, and the incidence of adverse effects is significant.

1540 nm fractional erbium:glass (Er:Glass) *laser* is one of the most reported nonablative fractional *lasers* for the treatment of both SR and SA. Fractional *lasers* emit light energy into the dermis through multiple microscopic columns surrounded by untreated areas [51]. They produce small columns of tissue destruction, termed as microscopic treatment zones (MTZs). Within these columns of tissue destruction, the production of new collagen and elastic fibers occurs. Fractionation is seen in both ablative and nonablative lasers [56]. A recent study reported the use of 1540 fractional Er:Glass *laser* in 51 patients with skin types II-IV. Subjects underwent 2 to 4 treatment sessions with 4-6 weeks intervals. After treatment sessions, non-blinded reviewers observed an overall improvement of 50% or greater for all subjects while blinded reviewers rated 14 randomly selected images and reported average to moderate (51-75%) improvement. Histologically, increased elastic fibers and new collagen formation were seen. Side effects were erythema and edema; however in 8 cases transient PIH was observed that completely resolved later [73]. Alves et al., studied the use of 1540 nm fractional Er:Glass *laser* in the treatment of corticosteroid-induced SR in four cases. Patients received treatment sessions at one month intervals. Significant improvement of SR was observed in two of the four patients after three sessions. The other two patients had similar improvement after four and six sessions, respectively. Side effects included only local erythema and edema. The authors suggest the fractional Er:Glass laser as a promising treatment modality for SR [74]. A different case series using this laser treated SD in 22 Asian women with two treatment sessions at 4 weeks intervals. The authors evaluated improvement by assessing clinical appearance and by performing histological studies. It is reported that 27% of subjects, all of whom had mature SA demonstrated marked improvement in appearance. An increase in epidermal and dermal thickness was seen in post-treatment biopsy specimens. Histologically, SR had more inflammatory cells and decreased collagen. The authors have advocated that this laser is most effective for late stage mature white *striae* owing to the significant induction of collagen production [75]. In other case series the 1550 nm erbium-doped fractional *laser* was used to treat SD. Adverse effects including transient erythema, edema and transient PIH were observed in this case series [72-76]. Most of these studies agree that this modality is generally safe and well-tolerated by patients. Additionally, clinical improvement of white *striae* was observed in many of these clinical trials.

10,600 nm fractional carbon dioxide (CO_2) *laser* has also been reported to be highly effective for ablating the epidermal layer and it can penetrate deep into the dermis. Also it has been shown that the fractional CO_2 *laser* induces neocollagenesis to a greater degree than the nonablative *lasers* due to its ability to stimulate collagen and elastin regeneration and remodeling [1]. However, due to high risk of pigmentary changes in dark skinned patients, caution is advised when treating patients with skin phototypes IV and higher [1,

51]. Lee et al., reported the use of fractional CO_2 *laser* in the treatment of SA in 27 women. The patients received one single session and were evaluated after three months. 59% of patients had marked or near total improvement in the clinical appereance of their *striae*. The treatment sessions were mostly without complication; however, posttreatment erythema, transient pruritus, hyperpigmentation, scaling or crusting, and oozing were observed in the treated area [80]. Yang et al., studied comparison of the nonablative fractional 1550 nm Er:Glass *laser* to the ablative fractional 10,600 nm CO_2 *laser* in 22 Korean female patients with abdominal atrophic *striae*. Patients received three treatment sessions at 4-week intervals with both lasers. It was shown that both lasers produced statistically significant improvement in overall clinical appereance, skin elasticity, and width of the *striae*. The fractional CO_2 *laser* was more effective than the fractional nonablative Er:Glass *laser* according to the assessment by blinded physicans and scoring by the patients themselves; although the difference was not statistically significant [81]. Future randomized controlled trials with larger sample sizes are needed to develop laser parameters that maximize positive results while minimizing the risks.

CONCLUSION

Currently, there is no single treatment modality that can significantly improve the appearance of SD. From personal clinical experience, we suggest the clinicians to consider utilizing a combination treatment modality for better results, with topical agents, mechanical techniques and/or laser and light devices, instead of a single treatment modality.

REFERENCES

[1] Ross, Nicholas A., and Derek Ho, Juliya Fisher, Andrew Mamalis, Edward Heilman, Nazanin Saedi, Jared Jagdeo. 2017. "Striae Distensae: Preventative and Therapeutic Modalities to Improve Aesthetic Appearance." *Dermatologic Surgery* 43:635-48. doi: 10.1097/DSS.0000000000001079.

[2] Chang, Anne L. S., and Yolanda Z. Agredano, Alexa B. Kimball. 2004. "Risk factors associated with striae gravidarum." *Journal of the American Academy of Dermatology* 51:881-5. Doi: 10.1016/j.jaad.2004.05.030.

[3] AL-Himdani, S., and S. UD-Din, S. Glimore, A. Bayat. 2014. "Striae distensae: a compherensive review and evidence-based evaluation of prophylaxis and treatment." *The British Journal of Dermatology* 170:527-47. doi: 10.1111/bjd.12681.

[4] Kelekci, Kiymet H., and Sefa Kelekci, Emre Destegul, Ayhan Aksoy, Necdet Sut, Bulent Yilmaz. 2011. "Prematurity: is it a risk factor for striae distensae?" *International Journal of Dermatology* 50:1240-5. doi: 10.1111/j.1365-4632.2011. 04899.x.

[5] Dosal, Jacquelyn, and Marc Z. Handler, Carlos A. Ricotti, Janelle Vega, Antonella Tosti, Francisco A. Kerdel. 2012. "Ulceration of abdominal striae distensae (stretch marks) in a cancer patient." *Archives of Dermatology* 148:385–90. doi: 10.1001/archderm.148.3.385-c.

[6] Cordeiro, R. C., and A. M. de Moraes. 2009. "Urticariform striae distensae." *Journal of the European Academy of Dermatology and Venereology* 23:340–1. doi: 10.1111/j.1468-3083.2008.02881.x.

[7] Peterson, J. L., and S. L. McMarlin, S. I. Read. 1984. "Edematous striae distensae."*Archives of Dermatology* 120:1097–8.

[8] Kumar, Vivek, and Sreenivasa S. Iyengar. 2012, "Edematous striae distensae." *Internal and Emergency Medicine* 7:159–60. doi: 10.1007/s11739-012-0782-0.

[9] Tsuji, Takuo, and Motokazu Sawabe. 1993. "Hyperpigmentation in striae distensae after bleomycin treatment." *Journal of the American Academy of Dermatology* 28:503–5.

[10] Verma, S. B. 2009. "Vitiligo precipitated by striae: a little known entity." *Journal of the European Academy of Dermatology and Venereology* 23:357–8. doi: 10.1111/j.1468-3083.2008.02844.x.

[11] Cordeiro, R. C., and A. M. Moraes. 2008. "Ulceration of striae distensae in a patient with systemic lupus erythematosus." *Journal of the European Academy of Dermatology and Venereology* 22:390–2. doi: 10.1111/j.1468-3083.2007.02343.x.

[12] Peters, Katherine B., and Thomas E. Coyle, James J. Vredenburgh, Annick Desjardins, Henry S. Friedman, David A. Reardon. 2011. "Ulceration of striae distensae in high-grade glioma patients on concurrent systemic corticosteroid and bevacizumab therapy." *Journal of Neuro-oncology* 101:155–9. doi: 10.1007/ s11060-010-0239-0.

[13] Wheeler, Helen, and Jason Black, Suzanne Webb, Han Shen. 2012. "Dehiscence of corticosteroid induced abdominal striae in a 14-year-old boy treated with bevacizumab for recurrent glioblastoma." *Journal of Child Neurology* 27:927–9. doi: 10.1177/0883073811428007.

[14] Nakajima, Kiyokazu, and Yasuyuki Kai, Keigo Yasumasa, Toshirou Nishida, Toshinori Ito, Riichiro Nezu. 2006. "Subcutaneous emphysema along cutaneous striae after laparoscopic surgery: a unique complication." *Surgical Laparoscopy, Endoscopy & Percutaneous Techniques* 16:119–21.

[15] Verma, S. B. 2009. "Striae: stretching the long list of precipitating factors for 'true koebnerization' of vitiligo, lichen planus and psoriasis." *Clinical and Experimental Dermatology* 34:880-3. doi: 10.1111/j.1365-2230.2009.03312.x.

[16] Salter, Sharon A., and Ritu S. Batra, Thomas E. Rohrer, Neeraj Kohli, Alexa B. Kimball. 2006. "Striae and pelvic relaxation: two disorders of connective tissue with a strong association." *The Journal of Investigative Dermatology* 126:1745–8. Doi: 10.1038/sj.jid.5700258.

[17] Glesby, Marshal J., and Reed E. Pyeritz. 1989. "Association of mitral valve prolapse and systemic abnormalities of connective tissue. A phenotypic continuum." *JAMA* 262:523–8.

[18] Sheikhzadeh, S., and M. L. Kusch, M. Rybczynski, C. Kade, B. Keyser, A. M. Bernhardt, M. Hillebrand, T. S. Mir, B. Fuisting, P. N. Robinson, J. Berger, V. Lorenzen, J. Schmidtke, S. Blankenberg, Y. von Kodolitsch. 2012. "A simple clinical model to estimate the probability of Marfan syndrome." *QJM* 105:527–35. doi: 10.1093/qjmed/hcs008.

[19] Atwal, G. S., and L. K. Manku, C. E. Griffiths, D. W. Polson. 2006. "Striae gravidarum in primiparae." *The British Journal of Dermatology* 155:965–9. Doi: 10.1111/j.1365-2133.2006.07427.x.

[20] White, D. J., and P. L. Schnur. 1995. "Striae distensae after augmentation mammoplasty." *Annals of Plastic Surgery* 34:16–22.

[21] Chan, W. Y., and S. Akhtar, A. R. Phipps. 2006. "Striae distensae in tissue-expanded skin in the upper arm." *Annals of Plastic Surgery* 57:240–1. Doi: 10.1097/01.sap.0000227498.84223.75.

[22] Ergun, Selma S., and R. Hakan Ozcan, Yasemin B. Kural. 2007. "Striae distensae: a rare complication resulting from overinflation of the tissue expander." *Aesthetic Plastic Surgery* 31:606–7. Doi: 10.1007/s00266-007-0033-3.

[23] Guimaraes, Paulo A., and Alessandro Haddad, Miguel Sabino Neto, Fabiana C. Lage, Lydia M. Ferreira. 2013. "Striae distensae after breast augmentation: treatment using the nonablative fractionated 1550-nm erbium glass laser." *Plastic and Reconstructive Surgery* 131:636–42. doi: 10.1097/PRS.0b013e31827c7010.

[24] Elsaie, Mohamed L., and Leslie S. Baumann, Lotfy T. Elsaaiee. 2009. "Striae Distensae (Stretch marks) and Different Modalities of Therapy: An Update." *Dermatologic Surgery* 35:563-73. doi: 10.1111/j.1524-4725.2009.01094.x.

[25] Hague, Adam, and Ardeshir Bayat. 2017. "Therapeutic targets in the management of striae distensae: A systematic review." *Journal of the American Academy of Dermatology* 77:559-568. doi: 10.1016/j.jaad.2017.02.048.

[26] Kang, Sewon, and Kwang J. Kim, Christopher E. Griffiths, Tai-Yuen Wong, Harvinder S. Talwar, Gary J. Fisher, David Gordon, Ted A. Hamilton, Charles N. Ellis, John J. Voorhees. 1996. "Topical tretinoin (retinoic acid) improves early stretch marks," *Archives of Dermatology* 132:519-26.

[27] Kang, S. 1998. "Topical tretinoin therapy for managemant of early striae." *Journal of the American Academy of Dermatology* 39:90-2.

[28] Sparavigna, A., and M. Setaro, G. Mamini, C. Rigoni. 2005. "Boswellic acid based cream is effective and well tolerated treatment for striae distensae." *J. Appl. Cosmetol.* 23:93-104.

[29] Draelos, Z. D., and M. H. Gold, M. Kaur, B. Olayinka, S. L. Grundy, E. J. Pappert, B. Hardas. 2010. "Evaluation of an onion extract, Centella asiatica, and hyaluronic acid cream in the appearance of striae rubra." *Skinmed* 8:80-6.

[30] Morganti, P., and P. Palombo, G. Fabrizi, M. Palombo, S. Persechino. 2001. "Biweekly in office treatment of striae distensae: a long term daily use of topical vitamin C." *J. Appl. Cosmetol.* 19:107-12.

[31] Ud-Din, Sara, and Sarah-Louise McAnelly, Alison Bowring, Sigrid Whiteside, Julie Morris, Iskander Chaudhry, Ardeshir Bayat. 2013. "A double-blind controlled clinical trial assessing the effect of topical gels on striae distensae (stretch marks): a non-invasive imaging, morphological and immunohistochemical study." *Archives of Dermatological Research* 305:603-17. doi: 10.1007/s00403-013-1336-7.

[32] Taavoni, Simin, and Farzaneh Soltanipour, Hamid Haghani, Masoomeh Kheirkhah. 2011. "Effects of olive oil on striae gravidarum in the second trimester of pregnancy." *Complementary Therapies in Clinical Practice* 17:167–9.

[33] Timur Tashan, Sermin, and Ayse Kafkasli. 2012. "The effect of bitter almond oil and massaging on striae gravidarum in primiparous women." *Journal of Clinical Nursing* 21:1570–6. doi: 10.1111/j.1365-2702.2012.04087.x.

[34] Mazzarello, Vittorio, and Francesco Farace, Pasquale Ena, Grazia Fenu, Pietro Mulas, Luisella Piu, Corrado Rubino. 2012. "A superficial texture analysis of 70% glycolic acid topical therapy and striae distensae. " *Plastic and Reconstriuctive Surgery* 129:589–90. doi: 10.1097/PRS.0b013e3182419c40.

[35] Adatto, M. A., and P. Deprez. 2003. "Striae treated by a novel combination treatment-sand abrasion and a patent mixture containing 15% trichloracetic acid followed by 6–24 hrs of a patent cream under plastic occlusion." *Journal of Cosmetic Dermatology* 2:61–7. doi: 10.1111/j.1473-2130.2004.00023.x.

[36] Deprez, Philippe. 2000. "Easy peel for the treatment of stretch marks." *International Journal of Cosmetic Surgery and Aesthetic Dermatology* 2:201–4. Doi: 10.1089/153082000750062894.

[37] Ash, K., and J. Lord, M. Zukowski. 1998. "Comparison of topical therapy for striae alba (20% glycolic acid/0.05% tretinoin versus 20% glycolic acid/10% L-ascorbic acid)." *Dermatologic Surgery* 24:849–56.

[38] Cook, Kim K., and William R. Cook Jr. 2000. "Chemical peel of nonfacial skin using glycolic acid gel augmented with TCA and neutralized based on visual staging." *Dermatologic Surgery* 26:994–9.

[39] Zeitter, S., and Z. Sikora, S. Jahn, F. Stahl, S. Strauß, A. Lazaridis, K. Reimers, P. M. Vogt, M. C. Aust. 2014. "Microneedling: matching the results of medical

needling and repetitive treatments to maximize potential for skin regeneration." *Burns* 40:966–73. doi: 10.1016/j.burns.2013.12.008.

[40] Aust, M. C., and K. Reimers, H. M. Kaplan, F. Stahl, C. Repenning, T. Scheper, S. Jahn, N. Schwaiger, R. Ipaktchi, J. Redeker, M. A. Altintas, P. M. Vogt. 2011. "Percutaneous collagen induction-regeneration in place of cicatrisation?" *Journal of Plastic, Reconstructive & Aesthetic Surgery* 64:97–107. doi: 10.1016/j.bjps. 2010.03.038.

[41] Khater, Mohamed H., and Fathia M. Khattab, Manal R. Abdelhaleem. 2016. "Treatment of striae distensae with needling therapy versus CO fractional laser." *Journal of Cosmetic and Laser Therapy* 18:75–9. doi: 10.3109/14764172. 2015.1063665.

[42] Aust, Matthias C., and Karsten Knobloch, Peter M. Vogt. 2010. "Percutaneous collagen induction therapy as a novel therapeutic option for striae distensae." *Plastic and Reconstructive Surgery* 126:219e–20e. doi: 10.1097/PRS.0b013e 3181ea93da.

[43] Park, Kui Y., and Hyun K. Kim, Sung E. Kim, Beom J. Kim, Myeung N. Kim. 2012. "Treatment of striae distensae using needling therapy: a pilot study." *Dermatologic Surgery* 38:1823–8. doi: 10.1111/j.1524-4725.2012.02552.x.

[44] Nassar, Amani, and Soheir Ghomcy, Yosria El Gohary, Fatma El-Desoky. 2016. "Treatment of striae distensae with needling therapy versus microdermabrasion with sonophoresis." *Journal of Cosmetic and Laser Therapy* 18:330–4. doi: 10.1080/14764172.2016.1175633.

[45] Luis-Montoya, P., and P. Pichardo-Velazquez, M. T. Hojyo-Tomoka, J. Dominguez-Cherit. 2005. "Evaluation of subcision as a treatment for cutaneous striae." *Journal of Drugs in Dermatology* 4:346–50.

[46] Karimipour, Darius J., and Sewon Kang, Timothy M. Johnson, Jeffrey S. Orringer, Ted Hamilton, Craig Hammerberg, John J. Voorhees, Gary Fisher. 2005. "Microdermabrasion: a molecular analysis following a single treatment." *Journal of the American Academy of Dermatology* 52:215–23. Doi: 10.1016/j.jaad. 2004.10.008.

[47] Abdel-Latif, A. M., and A. S. Albendary. 2008. "Treatment of striae distensae with microdermabrasion: a clinical and molecular study." *Journal of Egyptian Women's Dermatologic Society* 5:24–30.

[48] Ibrahim, Zeinab A., and Rania A. El-Tatawy, Marwa A. El-Samongy, Dareen A. Ali. 2015. "Comparison between the efficacy and safety of platelet-rich plasma vs. microdermabrasion in the treatment of striae distensae: clinical and histopathological study." *Journal of Cosmetic Dermatology* 14:336–46. doi: 10.1111/jocd.12160.

[49] Bitencourt, Shanna, and Adroaldo Lunardelli, Robson H. Amaral, Henrique B. Dias, Emerson S. Boschi, Jarbas R. de Oliveira. 2016. "Safety and patient

subjective efficacy of using galvanopuncture for the treatment of striae distensae." *Journal of Cosmetic Dermatology* 15:393–8. doi: 10.1111/jocd.12222.

[50] Gamil, Hend D., and Samia A. Ibrahim, Howyda M. Ebrahim, Waleed Albalat. 2018. "Platelet-Rich Plasma Versus Tretinoin Treatment of Striae Distensae. A Comparative Study." *Dermatologic Surgery* 44:697-704. doi: 10.1097/DSS.00000 00000001408.

[51] Savas, J. A., and J. A. Ledon, K. Franca, K. Nouri. 2014. "Lasers and lights for the treatment of striae distensae." *Lasers in Medical Science* 29:1735-43. doi: 10.1007/s10103-013-1342-1.

[52] Hernandez-Perez, Enrique, and Emilio Colombo-Charrier, Erick Valencia-Ibiett. 2002. "Intense pulsed light in the treatment of striae distensae." *Dermatologic Surgery* 28:1124–30.

[53] Trelles, M. A., and J. L. Levy, I. Ghersetich. 2008. "Effects achieved on stretch marks by a nonfractional broadband infrared light system treatment." *Aesthetic Plastic Surgery* 32:523–30. doi: 10.1007/s00266-008-9115-0.

[54] Shokeir, Hisham, and Ahmed El Bedewi, Safinaz Sayed, Ghada El Khalafawy. 2014. "Efficacy of pulsed dye laser versus intense pulsed light in the treatment of striae distensae." *Dermatologic Surgery* 40:632–40. doi: 10.1111/dsu.00000000 00000007.

[55] Al-Dhalimi, Muhsin A., and Ali A. Abo Nasyria. 2013. "A comparative study of the effectiveness of intense pulsed light wavelengths (650 nm vs 590 nm) in the treatment of striae distensae." *Journal of Cosmetic and Laser Therapy* 15:120–5. doi: 10.3109/14764172.2012.748200.

[56] Aldahan, Adam S., and Vidhi V. Shah, Stephanie Mlacker, Sahal Samarkandy, Mohammed Alsaidan, Keyvan Nouri. 2016. "Laser and Light Treatments for Striae Distensae: A Comprehensive Review of the Literature." *American Journal of Clinical Dermatology* 17:239-56. doi: 10.1007/s40257-016-0182-8.

[57] Sadick, Neil S., and Cynthia Magro, Alison Hoenig. 2007. "Prospective clinical and histological study to evaluate the efficacy and safety of a targeted highintensity narrow band UVB/UVA1 therapy for striae alba." *Journal of Cosmetic and Laser Therapy* 9:79–83. doi: 10.1080/14764170701313767.

[58] Harmelin, Yona, and Dominique Boineau, Nathalie Cardot-Leccia, Eric Fontas, Philippe Bahadoran, Anne-Lise Becker, Henri Montaudié, Emeline Castela, Christophe Perrin, Jean-Philippe Lacour, Thierry Passeron. 2016. "Fractionated bipolar radiofrequency and bipolar radiofrequency potentiated by infrared light for treating striae: a prospective randomized, comparative trial with objective evaluation." *Lasers in Surgery and Medicine* 48:245–53. doi: 10.1002/lsm.22458.

[59] Naeini, Farahnaz F., and Shadi Behfar, Bahareh Abtahi-Naeini, Shima Keyvan, Mohsen Pourazizi. 2016. "Promising option for treatment of striae alba:

fractionated microneedle radiofrequency in combination with fractional carbon dioxide laser." *Dermatology Research and Practice* 2016:2896345.

[60] Manuskiatti, Woraphong, and Einapak Boonthaweeyuwat, Supenya Varothai. 2009. "Treatment of striae distensae with a TriPollar radiofrequency device: a pilot study." *The Journal of Dermatological Treatment* 20:359–64. doi: 10.3109/09546630903085278.

[61] Suh, Dong-Hye, and Ka-Yeun Chang, Ho-Chan Son, Ji-Ho Ryu, Sang-Jun Lee, Kye-Yong Song. 2007 "Radiofrequency and 585- nm pulsed dye laser treatment of striae distensae: a report of 37 Asian patients." *Dermatologic Surgery* 33:29–34. Doi: 10.1111/j.1524-4725.2007.33004.x.

[62] Ryu, Han-Won, and Sung-Ae Kim, Hye R. Jung, Young-Wook Ryoo, Kyu-Suk Lee, Jae-We Cho. 2013. "Clinical improvement of striae distensae in Korean patients using a combination of fractionated microneedle radiofrequency and fractional carbon dioxide laser." *Dermatologic Surgery* 39:1452–8. doi: 10.1111/dsu.12268.

[63] Kim, In S., and Kui Y. Park, Beom J. Kim, Myeung N. Kim, Chan W. Kim, Sung E. Kim. 2012. "Efficacy of intradermal radiofrequency combined with autologous platelet-rich plasma in striae distensae: a pilot study." *International Journal of Dermatology* 51:1253–8. doi: 10.1111/j.1365-4632.2012.05530.x.

[64] Suh, Dong-Hye, and Sang-Jun Lee, Jong-Ho Lee, Hyun-Ju Kim, Min-Kyung Shin, Kye-Yong Song. 2012. "Treatment of striae distensae combined enhanced penetration platelet-rich plasma and ultrasound after plasma fractional radiofrequency." *Journal of Cosmetic and Laser Therapy* 14:272–6. doi: 10.3109/14764172.2012.738916.

[65] Goldberg, David J., and Dale Sarradet, Mussarrat Hussain. 2003. "308-nm Excimer laser treatment of mature hypopigmented striae." *Dermatologic Surgery* 29: 596–8.

[66] Alexiades-Armenakas, Macrene R., and Leonard J. Bernstein, Paul M. Friedman, Roy G. Geronemus. 2004. "The safety and efficacy of the 308-nm excimer laser for pigment correction of hypopigmented scars and striae alba." *Archives of Dermatology* 140:955–60. doi: 10.1001/archderm.140.8.955.

[67] Ostovari, Nima, and Nelda Saadat, Sohelina Nasiri, Hamideh Moravvej, Parviz Toossi. 2010. "The 308-nm excimer laser in the darkening of the white lines of striae alba." *The Journal of Dermatological Treatment* 21:229–31. doi: 10.3109/09546631003592044.

[68] McDaniel, David H., and Keith Ash, Mark Zukowski. 1996. "Treatment of stretch marks with the 585-nm flashlamp-pumped pulsed dye laser." *Dermatologic Surgery* 22:332–7.

[69] Jimenez, Gloria P., and Francisco Flores, Brian Berman, Zeenat Gunja-Smith. 2003. "Treatment of striae rubra and striae alba with the 585-nm pulsed-dye laser." *Dermatologic Surgery* 29:362–5.

[70] Longo, M., and M. G. Postiglione, O. Marangoni, M. Melato. 2003. "Two-year follow up results of copper bromide laser treatment of striae." *Journal of Clinical Laser Medicine & Surgery* 21:157–60. doi: 10.1089/104454703321895617.

[71] Goldman, Alberto, and Flavia Rossato, Clarissa Pratti. 2008. "Stretch marks: treatment using the 1,064 nm Nd:YAG laser." *Dermatologic Surgery* 34:1–7. doi: 10.1111/j.1524-4725.2008.34129.x.

[72] Tay, Yong-Kwang, and Colin Kwok, Eileen Tan. 2006. "Non-ablative 1,450-nm diode laser treatment of striae distensae." *Lasers in Surgery and Medicine* 38:196–9. Doi: 10.1002/lsm.20281.

[73] De Angelis, Francesca, and Larissa Kolesnikova, Franco Renato, Giuseppina Liguori. 2011. "Fractional nonablative 1540-nm laser treatment of striae distensae in Fitzpatrick skin types II to IV: clinical and histological results." *Aesthetic Surgery Journal* 31:411–419. doi: 10.1177/1090820X11402493.

[74] Alves, Renata O., and Maria F. Boin, Elisete I. Crocco. 2015. "Striae after topical corticosteroid: treatment with nonablative fractional laser 1540nm." *Journal of Cosmetic and Laser Therapy* 17:143–7. doi: 10.3109/14764172.2014.1003243.

[75] Bak, Hana, and Beom J. Kim, Woo J. Lee, Jang S. Bang, Sun Y. Lee, Jee H.. Choi, Sung E. Chang. 2009. "Treatment of striae distensae with fractional photothermolysis." *Dermatologic Surgery* 35:1215–20. doi: 10.1111/j.1524-4725.2009.01221.x.

[76] Stotland, M, and A. M. Chapas, L. Brightman, S. Sukal, E. Hale, J. Karen, L. Bernstein, R. G. Geronemus. 2008. "The safety and efficacy of fractional photothermolysis for the correction of striae distensae." *Journal of Drugs in Dermatology* 7:857–61.

[77] Guimaraes, Paulo A., and Alessandra Haddad, Miguel S. Neto, Fabiana C. Lage, Lydia M. Ferreira. 2013. "Striae distensae after breast augmentation: treatment using the nonablative fractionated 1550-nm erbium glass laser." *Plastic and Reconstructive Surgery* 131:636–42. doi: 10.1097/PRS.0b013e31827c7010.

[78] Kim, Beom J., and Dong H. Lee, Myeung N. Kim, Kye Y. Song, Wan I. Cho, Chang K. Lee, Jo Y. Kim, Oh S. Kwon. 2008. "Fractional photothermolysis for the treatment of striae distensae in Asian skin." *American Journal of Clinical Dermatology* 9:33–7. Doi: 10.2165/00128071-200809010-00003.

[79] Katz, Tracy M., and Leonard H. Goldberg, Paul M. Friedman. 2009. "Nonablative fractional photothermolysis for the treatment of striae rubra." *Dermatologic Surgery* 35:1430–3. doi: 10.1111/j.1524-4725.2009.01252.x.

[80] Lee, Sang E., and Jong H. Kim, Sang J. Lee., Jung E. Lee, Jin M. Kang, Young K. Kim, Dongsik Bang, Sung B. Cho. 2010. "Treatment of striae distensae using an ablative 10,600-nm carbon dioxide fractional laser: a retrospective review of 27 participants." *Dermatologic Surgery* 36:1683–1690. doi: 10.1111/j.1524-4725.2010.01719.x.

[81] Yang, You J., and Ga-Young Lee. 2011. "Treatment of striae distensae with nonablative fractional laser versus ablative CO_2 fractional laser: a randomized controlled trial." *Annals of Dermatology* 23:481–489. doi: 10.5021/ad.2011.23.4.481.

In: Cutaneous Scars: Biology, Clinics and Management ISBN: 978-1-53615-657-7
Editors: Berna Aksoy, Hasan Mete Aksoy et al. © 2019 Nova Science Publishers, Inc.

Chapter 28

HAIR TRANSPLANTATION FOR SCARS IN HAIR BEARING SKIN

Ekrem Civas*
Dermatology Specialist, Private Civas Clinic, Ankara, Turkey

ABSTRACT

Appropriate patient selection as well as correct planning can lead to better hair transplantation results in cicatricial alopecia (scars in hair bearing skin) patients. Currently, there is no medical treatment that can regenerate lost hair. Unfortunately stem cell is not yet available as a treatment option. The most important criterion in primary cicatricial alopecia is that the scar should be in the stable period during the procedure. It is recommended that such patients undertake the procedure at least one year after the stabilization period. In patients who are eligible for primary scar excision, the best cosmetic results can be obtained by performing hair transplantation on the remaining scar after excision.

Keywords: cicatricial alopecia, FUE, FUT, hair transplantation

1. INTRODUCTION

Cicatricial alopecias (syn. scarring alopecias; permanent alopecias) are an uncommon and clinically diverse set of disorders that result in permanent and irreversible hair loss in the scalp, often leading to major disfigurement, discomfort, and psychological distress. Clinically, this form of irreversible hair loss is characterized by the

*Corresponding Author's Email: ekremcivas@yahoo.com.

disappearance of visible follicular ostia within an area of alopecia. *Cicatricial alopecia* is one of the most difficult diseases that is encountered by dermatologists in daily practice to diagnose and treat. Patients are psychologically affected by the presence of a visible scar on the scalp. This may in turn lead to lack of self-confidence [1].

Cicatricial alopecias are categorized into 3 classes;

1. Primary cicatricial alopecia (PCA),
2. Secondary cicatricial alopecia (SCA),
3. Developmental or hereditary cicatricial alopecia.

The main clinical characteristics of *cicatricial alopecias* are; depletion of visible follicular ostia on the scar, atrophy of the epidermis in some cases, and lack of pilosebaceous structures which are replaced by fibrous tracts [2].

2. EPIDEMIOLOGY

There is very limited data available on the epidemiology of *cicatricial alopecia*. One study shows that only about 7.3% of all hair loss cases are caused by *cicatricial alopecia*, and females are more commonly affected than males [3, 4].

Primary *cicatricial alopecia* is much more prevalent than secondary in the ratio of 4:1. The most common causes of PCA were pseudopelade of Brocq (PPB) (40.6%), lichen planopilaris (LPP) (12.6%) and folliculitis decalvans (FD) (11.2%) respectively [2]. Primary *Cicatricial Alopecia* is not uncommon. It accounts for about 7% of the patients who applied with hair loss to hair diseases clinic. In secondary *cicatricial alopecia*, unlike primary *cicatricial alopecia*, the follicle bulge may not completely be destroyed at the beginning; for this reason, the damage on the hair follicle can be reversed by effective treatment during the initial periods of the disease [3, 4].

3. CLASSIFICATION

3.1. Primary Cicatricial Alopecia (PCA)

Primary *cicatricial alopecia* (PCA) is in the category of hair loss diseases where the hair follicle is completely destroyed and is replaced by fibrous tissue. PCA is irreversible since the epithelial stem cells in the bulge of the outer root sheath are destroyed and hence it is impossible to regenerate new hair [3, 5].

Clinical findings related to PCA are diffuse or perifollicular erythema, follicular hyperkeratosis, pigment changes, tufting and pustules.

Table 1. Primary cicatricial alopecias [6].

Lymphocytic Primary Cicatricial Alopecia 1. Discoid lupus erythematosus [DLE] 2. Lichen planopilaris (LPP) (a) Classic LPP (b) Frontal fibrosing alopecia (FFA) (c) Graham-Little syndrome 3. Classic pseudopelade of Brocq (PPB) 4. Central centrifugal cicatricial alopecia (CCCA) 5. Alopecia mucinosa (AM) 6. Keratosis follicularis spinulosa decalvans (KFSD)
Neutrophilic Primary Cicatricial Alopecia. 1. Folliculitis decalvans (FD) 2. Dissecting cellulitis/folliculitis (perifolliculitis capitis abscedens et suffodiens)
Mixed Cicatricial Alopecia. 1. Folliculitis (acne) keloidalis 2. Folliculitis (acne) necrotica 3. Erosive pustular dermatosis

The patients develop one or more patches, and follicular openings disappear in the scarred regions. The skin appears shinier. In the advanced stages, scar lesions histologically resemble each other – known as pseudopelade of Brocq. The group of PCA can precisely be distinguished during the early stages of inflammation [3, 5].

Diagnosis of primary cicatricial alopecia can be done by dermoscopic examination, reflectance confocal microscopy, histopathology and direct immunofluorescence study [6].

Table 2. Causes of Secondary Cicatricial Alopecia [5]

Genodermatoses and developmental defects with permanent alopecia
Physical and chemical injury
Infections
Inflammatory dermatoses
Drugs
Neoplastic

3.2. Secondary Cicatricial Alopecia (SCA)

Even though Secondary *Cicatricial Alopecia* (SCA) is irreversible, destruction of the follicle is caused by extrinsic factors that do not directly target the follicle itself such as burns, radiation, and trauma. The size of the scar and the extent of skin damage vary according to the severity or depth of injury. Loss of follicular orifices is the most common characteristic of SCA. Late stage and localized SCA can only possibly be distinguished with the help of patient's history [5, 7].

4. Surgical Treatment Methods

In *cicatricial alopecia*, the only way to restore hair back on the scar region is through stem cell therapy or through *hair transplantation*. Unfortunately, the treatment of hair loss through stem cell technology is not yet possible. Surgical correction of the *cicatricial alopecia* can be performed in 3 ways:

1. Surgical excision
2. *Hair Transplantation*
3. Surgical excision and *hair transplantation*

This section will mainly emphasize the treatment of scalp lesions with *hair transplantation* [8].

5. Hair Transplantation in the Cicatricial Alopecias

5.1. Appropriate Candidate Selection

SCAs are considered stable after scar formation is complete. When planning treatment for these patients, the patient is only evaluated in terms of risks of the procedure and results that can be achieved with surgery. If satisfactory results are likely to be obtained, then the patient is accepted as an appropriate candidate for surgical treatment.

In PCA, it is necessary to evaluate the disease activity before deciding that the patient is a suitable candidate for surgery. Itching and pain in the lesion may be a sign that the disease is still active. Additionally, perifollicular erythema, pustules, and perifollicular scaling during examination can also indicate that the disease is active [6, 8, 9].

At this point, there is no precise information about when the PCA scar formation becomes completed and when disease becomes inactive. *Hair transplantation* for PCA is still a controversial topic of discussion. There are limited publications about it and most of the available information derives from only case reports. Some publications state that a patient in the stable condition should wait at least 1 year before hair transplantation, while others suggest 2 years. From my own experience, the patient should wait at least 2 years [6, 8, 10, 11].

Even if the patient is considered to be in the stable stage, careful clinical and dermoscopic examination should be performed. If the disease is suspected to be active a test session with 200 grafts should be performed on a small scarred area. After the test session, the patient should undergo regular checks for 6 months. Erythema, itching and hair loss on the donor or recipient area may be signs of reactivation. Medical treatment should be started in patients who are thought to be reactivated. Patients without reactivation for 6 months can be accepted as stable and the surgical procedure can be planned.

In both primary and secondary *cicatricial alopecia*, the patient expectations play a very important role in patient selection. Before the surgery, the treating doctor should explain the expected hair density on the scar tissue and the resulting decreased hair density of the donor areas to the patient in detail. Patients who do not have realistic expectations are not good candidates for the procedure.

5.2. Planning

Planning is the most important key to a successful classic or *cicatricial alopecia* hair transplant. Before the procedure, the size of the scar, scar tissue characteristics, donor capacity, patient's expectations and priorities should be taken into account.

In addition, male patients should be examined for the possibility of Androgenetic Alopecia (AGA) in the future. Genetic history of the patient and signs of miniaturization should be examined carefully. In areas where there is a possibility of future hair loss, transplanted scarred areas will be seen from outside as individual islands of hairy scalp in regions with no hair, which can disrupt the natural look.

5.3. Clinical Evaluation before the Procedure

5.3.1. Primary Cicatricial Alopecia

Proper diagnosis of PCA can be done through medical history, physical examination of the scalp and skin biopsies [1]. Symptoms such as pruritus and pain may indicate that the disease is in the active phase. Erythema, follicular hyperkeratosis, pigment changes, tufting, and pustules are among the clinical indications of the active disease [6, 11].

Clinical findings pointing to PCA may be diffuse or perifollicular erythema, follicular hyperkeratosis, pigment changes, tufting and pustules. Hair transplantion is suitable for patients with suitable occipital donor area but the disease must be in its burn out stage – with no inflammation or progression for at least 2 years without any treatment [1, 6, 11].

5.3.2. Secondary Cicatricial Alopecia

5.3.2.1. Scar Characteristics

Scars can be either atrophic or hypertrophic. In atrophic scars, the thickness of the scar and vascular circulation should be examined. Graft survival will be low in scars that have poor circulation. To understand the circulation level, Dr. Unger recommends making a few incisions with a 19G needle under local anesthesia and monitoring bleeding. A scar tissue with good bleeding is a suitable candidate recipient site for hair transplantation. Patients with poor bleeding should be considered as bad candidates in terms of vascular circulation. For such patients, an initial *hair transplantation* session with low graft density should be planned [8].

5.3.2.2. Excision or Transplantation?

Where possible, primary excision should always be the first choice. For patients who have large lesions or those who do not have enough donor hair to cover the whole scar, excision can be done first then *hair transplantation* is performed to cover the remaining scar area. *Hair transplantation* should always be the most preferred option for patients who have scars in openly visible areas such as the hairline because excision could leave an additional scar (Figure 1) [8, 12, 13].

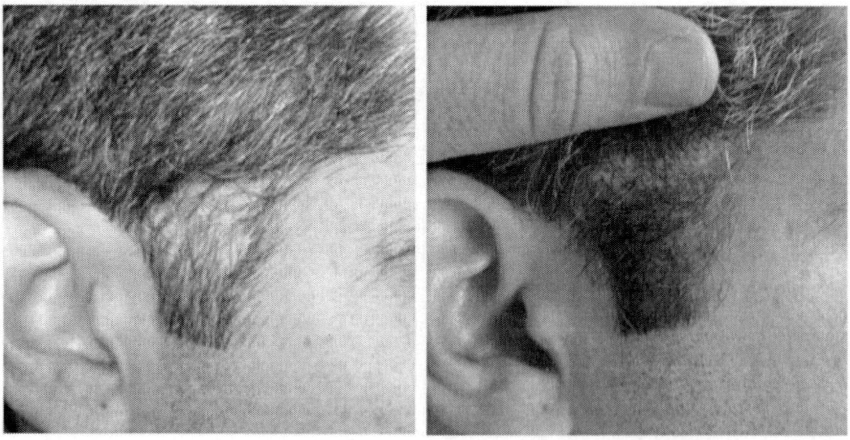

Figure 1. Long term result of hair transplantation for coverage of an openly visible secondary cicatricial alopecia site.

5.4. Surgical Technique for Hair Transplantation

There are three main stages of the *hair transplantation* surgery: anesthesia, graft extraction and graft implantation.

5.4.1. Anesthesia

Depending on the location of the scar and the number of grafts needed, anesthesia can be performed in a small area in the form of infiltration anesthesia. In cases of large scars or large number of grafts needed, ring block or nerve block anesthesia can be done on the whole donor and recipient areas. Effective and safe cranial nerve analgesia can be achieved with blocking of sensory scalp nerves; supraorbital nerve, supratrochlear nerve, zygomaticotemporal nerve, auriculotemporal nerve, lesser occipital nerve and greater occipital nerves [14].

Short duration local anesthetics such as lidocaine and prilocaine and long lasting local anesthetics such as bupivacaine can be used in combination for anesthesia. Adding epinephrine to the local anesthetics prolongs the duration of the anesthetic effect. Addition of epinephrine also reduces the risk of toxicity and bleeding [14].

5.4.2. Tumescent

Tumescent is applied differently on the donor area where the follicles are obtained and the recipient area where the grafts are implanted. The most important advantage of tumescent fluid is to control hemostasis in both donor and recipient areas. In cicatricial alopecia, the ratio of epinephrine used in the tumescent solution is very crucial. The ratio of epinephrine used should be determined according to the blood circulation of the scar tissue. Addition of epinephrine to tumescent solution can cause graft or tissue necrosis when scars have poor circulation. For normal tissue, 1/100,000 is used, the ratio can be reduced down to 1/250,000 in scarred tissue. In fact for some scars there's no need to use epinepherine [14, 15].

5.4.3. Extraction of Grafts

Grafts can be obtained by 2 different methods; strip technique or *FUT* (Follicular unit transplantation) and extraction of grafts one by one through *FUE* technique (Follicular unit extraction/excision).

5.4.3.1. FUT

Separation of the Follicular units (FU) under the microscope is performed after a hair bearing skin strip is excised from the scalp. The strip length and width vary according to the number of grafts required [8, 16].

The following conditions must be considered before *FUT* operation.

1. Patients with scars on the donor area: Scarring in the donor area is common, especially in patients with primary *cicatricial alopecia*. Therefore, the strip from the donor area may not contain enough grafts. However, strip excision can be considered if primary scar excision is performed.
2. *FUT* comes with the risk of creating a new scar in the donor area. Patients may not prefer this option.
3. The *FUT* procedure may not be appropriate for patients in need of a small test session because this will be extremely traumatic.
4. For patients with androgenetic alopecia who need high number of grafts, with an unaffected donor area; *FUT* may be considered in the first session then *FUE* is performed afterwards [8, 16].

5.4.3.2. FUE

In *FUE* after a 3-4 mm deep incision is made around the follicular unit, extraction is done by using forceps. This process is preferably termed as Follicular Unit Excision instead of Follicular Unit Extraction [17, 18].

The *FUE* technique can be performed by three methods; manual, motor assisted and robotic. The choice of technique is up to the physician's preference [15, 17].

5.4.3.2.1. Manual FUE

The graft extraction procedure is done manually with the help of a punch. To reduce transsection rates, Dr. Harris defined a 3-step *FUE* method. After making a 1mm deep cut with sharp punch, a blunt punch is used to deepen the incision. Finally, the extracted FUs are collected by forceps. Blunt punch is used to reduce the rate of transection. In recent years, punches have also become specialized according to the skin structure of the patient and the technique of the surgeon [17, 19].

5.4.3.2.2. Motorized FUE

This process uses the punch together with the motor in the desired rotation direction and speed. It allows the surgeon to better control the punch. In the early days, the motor method was not used very often because of the high rates of transsection of the grafts and because it did not allow sharp and blunt punches to be used at the same time. However it has been widely used as a consequence of increased experience and production of increasingly standardized punches, especially after 2010. Today it's easy to obtain about 1500 grafts in an hour with the help of the motor technique. The only difference between manual and motorized *FUE* method is that in motorized *FUE*, the incision is made with the help of the motor. The grafts are then harvested in the same manner with the aid of forceps [17, 20, 21].

5.4.3.2.3. Robotic FUE

Robotic *FUE* was approved by the FDA in 2011. The robot, remotely controlled by the physician helps extract grafts by using *FUE* method. After a sharp punch makes an incision 1mm deep, then the blunt punch is advanced down to the fat tissue. Thanks to special software, the system-operating surgeon can adjust the entry angle much more easily.

In addition, visible scar formation risks and overharvesting are reduced since the system requires a minimum distance of 1.6 mm between extracted follicular groupings. The rates of graft transection and daily graft extraction numbers are not yet at the desired level. Since the doctor and the technician have to actively participate in the process, they have not yet fully removed the need for a technician [22].

5.4.3.2.4. Advantages of the FUE Method in Cicatricial Alopecia Patients

1. There is no significant formation of new scarring: The punches used in the *FUE* method are only 1 mm or less in diameter and resulting scars are only noticeable when looked at very closely.
2. There is availability of alternative donor sites (such as chest, beard). Body hair may be used as donor when there is insufficient occipital donor in cicatricial alopecia patients.
3. You can obtain as many grafts as needed for small recipient areas (Figure 2).
4. Grafts can be obtained from stable unscarred areas in partially scarred donor sites [17].

5.4.4. Recipient Area Preparation

This stage consists of anesthesia and tumescent administration and opening of the channels. Adrenaline dosage should be determined according to the scar circulation and scar quality for both primary and secondary cicatricial alopecia. It is recommended that the adrenaline dosage should be reduced or adrenaline even should not be used when scars that have bad vascular circulation or excessively atrophic scars are treated. Otherwise the graft survival rate may be reduced [8, 15].

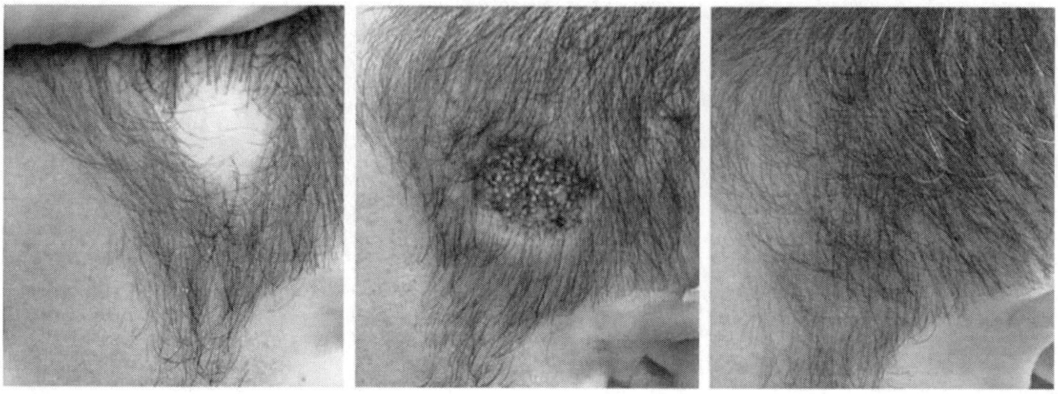

Figure 2. The immediate and long term result of hair transplantation for secondary cicatricial alopecia with transplantation of 100 grafts obtained by using FUE technique.

5.4.5. Opening of Channels

For scars with poor circulation and atrophic scars, channel density should be kept low in the first session. High density of channels may lead to both graft and tissue necrosis. The channel width and depth must be adjusted according to the size of the grafts. The size of the incision sites depends on the scar characteristics. To prevent grafts from popping out, smaller sites are required for scars with little laxity and dermal recoil. Large sites should be made for tight scars with poor laxity and more fibrous tissue with high recoil [8, 23].

Channels should be opened in angles parallel to the existing hair. If there is no hair around the scar tissue, the channels should be opened at 30-45 degrees in accordance with existing scalp hair [8, 13, 23].

Transplantation of grafts on scars that are located on the hairline should be planned according to the patient's current hairline. However, it is important to be cautious about patients who have a family history of hair loss or those patients who show signs of miniaturization. When the patient's hairline recedes as a result of genetic hair loss, the remaining transplanted hair on the scar will cause an unnatural appearance [8, 13, 23].

5.4.6. Graft Implantation

It is usually performed by two or three technicians with the use of forceps. Although automatic implanters have been produced for this purpose in recent years, manual method is still preferred because these automatic implanters may cause graft damage. Attention should be paid to graft hydration during the implantation. An experienced technician can transfer 400-500 grafts per hour.

5.5. Postoperative Period

Unlike classical hair transplantation patients, scarred patients should be followed more carefully, especially in terms of risk of necrosis. The first wash can be done 24-48 hours after the surgery. They should particularly be instructed to be extremely careful for the first 10 days for the development of infection and necrosis [8, 24].

6. Other Surgical Methods

Small, flexible scars can be excised in the form of simple primary scar excision, and in the same way, large and taut scars which cannot be excised primarily can be excised after sufficient skin flexibility is obtained by using an expander or extender. If necessary, hair transplantation can be planned on the remaining scars after excision. Hair transplantation should be performed 3-6 months after scar excision [8, 13].

Conclusion

Unfortunately, for scars in hair bearing sites, there is no medical treatment that can remove or conceal the scar. Optimal results can only be obtained with use of surgery for appropriate patients and with good planning. In PCA the most important determinant for successful surgical results is whether the disease is stabilized or not. However, the issue of whether the disease will reactivate after a long period of stabilization is not exactly clear. Hair transplantation surgical treatment approaches of PCA patients who are believed to be definitively stable is not different from those of SCA.

The limit of surgical treatment will be determined by the size of the area to be covered and the amount of donor available. In cases where the donor is inadequate, if possible excision can be done first, followed by hair transplant. Primary excision should be the first choice in appropriate patients. In unsuitable patients, excision then hair transplantation can provide maximum aesthetic results.

References

[1] Shapiro, Jerry. 2008. 'Cicatricial alopecias.' Dermatologic Therapy 21:211 doi: 10.1111/j.1529-8019.2008.00201.

[2] Dogra, Sunil, and Rishu Sarangal. 2013. 'What's new in cicatricial alopecia?' Indian *Journal of Dermatology Venereology Leprology* 79:576-90 Doi: 10.4103/0378-6323.116726.

[3] Filbrandt, Rebecca, and Nicholas Rufaut, Leslie Jones, and Rodney Sinclair. 2013. 'Primary cicatricial alopecia: diagnosis and treatment.' *Canadian Medical Association Journal* 185:1579–85. doi: 10.1503/cmaj.111570.

[4] Gordon, Katherine A., and Antonella Tosti. 2011. 'Clinical Alopecia: evaluation and treatment.' *Cosmetic and Investigational Dermatology* 4:101–6 doi: 10.2147/CCID.S10182.

[5] Finner, Andreas M., and Nina Otberg, Jerry Shapiro. 2008. 'Secondary cicatricial and other permanent alopecias.' *Dermatologic Therapy* 21:279-94. Doi: 10.1111/j.1529-8019.2008.00210.x.

[6] Otberg, Nina, and Wen-Yu Wu, Kevin J. McElwee, Jerry Shapiro. 2008. 'Diagnosis and management of primary cicatricial alopecia: part I.' *Skinmed* 7:19-26.

[7] Kutlubay, Zekai, and Murat Kucuktas, Burhan Engin. 2013. 'Hair Transplantation in the Cicatricial Alopecias.' *Hair: Therapy & Transplantation* 3:109. doi:10.4172/2167-0951.1000109.

[8] Unger, Walter, and Robin Unger, Wesley Carlos. 2008. 'The surgical treatment of cicatricial alopecia.' *Dermatologic Therapy* 21:295–311. doi: 10.1111/j.1529-8019.2008.00211.x.

[9] Toledo-Pastrana, Tomás, and María J. G. Hernández, Francisco M. Camacho Martínez. 2013. 'Perifollicular Erythema as a Trichoscopy Sign of Progression in Frontal Fibrosing Alopecia.' *International Journal of Trichology* 5:151-3. doi: 10.4103/0974-7753.125616.

[10] Jimenez, Francisco, and Enrique Poblet. 2013. 'Is Hair Transplantation Indicated in Frontal Fibrosing Alopecia? The Results of Test Grafting in Three Patients.' *Dermatologic Surgery* 39:1115-8. DOI: 10.1111/dsu.12232

[11] Civaş, Ekrem, and Andac Aykan, Berna Aksoy, Muhitdin Eski. 2018. 'Surgical correction of primary cicatricial alopecia: Experience with nine patients.' Turkderm *-Turkish Archives of Dermatology and Venereology* 52:85-90. Doi: 10.4274/turkderm.20270.

[12] Jeong, Seong-Ho, and Sang-Hwan Koo, Seung-Kyu Han, W. K. Kim. 2010. 'An Algorithmic Approach for Reconstruction of Burn Alopecia.' *Annals of Plastic Surgery* 65:330-7. doi: 10.1097/SAP.0b013e3181d2487a.

[13] Shao, Huawei, and Hu Hang, Jin Yunyun, Jiang Hongfei, Han Chunmao, Jufang Zhang, Haiyan Shen, Fei Zhu, Ming Jia, Yuyan Wang, Xiaobo Guo. 2014. 'Follicular unit transplantation for the treatment of secondary cicatricial alopecia.' *Plastic Surgery* 22:249–253. DOI: 10.1111/dsu.12232

[14] Civas, Ekrem. 2011. 'Dermatokozmetik Cerrahilerde Skalp Blokları. Scalp Block in Dermatologic Surgery.' Turkiye Klinikleri Journal of Cosmetic Dermatology - Special Topics 4:19-22.

[15] Bernstein, Robert M., and William R. Rassman. 2000. 'Limiting epinephrine in large hair transplant sessions.' Hair Transplant Forum International 10:39-42.

[16] Callender, Valerie D., and Christina N. Lawson, Oge C. Onwudiwe 2014. 'Hair transplantation in the surgical treatment of central centrifugal cicatricial alopecia.' Dermatologic Surgery 40:1125-31. doi: 10.1097/DSS.0000000000000127.

[17] Civas, Ekrem. 2010. 'FUE Yöntemi ile Köklerin Elde Edilmesi. Follicullar Unit Extraction (FUE).' *Turkiye Klinikleri Journal of Cosmetic Dermatology - Special Topics* 3:55-7.

[18] Mejia, Ricardo. 2018. 'Redefining the "E" in FUE: Excision = Incision + Extraction.' *Hair Transplant Forum International* 28:5-7.

[19] Civas, Ekrem, and H. Mete Aksoy, Erol Koc, Berna Aksoy. 2009. 'Evaluation of three instruments used in FUE.' *Hair Transplant Forum International* 19:14-15.

[20] Dua, Aman, and Kapil Dua. 2010. 'Follicular Unit Extraction Hair Transplant.' *Journal of Cutaneous and Aesthetic Surgery* 3(2):76–81. doi: 10.4103/0974-2077.69015.

[21] Bicknell, Lindsay M., and Natalie Kash, Chitra Kavouspour, Rashid M. Rashid. 2014. 'Follicular unit extraction hair transplant harvest: a review of current recommendations and future considerations.' *Dermatology Online Journal* 20(3). pii: doj_21754.

[22] Avram, Marc R., and Shannon A. Watkins. 2014. 'Robotic Follicular Unit Extraction in Hair Transplantation.' *Dermatologic Surgery* 40:1319-27. doi: 10.1097/DSS.0000000000000191.

[23] Aksoy, H. Mete, and Berna Aksoy. 2010. 'Alıcı Bölgenin Hazırlanması: Kanalların Açılması. Preparation of Recipient Area: Recipient Site Creation.' *Turkiye Klinikleri Journal of Cosmetic Dermatology - Special Topics* 3:60-5.

[24] Bernstein, R. M. 2015. 'Chapter 30. Follicular Unit Hair Transplantation.' In Surgery of the Skin: Procedural Dermatology edited by, Robinson, J. K., and C. W. Hanke, D. M. Siegel, A. Fratila, 503-33. *London UK: Mosby Elsevier Inc*. Doi: 10.1016/B978-0-323-26027-5.00030-9.

About the Editors

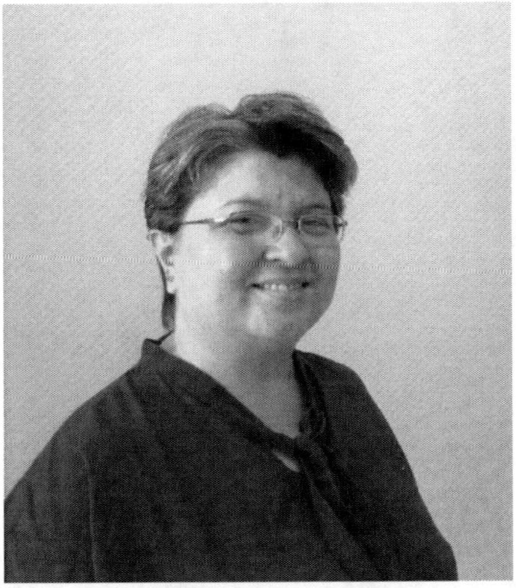

Berna Aksoy, MD

Assoc. Professor, Chief, Department of Dermatology, Faculty of Medicine, Bahcesehir University, Istanbul, Turkey; Dermatology Clinic, VM Medicalpark Hospital, Kocaeli, Turkey

Dr. Berna Aksoy, MD received her medical training at Hacettepe University Faculty of Medicine, Ankara, Turkey. Dr. Aksoy graduated as doctor of medicine in 1999. Dr. Aksoy did her dermatology residency and specialty training at the Department of Dermatology of Hacettepe University Faculty of Medicine. She graduated as dermatologist in 2003. She got dermatology board certification in 2012. Dr. Aksoy became Associate Professor in Dermatology in 2018. Dr. Aksoy performed many clinical and experimental scientific studies in the field of Dermatology. As a result of her scientific efforts Dr. Aksoy currently has 34 international scientific publications and 36 scientific paper presentations at international congresses. Dr. Aksoy also has 52 national scientific publications and 108 scientific paper presentations at national congresses. She wrote 4 international and 2 national books/book chapters as well. Dr. Aksoy's Google Scholar H-index is 9 and her Web of Science H-index is 7. Dr. Berna Aksoy MD is specifically interested in the following subjects: Acne and rosacea, psoriasis, eczema, hair disorders, nail disorders and surgery, dermatoimmunology, psychodermatology, life quality, dermatologic surgery, scar biology, scar treatment, wound healing, chronic wounds, dermato-oncology, non-melanoma skin cancer biology and treatment.

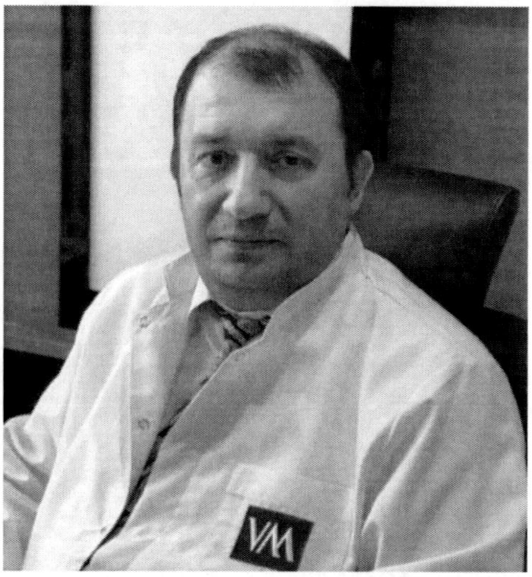

Hasan Mete Aksoy, MD

Assist. Professor, Department of Plastic, Reconstructive and Aesthetic Surgery, Faculty of Medicine, Bahcesehir University, Istanbul, Turkey; Plastic, Reconstructive Aesthetic Surgery Clinic, VM Medicalpark Hospital, Kocaeli, Turkey

Dr. Hasan Mete Aksoy, MD received his medical training at Hacettepe University Faculty of Medicine, Ankara, Turkey. He worked as research fellow at Fels Research Institute for Molecular Biology and Cancer, Temple University School of Medicine, Philadelphia, Pennsylvania (U.S.A.) under supervision by Dr. Sidney Weinhouse, PhD, Professor of Biochemistry in 1990. Dr. Aksoy graduated as doctor of medicine in 1991. Dr. Aksoy did his plastic surgery residency and specialty training at the Department of Plastic and Reconstructive Surgery of Hacettepe University Faculty of Medicine. He graduated as plastic surgery specialist in 2000. Dr. Aksoy performed many clinical and experimental scientific studies in the field of plastic surgery. As a result of his scientific efforts Dr. Aksoy currently has 39 international scientific publications and 39 scientific paper presentations at international congresses. He also has 30 national scientific publications and 63 scientific paper presentations at national congresses. He wrote 3 books/book chapters as well. Dr. Aksoy's Google Scholar H-index is 13 and his Web of Science H-index is 8. Dr. Hasan Mete Aksoy, MD is specifically interested in the following subjects: Aesthetic and functional nose surgery, aesthetic breast surgery, aesthetic ear surgery, scar biology, scar treatment, non-melanoma skin cancer biology, non-melanoma skin cancer treatment, finger-tip reconstruction, nail surgery, wound healing, chronic wounds.

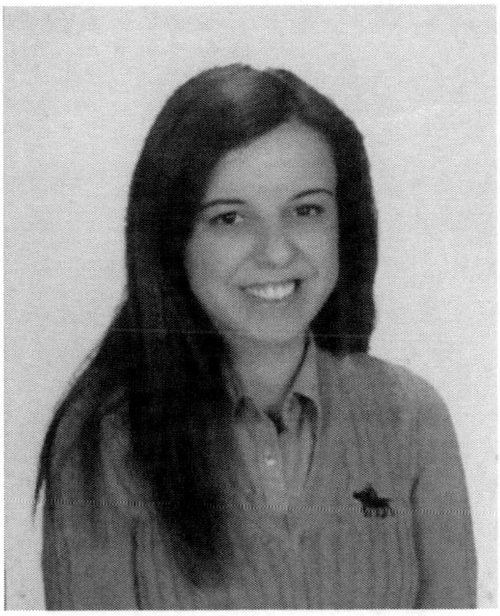

Asli Tatliparmak, MD

Assist. Professor, Department of Dermatology, Faculty of Medicine,
Bahcesehir University, Istanbul, Turkey;
Dermatology Clinic, Bahcesehir Liv Hospital, Istanbul, Turkey

Dr. Asli Tatliparmak, MD, received her medical training at Ege University Faculty of Medicine, Izmir, Turkey. Dr. Tatliparmak graduated as doctor of medicine in 2006. Dr. Tatliparmak did her dermatology residency and specialty training at the Department of Dermatology of Ege University Faculty of Medicine. She graduated as dermatologist in 2012. Dr. Tatliparmak performed many clinical and experimental scientific studies in the field of dermatology. As a result of her scientific efforts Dr. Tatliparmak currently has 13 international scientific publications and 4 scientific paper presentations at international congresses. Dr. Tatliparmak also has 13 national scientific publications and 29 scientific paper presentations at national congresses. She wrote 3 international books/book chapters as well. Dr. Tatliparmak's Google Scholar H-index is 5 and her Web of Science H-index is 2. Dr. Asli Tatliparmak, MD is specifically interested in the following subjects: Acne and rosacea, psoriasis, eczema, hair disorders, nail disorders and surgery, skin infections, dermatologic surgery, scar biology, scar treatment, wound healing, chronic wounds, dermato-oncology, non-melanoma skin cancer biology and treatment.

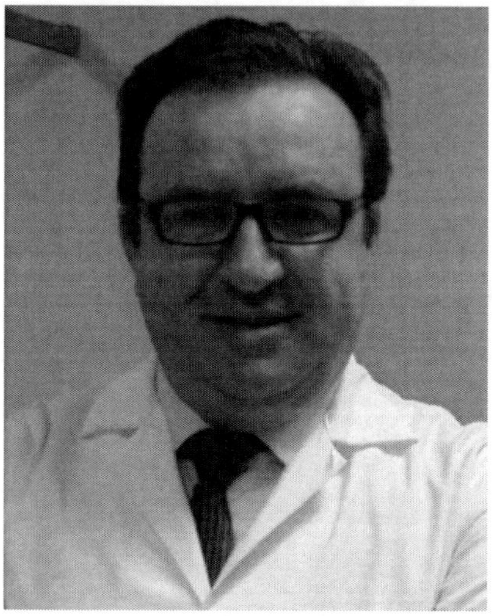

Erol Koc, MD

Professor, Dermatology Clinic, Medicalpark Hospital, Ankara, Turkey

Dr. Erol Koc, MD, graduated from Gulhane Military Medical Faculty in 1991. He completed his specialist training at the Department of Dermatology of Gulhane Military Medical Faculty between1994-1997. He became Associate Professor in 2010 and became Professor in 2015. As a result of his scientific efforts Dr. Koc currently has 37 international scientific publications and 48 national scientific publications. He also has 28 scientific paper presentations at international congresses and 64 presentations at national congresses. He wrote 4 international and 4 national books/book chapters as well. His Google Scholar H-index is 15 and her Web of Science H-index is 12. He retired from Gulhane Military Medical Faculty in 2014. He worked in Department of Dermatology of Bahcesehir University School of Medicine from 2014 to 2017. He is currently Dermatology and Cosmetology Department Coordinator in Medicalpark Hospital, Ankara, Turkey. He is specifically interested in the following subjects: Psoriasis, biological treatment, acne, cosmetics, botulinum toxin, filler applications, lasers, facial and skin rejuvenation systems, face lift with thread, lipolysis and mesotherapy. He is also a member of many national and international organizations, gave speeches as invited speaker at national and international conferences and symposiums, and served as organiser and trainer in various workshops.

INDEX

#

A

B

C

F

G

H

I

K

L

M

N

O

P

Q

R

S

T

U

V

W

X

Y

Z

Related Nova Publications

Scars and Scarring: Causes, Types and Treatment Options

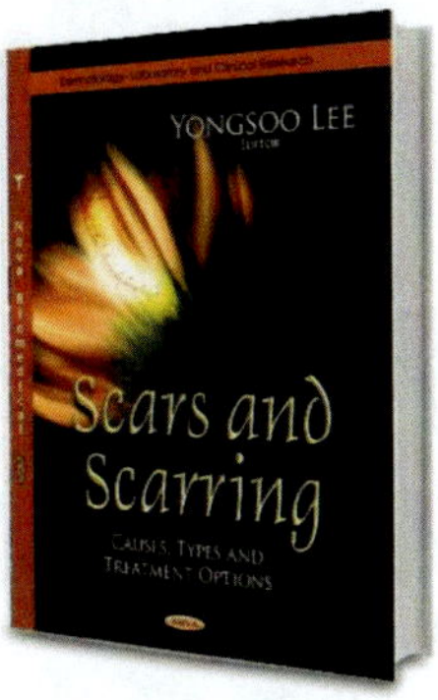

Editor: Yongsoo Lee

Series: Dermatology - Laboratory and Clinical Research

Book Description: In the era in which human beings began seeking aesthesis, numerous options for scar treatments have been invented. Not all, but almost all of the useful treatment options are described in this book, along with the latest discoveries of scar pathogenesis.

Hardcover ISBN: 978-1-62808-005-6
Retail Price: $179

An Essential Guide to Astaxanthin: Dietary Sources, Properties and Health Benefits

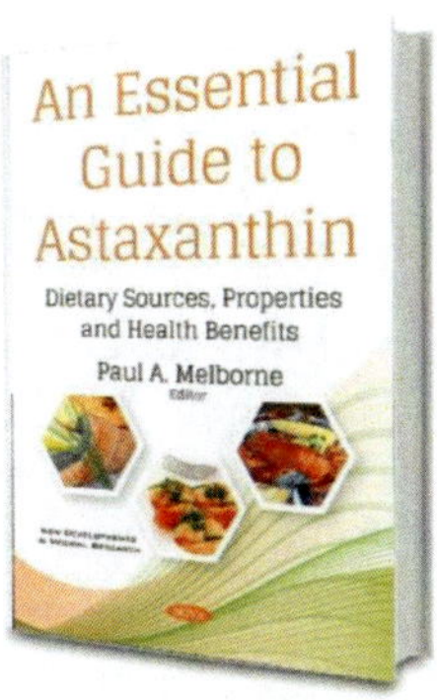

Editor: Paul A. Melborne

Series: Biochemistry Research Trends

Book Description: *An Essential Guide to Astaxanthin: Dietary Sources, Properties and Health Benefits* begins with a review of published studies regarding the efficacy and application of natural astaxanthin in aquaculture and human health, respectively.

Softcover ISBN: 978-1-53615-571-6
Retail Price: $82

To see complete list of Nova publications, please visit our website at www.novapublishers.com

Related Nova Publications

SENSORY INTEGRATION: DEVELOPMENT, DISORDERS AND TREATMENT

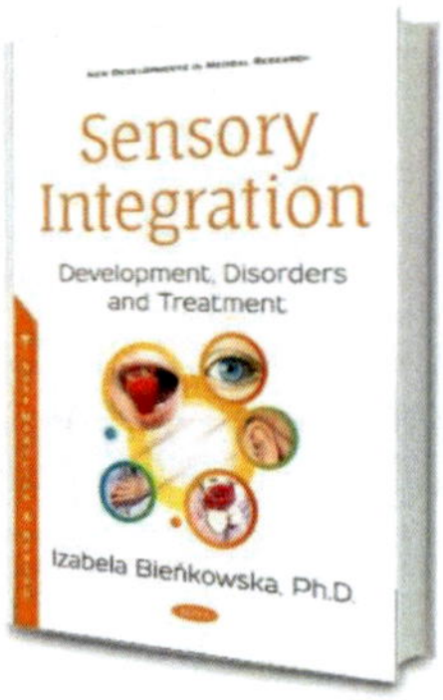

AUTHOR: Izabela Bieńkowska, PhD

SERIES: New Developments in Medical Research

BOOK DESCRIPTION: This book attempts to address and answer questions about different types of disorders in particular developmental spheres in children with learning and behavioral problems. It suggests how a child with sensory integration disorders can be helped in therapy and via other means using methods supporting disturbed sensory integration and other methods supporting the child's development.

SOFTCOVER ISBN: 978-1-53615-454-2
RETAIL PRICE: $95

RECOLLECTIONS OF PIONEERS IN XENOTRANSPLANTATION RESEARCH

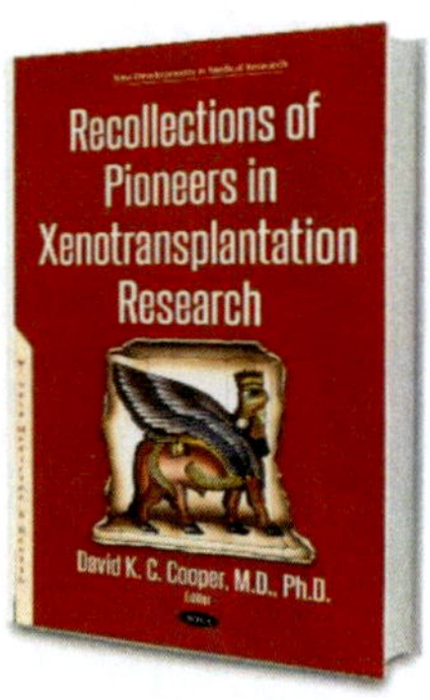

EDITOR: David K. C. Cooper

SERIES: New Developments in Medical Research

BOOK DESCRIPTION: The book provides a historical record of the research that has contributed to an advance in medicine that has been called "the next great medical revolution." Within a few years, this new form of therapy is likely to impact every family in the developed world.

HARDCOVER ISBN: 978-1-53613-945-7
RETAIL PRICE: $195

To see complete list of Nova publications, please visit our website at www.novapublishers.com